MANAGEMENT AND PRACTICE

IN HEALTH AND HUMAN SERVICE ORGANISATIONS

LYNDA BERENDS
KAREN CRINALL

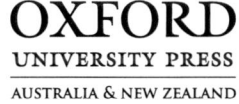

OXFORD
UNIVERSITY PRESS
AUSTRALIA & NEW ZEALAND

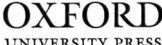

OXFORD
UNIVERSITY PRESS

Oxford University Press is a department of the University of Oxford.

It furthers the University's objective of excellence in research, scholarship, and education by publishing worldwide. Oxford is a registered trademark of Oxford University Press in the UK and in certain other countries.

Published in Australia by
Oxford University Press
253 Normanby Road, South Melbourne, Victoria 3205, Australia

© Lynda Berends and Karen Crinall 2014

The moral rights of the authors have been asserted.

First published 2014
Reprinted 2015 (D)

National Library of Australia Cataloguing-in-Publication entry

Author: Berends, Lynda, author.

Title: Management and practice in health and human service
        organisations / Lynda Berends; Karen Crinall.
ISBN: 9780195524154 (paperback)

Notes: Includes bibliographical references and index.
Subjects: Health services administration.
            Social work administration.

Other Authors/Contributors: Crinall, Karen, author.

Dewey Number: 362.11068

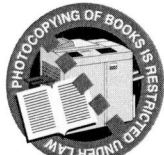
Edited by Kirsten Rawlings
Text design by Aisling Gallagher
Typeset by diacriTech, Chennai, India
Proofread by Geraldine Corridon
Indexed by Nikki Davis
Printed and bound in Australia by Ligare Book Printers, Pty Ltd
Cover Images: Getty Images/Yagi Studio; Nanamee/Kappa; Nanamee/Travis Stearns
            Nanamee/Visual Freaks; Shutterstock/Morphart Creation.

MANAGEMENT AND PRACTICE

IN HEALTH AND HUMAN SERVICE ORGANISATIONS

Contents

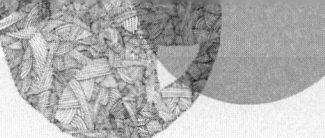

List of Figures and Tables

List of Case Examples, Practice Examples and Practitioner Profiles

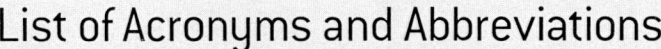

List of Acronyms and Abbreviations

AASW	Australian Association of Social Workers
ACWA	Australian Community Workers Association
AIHW	Australian Institute of Health and Welfare
CEO	chief executive officer
COAG	Council of Australian Governments
CSO	Community Service Organisation
DHS	Department of Human Services
DSE	Department of Sustainability and Environment (now DEPI—Department of Environment and Primary Industries)
DVA	Diversity Council of Australia
FFA	force field analysis
FTE	full time equivalent
GCASA	Gippsland Centre Against Sexual Assault
GONGO	government operated non-government organisation
GST	Goods and Services Tax
HR	human relations
HWA	Health Workforce Australia
NFP	not for profit
NGO	non-government organisation
NPM	new public management
OWL	Older Wiser Lifestyles
PEST	political, economic, social and technological
PESTLE	political, economic, social, technological, legal and environmental
QANGO	quasi-autonomous non-government organisation
QIC	Quality Improvement Council
QIP	Quality Innovation Performance
SPELT	social, political, economic, legal and technological
SWOC	strengths, weaknesses, opportunities, challenges
SWOT	strengths, weaknesses, opportunities, threats
TQM	Total Quality Management

Preface

Over the past three decades fundamental changes have occurred in the way health and human service organisations are required to deliver services, how they are resourced and administered, and how they are held accountable. Multifaceted funding arrangements pose management challenges, while at the same time policy shifts and community interest in the provision of effective responses to social problems and the needs of individual service users create escalating expectations (Reeve, 2005). This sector is now one of the most rapidly growing workforces in Australia, and yet little is known about the training needs, trends and challenges that exist and continue to emerge (Healy, 2009). Additionally, we do not know enough about the knowledge, skills and attributes required of its managers and leaders (Liang et al., 2012). This text aims to address some of these concerns by contributing to the knowledge base and skill development required for effective service delivery and organisational success, in the increasingly complex and demanding community services environment.

In this preface we explain the need for and origin of the text, and the centrality of practice perspectives in determining the approach we have used. We outline our goals and provide a brief overview of each chapter. The preface closes with a brief description about us: our backgrounds, interests, and hopes regarding the usefulness of this book.

ABOUT THE TEXT

Through our work with health and human service organisations we encountered many instances highlighting the complex and rapidly changing role of managers, and at the same time found a dearth of current, Australian-focused texts addressing this area. We also saw demand for literature that was informed by the experiences of community sector organisations in the wake of the turbulent period of rapid and profound change accompanying the introduction of managerialism to the not-for-profit sector. We determined that there was a place for a text addressing issues relating to management and leadership in health and human service organisations, with a particular focus on strategies for organisational success. In order to develop an evidence base on which to build this knowledge, and to ensure a practice-relevant resource, we commenced by exploring management perspectives on 'what matters' in organisational leaders' day-to-day roles and for the longer term.

Our research

We surveyed thirty-one managers from twenty-seven health and human services and found that their roles were diverse and demanding. Of a list of twenty issues ranging from 'community engagement' and 'external policy requirements' to 'program planning', most respondents reported that these items were important, while fewer regarded them as both important *and* challenging. Issues that were identified as important or extremely important by over 90% of respondents include budgets/financial management, external policy requirements, service delivery, community engagement, evaluation, strategic planning and program planning. These survey findings were further interrogated through six in-depth case study interviews with a selection of survey respondents.

The interviews explored the reasons why managers considered these issues to be critical. Participants also described successful strategies for managing organisational change, for responding effectively to external policy and funding expectations, for ensuring quality standards, and for planning, policy development and program implementation. The critical issues identified by managers, along with an extensive literature search and our own knowledge of the practice sector, culminated in the topics in this text. We are confident that the content is relevant to managers, leaders and practitioners in health and human service organisations because it has been shaped and informed by their knowledge and experience.

A practice approach

The format we have used is designed to support both those aspiring to be managers and leaders, as well as those already in these roles. Importantly, practitioner profiles throughout illustrate the nature of the work, the skills and challenges involved, and the lessons that have been learnt. These profiles include managers in small stand-alone organisations and those in community health and welfare settings. Their areas of expertise range from homelessness and disability to substance use and mental health problems. We have included practitioners from mainstream services and those operating in Aboriginal programs in Australia, and an integrated Māori-Pākehā service model in New Zealand.

The practitioners have contributed heartfelt reflections on their experiences, from an applied perspective, and they provide invaluable advice on how to operate effectively within a complex and dynamic practice environment. The thriving and evolving nature of management in the sector is highlighted throughout.

Aims

Our overall goal is to provide future and current managers and leaders in health and human service organisations with a well-researched, relevant and accessible resource that identifies and addresses skills and strategies for good management and leadership. A key aim is to explore successful and innovative strategies that are being applied, but which have not been well documented or widely shared, along with the consideration of management theory in the context of health and human service operations.

The book is divided into three sections: context and structure; planning and practice; and connection and engagement. While we have organised the topics according to our own logic, chapters may be read in any order, dependent on the needs of the reader. The following overview may help guide you to sections and chapters that are particularly relevant.

CHAPTER OVERVIEWS

Part 1, 'Context and Structure', is primarily concerned with the institutional, economic, governmental and professional factors that structure and contextualise health and human services, and the influence of these on the internal functioning of organisations.

We discuss external elements that define and circumscribe the political, social and economic climate within which health and human services operate. The internal roles, functions and processes that are necessary for ensuring that organisations are able to respond to external demands, and deliver ethical and effective services, are also examined. Emphasis is placed on the interconnectedness and interdependence of internal processes and external requirements.

Chapter 1, 'Contextualising Management in Health and Human Service Organisations', offers a historical overview of the ideas that inform contemporary management and leadership in health and human service organisations. We look at some of the continuities in approaches to management over time. Concepts are introduced that are helpful for understanding and addressing contemporary management and practice issues, in particular the role of power in management and organisation.

Chapter 2, 'External Factors that Shape Health and Human Services', then examines how external policy and funding demands shape and legitimise health and human service organisations. We outline the origin and nature of health and human services in Australia before exploring the onset of new public management and how organisations have adjusted to this environment. An outline of funding streams and views on equity and effectiveness adds to this representation of how external factors impact health and human service organisations.

In Chapter 3, 'Organisational Culture and Operation', our focus shifts to the organisation itself. We explore organisational culture and the importance of a healthy workplace in supporting shared values and effective operations. Organisational ethics are considered, in terms of the multiple sets of obligations that managers encounter and the role of professional associations. Diversity and discrimination are defined and the legislative framework in Australia is introduced, before practical strategies against discrimination and for diversity are described. The chapter closes with an introduction to policy development, implementation and monitoring.

The roles, functions and tasks of management, leadership and governance, and relationships between them, are described in detail in Chapter 4, 'Management, Leadership and Governance'. Our research has shown the importance of concentrating on the specific practices required of health and human services managers and leaders. The chapter draws on and consolidates ideas from the wider management literature, while attending to the values that distinguish health and human service organisations. We promote a participatory approach that fosters leadership across all organisational levels.

Part 2, 'Planning and Practice', is about the organisational and interpersonal processes that are necessary for fostering productive and effective teams, programs and services. The chapters in this section attend to workforce support and development, organisational planning processes, and project management and evaluation. The final chapter offers a practice-oriented perspective on financial management and accreditation.

Chapter 5, 'Workforce Support and Development', is concerned with human resource management, supervision and performance management. We describe characteristics of the workforce, along with ongoing challenges and associated developments. We then detail processes for staff recruitment, development, appraisal and review; consider how to manage underperforming staff; and look at processes for discipline, incompetence and dismissal. The final part of this chapter considers how professional associations and industrial organisations impact workplace conditions.

Chapter 6, 'Strategic Planning for Practice', explores the interlocking planning frameworks that shape and determine organisational direction, growth and success. Particular attention is given to tools for developing a comprehensive strategic plan, to ensure that the process is participatory, and for translating planning into action. The place of emergent planning in the contemporary health and human service environment is also discussed.

Project management and evaluation is the focus of Chapter 7 and we start by exploring the project manager's role and processes for project planning. Next, planning for implementation and mechanisms supporting project success, such as team configuration and project communication, are described. The purpose and usefulness of project evaluation are addressed in the final part of the chapter, with a particular focus on using a collaborative approach to maximise the relevance of evaluation. We outline two examples from our work that illustrate the potential success of this approach.

Chapter 8, 'Financial Management and Quality Accreditation', explores fundamental processes for financial management, with a particular emphasis on tools to assist with budget planning and accountability. Strategies for funds acquisition are explored. We also attend to preparing grant proposals that are matched to the expectations of funding guidelines, and the importance of inter-agency partnerships and collaborations. The final part of the chapter is an introduction to accreditation and we include management tips to facilitate a positive engagement in this process.

Part 3, 'Connection and Engagement', is concerned with links between stakeholders in health and human service organisations. Our research found that managers hold strong beliefs about the importance of community engagement for ethical and effective service provision, and that they consider this to be a central part of their role. While there is some tension between this orientation and claims about the role and function of managers in the business sector, we, along with others, see this as core to the values that drive and underpin health and human services.

We begin this section by examining management in a climate of change, recognising that this is the norm in today's health and human services environment. Next, approaches for fostering community engagement are considered. We explore a variety of understandings and meanings of community, with a focus on fostering diversity. The final chapter draws together the topics we have considered throughout the text, with insights from practitioners we encountered previously.

Chapter 9, 'Change Management', identifies different types of organisational change, with particular attention to working with the two primary forms: planned and emergent. We explore strategies for managing change effectively within a complex and fluid policy and funding climate, while retaining our emphasis on participatory and flexible approaches. Popular change management approaches, and the trend towards attending to emotion as a key factor in successfully bringing about organisational change are discussed.

Chapter 10, 'Communication, Community Engagement and Collaboration', explores the intertwined relationship between these organisational actions, and their fundamental role in building positive service systems and healthy organisations. Processes and conditions for supporting effective communication and inclusive practices are discussed, with emphasis on the importance of engaging with diverse stakeholders and communities.

Chapter 11, 'Towards Effective Management and Practice in Health and Human Services', provides a summary of the key topics and points. Approaches for successful management and leadership are drawn together into a workable, flexible framework for informing and supporting organisational practice and well-being.

IN CLOSING

The broad goal of this text is to foster successful organisational practice through effective management and leadership—it is forward focused. While we draw on current practice imperatives to achieve this aim, the mechanisms we explore have a long history and they are relevant to present and future challenges in health and human services. We have profound respect for the commitment and capacity of managers in health and human services and hope this text is a useful resource for those practising and considering a career in this field.

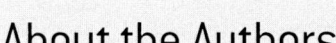

About the Authors

Lynda Berends is a health services researcher who specialises in the study of alcohol and other drug service delivery and system design, across acute and primary health sectors. Lynda is interested in the ways that organisational culture and settings impact service delivery, and client journeys into and through health and welfare services. She has worked with services and on behalf of state and national governments to evaluate pilot projects, review multi-site programs, and examine statewide systems in primary and acute health sectors across Australia and internationally. Lynda is a senior researcher at the National Drug and Alcohol Research Centre, University of New South Wales, and she has an extensive history with Turning Point Alcohol and Drug Centre, in Melbourne—an organisation that combines clinical practice with workforce development and research to explore service effectiveness. Lynda is the inaugural chair of the Health and Human Services Working Group, for the Alcohol and other Drugs Council of Australia, and she is on the council of the Australasian Professional Society on Alcohol and other Drugs.

Karen Crinall is a senior lecturer in Community Welfare and Counselling and Human Services Management, and the Research Coordinator and Deputy Head of the School of Applied Media and Social Sciences, Federation University of Australia. Karen's current research in the human services is concerned with the translation of policy into practice, regional and rural issues, and workforce leadership and capacity development. Karen has conducted a range of research and evaluation projects, and published in areas including women and homelessness, the Victorian integrated family violence service system reforms, Aboriginal leadership in community-based initiatives for addressing family violence, and strategies for reducing restrictive interventions and increasing safety in disability accommodation services. Karen's expertise locates in practice-led research that utilises participatory, creative and visual methods. Prior to taking up an academic position, Karen worked as a manager in youth crisis accommodation.

About the Contributors

Vanessa Bleier has been working in health and human services for seventeen years. She has worked in aged care and disability services, having originally started as a casual disability support worker and attendant carer while working her way through university, gaining a Bachelor of Arts and a Graduate Diploma in psychology. She has a husband and three kids, and moved to Gippsland from Melbourne seven years ago. Vanessa is passionate about people reaching their full potential, and that is what takes her to work every day. She has been a manager now for four years.

Fiona Boyle has completed a Bachelor of Arts (psychology and humanities), Bachelor of Social Welfare, and Diploma of Business Management in off-campus mode. This has allowed her to work in the areas of homelessness, victims of crime, children who have experienced family violence, children and young people displaying sexualised behaviours, and sexual assault. She has worked in various roles including case management, counsellor and senior clinician, and more recently has moved into a management role as CEO of the Gippsland Centre Against Sexual Assault.

Sue Carswell has a doctorate in social anthropology from Otago University and over eighteen years' research and evaluation experience working for government agencies, community organisations and universities. For the last nine years she has worked as an independent research and evaluation consultant based in Christchurch, New Zealand. Primarily working in the justice and human service sectors, Sue's focus has been on identifying effective service delivery and interventions to inform policy and organisational development. Her particular areas of interest are family violence, care and protection of children, and offender rehabilitation and reintegration.

Leanne Coupland is a qualified social worker who trained in the UK. Leanne spent several years working in generic child and family services teams, before moving to Victoria, Australia, in 2005. Leanne was recruited by the Department of Human Services and worked in Victoria's child protection system during a period of significant legislative change—during this time Leanne worked closely with community service organisations to implement the changes required. Leanne now works for a community service organisation, involved in the delivery of child, youth and family services. She also teaches undergraduates at a local university.

Melissa Elliott is a quality and risk management professional with significant experience in quality systems, enterprise risk management and accreditation. Melissa has completed a Bachelor of Arts in Social Science, majoring in Aboriginal and Intercultural studies. Her experience in accreditation includes the implementation of organisational processes and policies to manage the implementation of and monitor compliance with various accreditation systems. Melissa has developed and implemented health service quality, risk management and clinical governance systems, frameworks and policies in alcohol and drugs as well as mental health services. Her former roles include responsibility for the day-to-day management of health services in community health and hospital settings. This includes monitoring service delivery targets, program reporting, attraction and retention of staff, roster coordination, and oversight of budget and delivery of quality clinical services. Melissa is passionate about supporting staff and organisational capacity to provide efficient, quality services that are aligned with evidence-based practice.

Marie Feeley has worked in the community services in Victoria for over twenty-five years. She was a unit manager in disability services within the Department of Human Services for approximately seven years, and before that worked in a non-government welfare agency for ten years as the team leader of a counselling service. Earlier Marie worked in a variety of roles within the disability sector, from direct support worker to senior management positions, for almost ten years. Marie is currently a senior clinician in a small non-government counselling organisation: a management role with responsibilities for program development and coordination, supervision, counselling, etc. Social justice values inform her practice.

Sharon Fisher has over twenty years' experience in executive and senior human service management, policy and strategic partnership development and direct service delivery within state, local government and community services sectors, having worked extensively and in a range of positions with Melbourne City Mission. Her earlier career spanned child care, housing and homelessness, youth development, student well-being and employment, education and training. In 2011, Sharon joined the Department of Human Services (DHS) as Manager Strategic Projects, Children Youth and Families, Gippsland Region. She has a deep appreciation of the culture and complexity of statutory care programs, such as Child Protection and Youth Justice, and particularly their interface with Disability and Housing services and the funded community sector. Sharon commenced as the Director for Outer Gippsland with DHS in January 2013.

Daryl Fitzgibbon is Clinical Manager at Western Region Alcohol and Drug Centre (WRAD). He has worked in health-related roles for the past thirty-eight years, starting his career in public health via the army, serving in both the medical and dental corps. After getting his nursing degree, he worked for five years as a palliative care nurse, before completing his psychiatric nursing degree and working predominantly in the Psychiatric Admissions and Assessment Area and Psychiatric Prison and, from 1992, in the Community Psychiatric Division of a local health service. After completing a dual diagnosis qualification, he became a member of the WRAD staff in 1999. Daryl has worked in all areas at WRAD, and has taken responsibility for improvements in clinical service provision over the past ten years, and for quality improvements in other areas within the organisation.

Laurie Harkin, AM, is Victoria's inaugural Disability Services Commissioner. His office commenced operation on 1 July 2007 in accordance with provisions of the *Disability Act 2006*. Commissioner Harkin brings extensive senior experience to this role, having worked in a range of social and community services, including disability services, over a period of three decades. During that time, Commissioner Harkin has been a senior executive within state and local government agencies, non-government services and in the private sector. In 2013, Commissioner Harkin was appointed as a member of the Order of Australia for significant service to the community, particularly through the care and protection of people with a disability.

Terry Huriwai is of Te Arawa and Ngati Porou tribal descent. He is a probation officer by trade but has worked in various roles (including operational, policy and research) in the addiction sector for over twenty years. He is currently an advisor in New Zealand's National Addiction Workforce Programme.

Rachael Mackay is a social work practitioner working in health promotion and training in the women's health sector. Rachael has worked in youth and family homelessness in northeast Victoria and Melbourne before relocating to the Northern Territory. In the NT Rachael worked as the chairperson of the peak body NT Shelter and as an aged care coordinator, before moving to a private training company. Rachael has worked in Australia and the UK as a child protection practitioner. For the past ten years she has specialised in family violence support, coordinating the pilot Bsafe Project, and training police and human services in the area of domestic and family violence.

Jodie Martin has been the CEO at Gippsland Women's Health Service since January 2012. She has over fifteen years' experience in the health and human services sector, having worked in community health and local government prior to working in women's health. Jodie has qualifications in social welfare and bio-medical science. She has an interest in sexual and reproductive health and, in particular, improving access to education and services for young people in rural areas.

Sharon O'Reilly has a nursing qualification and post-graduate qualifications in drug dependence, psychoanalytic psychotherapy and health services management. Sharon has over twenty years' experience working in the drug and alcohol sector in Victoria; she has worked across a range of service types and held management positions for the past fifteen years. Her current role is Clinical Services Manager for the Bayside Medicare Local, integrating specialist alcohol and drug services and community-based mental health services across the Bayside Medicare Local Catchment. Sharon has well-shaped clinical, management, planning and policy development experience. She is an active participant in the International Harm Reduction Association, the global alcohol harm reduction network, in addition to a number of local community and regional networks. She has an enduring passion and commitment to advocating for and ensuring the human rights of marginalised communities. Sharon is currently the vice president of the Victorian Alcohol and Drug Association.

Simon Ruth spent fourteen years in management roles with Peninsula Health and the Salvation Army in Victoria, where he managed a range of alcohol and drug services, youth services, Indigenous health and ambulatory care programs. Simon has served on a range of government advisory groups, including the Whole of Victorian Government Alcohol and Drug Strategy Expert Advisory Group and was, for five years, President of the Victorian Alcohol and Drug Association. Simon is currently Director of Services at the Victorian AIDS Council. He is a passionate advocate for effective consumer participation.

Jenny Smith is the CEO of the Council to Homeless Persons, the peak body for the specialist homelessness sector in Victoria. Jenny has over twenty years of experience in leadership and management in the public sector. She has worked at policy, management and service delivery levels in health, mental health and community health, within government and now in the community sector. Jenny is a social worker and family therapist and has completed Masters Degrees in social work as well as public policy and management. Jenny is also a graduate of the Australian Institute of Company Directors and a board director of St Mary's House of Welcome and the Victorian Mental Health Carers Network.

Cheryl Sobczyk is responsible for a broad range of programs encompassing primary health services including medical practice, allied health, chronic disease management, nursing, refugee health and alcohol and other drug services. She has a passion for assisting people from all walks of life and with portfolios of service coordination and clinical governance strives to enable and empower people to maximise their choice and experience of accessing health and well-being services. Her professional background is nursing and has been with Bendigo Community Health Service for more than 18 years joining the executive management team in 2009. Cheryl is the current President of the Victorian Alcohol and Drug Association.

Geoff Soma is the Director of the Western Region Alcohol and Drug Centre (WRAD) medical services and specialist drug and alcohol centre in Warrnambool, Victoria. Previously he was the Director of the Odyssey House therapeutic community in Christchurch, New Zealand. He has had almost thirty years in management roles in a variety of settings as well as clinical responsibilities. Geoff is interested in fundraising, media and marketing, advocacy, and maximising the strength and contributions of not-for-profit organisations in the community. He values the role of partnerships and has learnt from success and failures and listening to others. In Geoff's career, he has enjoyed having contact with and helping people.

Allyson Walker is Yorta Yorta and Wemba Wemba from the Riverina. Her father was born on the hospital veranda as Aboriginal women were not allowed into the wards. She left school at 17 and went back to be educated as an adult and single mother. She has two Diplomas and a Bachelor of Social and Community Welfare Work. She writes songs and plays the piano, and sang at the Kangoo Bambadin (concert for culture), headlined by Troy Cassar-Daley, and for the Yalukit Wilum Ngargee: People Place Gathering festival (St Kilda Festival). She has worked in various roles including Liaison Officer, Caseworker, Indigenous Community Development Broker, and Manager, Community Strengthening.

Acknowledgments

It has been a pleasure and a privilege to collaborate in exploring and documenting management challenges and directions, as well as strategies for working within Australia's vibrant and ever-developing health and human service organisations. We have learnt much from this experience, from the heartfelt and insightful profiles provided by practitioners, from reading and reflecting on research and practice wisdom already in circulation, and from the opportunity to reflect on our own experiences working alongside services as they strive to improve how they operate and to what effect. We are deeply grateful for this experience and we salute the efforts of the many people whose work has enriched this book, including our colleagues at work, and the individuals and organisations that have taken part in our research.

The support of Debra James and Shari Serjeant, from Oxford University Press, in the preparation of the text has been a lovely balance of gentle guidance and attention to timelines. This has been invaluable in assisting us to reach the end of a long and positive journey as authors and collaborators on this project.

We are especially thankful to our partners and loved ones, who have listened patiently while we recounted tales of the challenges and triumphs involved, and celebrated with us as milestones were encountered and resolved. Particular thanks go to John and Will, for your wise words and your silences.

PART
1

CONTEXT AND STRUCTURE

The practice cases in this part are:

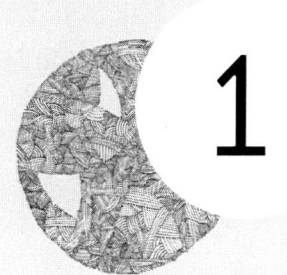

Contextualising Management in Health and Human Service Organisations

OVERVIEW

This chapter will:
- describe the development of key management theories and approaches
- propose definitions of power applicable to management in organisations
- explore the influence of management approaches developed in the profit sector on contemporary management in health and human services
- discuss organisational structures common to health and human services
- introduce management approaches that are appropriate to health and human services.

The historical background and organisational context of human services management and practice are discussed in this chapter. Key themes are identified and theoretical concepts that are helpful for understanding and addressing contemporary management and practice issues in health and human services are introduced.

KEY TERMS

administrative management
bureaucratic management
ecological systems theory
human relations management
Likert scale
McDonaldization
mechanistic organisations
organic organisations

participatory management
scientific management
situational leadership
Taylorism
Theory X and Theory Y management types
utilitarianism
welfarism

Organisation, management and power

Order and disorder are a matter of organisation. (Sun Tzu, 1991, p.36)

The strategic organisation and mobilisation of people and resources in order to complete seemingly impossible large-scale projects has ancient origins: the giant stone statues of Easter Island, Stonehenge in England, Machu Picchu in Peru, Angkor Wat in Cambodia and the pyramids in Egypt are but a few examples (Bartol et al., 2011). Centuries-old texts, which are still drawn upon today, such as *The Art of War* by Sun Tzu, *The Republic* by Plato and *The Prince* by Machiavelli, espouse philosophies for overpowering opponents, organising people and governing territories. These enduring monoliths and documents are evidence that civilisations across the history of the world have identified principles, instituted systematic approaches and formed operational guidelines for mobilising large numbers of people towards achieving immense accomplishments. A discomforting antecedent of contemporary management is slavery—used in all of the above-mentioned construction projects. This is because slavery gave rise to the concept of 'work as a consciously designed set of tasks under the control of an overseer' (Clegg et al., 2011, p.447).

These examples—and many more that you might identify yourself—illustrate the fundamental role of power and authority in facilitating or obstructing management and practice. From the outset of this text and, more importantly, in reference to your identity as a manager and leader, it is crucial to acknowledge the unavoidable and ever-present interrelationships between organisation, management, position and power. How leaders and managers understand power, their critical awareness of their own and others' privileges, and how they engage with and use power, determines whether or not they, and their organisations, are practising and performing ethically, effectively and efficiently.

Power

Working with power sits at the centre of the roles of managers and leaders. The way an organisation is structured determines its flow and direction, its operation and exercise and, importantly, the nature of its effects. It is important to be mindful that power has positive *and* negative, formal *and* informal influences. Without the exchange of power, health and human services would be unable to work with people to bring about positive change in their lives. The words of Mary Parker Follett (1868–1933) encourage careful reflection on the concept of power from a management perspective. Although written ninety years ago, they retain their relevance:

> No word is used more carelessly by us all than the word 'power'. I know no conception which needs today more careful analysis. We have not even decided whether power is a 'good' word or a 'bad' word … What is power? Is it influence, is it leadership, is it force? (Follett in Fox & Urwick, 1973, p.67)

Power can be understood in a wide variety of ways. It is commonly considered to be almost material, something that is possessed. People have *more* or *less* of it, depending on their structural position; it affords them with authority, and they can put it to use in constructive and/or destructive ways. Power can also be understood as an action—a drive or energy that impels. Rather than being a commodity that is traded backwards and forwards, power is seen as existing in actions and emerging through relationships (Tremain, 2005, p.4).

From this perspective, power is, in the first instance, a positive force that is evident in things becoming possible, such as freedom of choice. Paradoxically, making a choice is paired with repressive consequences—this is because each option is ultimately constraining, requiring conformity to certain behaviours and identities (Crinall et al., 2010). For example, if we choose to accept a position in an organisation (exercising our power to be self-determining), we make a commitment to behave in specific ways, and to conform to particular rules—of our own volition we make the choice to be constrained, thus power in this instance manifests as a limiting influence (Foucault, 1992).

Whichever meaning you adopt, Mary Parker Follett's question: 'What is power?' remains open. Try to keep these ideas about power in mind while you read about the development of management as a means of organising people and resources in order to achieve particular outcomes and goals. We will frequently return to consider power, and how it pertains to managing and leading health and human service organisations.

Linkage
In Chapter 4 we further explore power and authority. Suggested readings at the end of this chapter also address meanings of power in greater detail.

REFLECTION EXERCISE

Reflect on the above understandings of power. How do you define power? Can you think of examples of power as an object, and as an action?

We now take an abbreviated tour through some of the ideas and practices that provide the background to contemporary management approaches in the health and human services. Although the development of these management theories cannot be reduced to sole innovators, examples here are mainly limited to individuals. The reason for this is to highlight key concepts that inform these theories and to avoid watering down descriptions by trying to cover too many contributors in a contracted space.

Early theories about organisation and management for social well-being

The change from an agrarian to a factory-based workforce that accompanied the shift from a feudal to a capitalist economy during the industrial revolution across Great Britain, Europe and North America necessitated new approaches and technologies for organising populations, producing goods and supervising labour (Cree, 2010). Management was one of many new bodies of knowledge, along with sociology and psychology, that emerged from these profound changes during the early 1800s. In terms of management theory, this era is known as the pre-classical period, because the management ideas that were developed at this time were specific to particular problems, rather than management being treated as a separate domain of work, as it is now (Bartol et al., 2011).

Social work, along with many of the health professions, grew out of the social and living conditions that resulted from this intense period of rapid urbanisation. It is also worth noting that these professions represent a form of people management; they provide avenues for the exercise of power by organising people into categories and groups, and by promoting desirable, or normative, behaviours and living conditions.

Jeremy Bentham (1748–1832) is commonly credited with being the father of **utilitarianism**. Clegg et al. (2011) observe that his reform campaign was widespread: arguing for the abolition of slavery, the separation of church and state, equal rights for women, the decriminalisation of homosexual acts, and more humane working conditions (Clegg et al., 2011). He also promoted ideas that contributed to the development of **welfarism**. His reform approach was based on rational calculation and efficient planning; this included factories as efficient workspaces. Bentham designed an architectural management system to enable more effective supervision of workers, known as the Panopticon, which subsequently become a popular model for prisons (Foucault, 1979). The Panopticon enabled a single unseen observer to oversee the activities of many. Most significantly, the Panopticon created the psychological effect of being under constant surveillance, while never being able to see the observer or to know when they are watching.

The Panopticon is based on the principle that those contained within its space are made aware that they are constantly being watched, but cannot see who is watching them, or exactly when they are being observed. Therefore, to avoid reprisal, people are compelled to be self-disciplining, as they must behave at all times as if under surveillance. This form of people management endures in contemporary life, though now the domains in which we live, work and socialise extend beyond bricks and mortar into cyberspace, and our behaviours are monitored by electronic and digital devices, rather than concealed overseers. This is not limited to public or organisational workspaces but now includes what were once considered private domains, such as our homes and cars. Whenever we access the internet (Clegg et al., 2011), or when we use loyalty and reward cards, for example, our actions are being monitored and recorded by 'invisible' organisations, with the ultimate purpose of influencing our behaviour. Bentham's Panopticon and its effect on the way people are organised, and how they organise themselves, is important to keep in mind as we consider management technologies and strategies, and the way they enact power, especially **bureaucratic management** approaches.

Utilitarianism
The belief that the most ethical stance is to achieve the greatest good for the greatest number of people.

Welfarism
Attitudes and policies supporting the establishment of a welfare state.

Bureaucratic management
A theory of management based on the ideas of Max Weber, which proposes that the most effective and efficient way to run an organisation is to have a hierarchical structure, with clear role definitions and rigid lines of accountability.

REFLECTION EXERCISE

When you are next in your own work environment observe how workspaces are arranged, and the various physical structures and technologies that are used to remotely monitor the activity of workers. What effects does this form of power have: is it productive or oppressive? Who has access to the information that is gathered by observing worker activities? What is this information used for?

Robert Owen (1771–1858) was another Victorian-era reformer of working and social conditions. Owen advocated for investing in the well-being of employees, the outlawing of child labour, the regulation of working hours, and the provision of meals during the working day (Robbins et al., 2000). He is credited with having laid the foundations for the human relations management movement (Bartol et al., 2011), which is discussed in greater detail later in this chapter.

Charles Babbage (1792–1871) contributed to contemporary management practices by developing the first functional mechanical computer. Not only did this invention foreground the digital technologies we now use to manage and perform our lives and work, Babbage also observed that highly skilled workers often spend large amounts of time engaged in work requiring lesser expertise. Seeing this as inefficient, he promoted work and task specialisation. The Babbage Principle (a term coined in 1974 by Harry Braverman) was based on Babbage's ideas that skilled and highly paid workers should only be allocated demanding tasks, while those who are lower paid and less skilled should be given easier tasks. The Babbage Principle was influential in the development of **scientific management** (Bartol et al., 2011).

Scientific management
A management approach that is based on the belief that scientific research can aid organisational efficiency and productivity.

Administrative management

The **administrative management** approach was concerned with the development of management principles for the coordination of internal organisational activities (Bartol et al., 2011). Henri Fayol (1841–1925) is often identified as instigating the idea that management was something that could be learnt and should stand alone as a separate profession (Coulshed et al., 2006). He named five functions of management, which, although now modified, retain relevance today: planning, organising, commanding, coordinating and controlling (Clegg et al., 2011; Lewis et al., 2012).

Fayol introduced the notion of allowing workers in different departments to be able to communicate directly with each other, rather than having to observe a chain of command. The current organisational logic of breaking down workplace silos resonates with this innovation (Lewis et al., 2012). Fayol's management training program focused on fourteen principles for 'proper management, efficient organisations and happy employees' (Clegg et al., 2011, p.457). A number of these are particularly relevant for workers in health and human services:

1 Unity of direction—top-level positions are responsible for an organisation's vision and direction.
2 Specialisation of labour—work teams are divided into smaller groups to carry out particular functions, and build expertise in particular areas.
3 Unity of command—each worker reports to one supervisor only.
4 Order—all positions have clear job descriptions.
5 Span of control—the same person should supervise those who are doing similar work.

Source: adapted from Coulshed et al., 2006, p.25; Clegg et al., 2011, p.458

Administrative management
A theory of management that proposes that efficiency and effectiveness are achieved through the application of particular principles and practices across the whole organisation.

Linkage
We consider management functions in more detail in Chapter 4.

....

REFLECTION EXERCISE

These are no doubt familiar concepts arising from your own experience as an employee and/ or manager. Reflect on whether, and how, these principles are applied in your current practice context. How might this structuring of organisational practices direct the flow of power between employees at various levels?

──○

Scientific management

Taylorism
The principles of scientific management developed by Frederick Taylor, based on the idea that work processes can be completed more efficiently if they are broken into small, specialised tasks. Taylorism resulted in the development of the factory production line.

The scientific approach to management, also referred to as **Taylorism**, largely derives from the ideas of Fredrick W. Taylor (1856–1915). Rather than focusing on establishing rational principles for managing, Taylor was concerned with rationalising specific tasks (Coulshed et al., 2006). He pioneered 'time-and-motion' studies, and developed methods for enabling more efficient performance of tasks without increasing effort or workload. Taylor's methods are famous for increasing factory production rates and profits, while decreasing manufacturing costs. The assembly-line system developed by Taylor continues to be a boon in industry contexts, but even there it is criticised for devaluing workers as people and individuals, increasing absenteeism and causing monotony and boredom (Bartol et al., 2011).

In the contemporary health and human services sector, scientific management is evident in the principles of managerialism and economic rationalism. These principles are incorporated into many organisational processes and practices, for example, the concepts of efficiency and accountability, and the application of work analysis methods, such as logic models, performance indicators and quality audits (Coulshed et al., 2006; Lewis et al., 2012).

Linkage
Logic models, performance indicators and quality audits are discussed in greater detail in the chapters to come.

A close associate of Taylor's and a contributor to the development of scientific management whose name may be familiar to you is Henry Gantt, the inventor of the Gantt chart. Developed in the early 1900s, this planning tool is a horizontal bar chart that visually represents the scheduling of a project according to task, time, order of tasks, and key milestones.

Linkage
We look more closely at the Gantt chart in Chapter 7 when discussing project management tools.

Bureaucratic management

Bureaucratic management is frequently discussed in terms of bureaucracies, and identified as an organisational structure, rather than a management approach. It derives from the ideas of Max Weber (1864–1920), a German sociologist, who sought to understand what a functional and just organisational structure might entail. In the early twentieth century Weber conceived the 'ideal bureaucracy', and although his goal was directed at organisations, the model has been applied to the development of management practices. Weber's ideal bureaucracy functioned on processes of applying '*rational* means for the achievement of specific ends' (Clegg et al., 2011).

Characteristics of the ideal bureaucracy include the specialisation of labour, formal rules and procedures, impersonality, a clearly defined hierarchy, and career pathways (Bartol et al., 2011). Despite much criticism of bureaucratic management, bureaucracy has sustained as a dominant structure and organisational philosophy in large-scale health and human service organisations, particularly in the government sector (Lewis et al., 2012).

Bureaucratic approaches to management seek to minimise the capacity for individuals to influence organisational processes, relying instead on formal rules, policies and procedures. Promotion is based on merit and the achievement of key performance indicators, which have been *logically* determined and decisions are made according to *objective*, rather than *subjective*, criteria. People are subordinated to rules and processes, and the survival of the organisation is paramount.

Across the duration of a career in health and human services, it is difficult to avoid bureaucracies. Whether you are employed in a government department or a not-for-profit organisation, your work will be shaped by government policy, your organisation will have published standards and procedures, and your success in selection for a position will be based on key selection criteria. You will be expected to work towards achieving the goals and vision of the organisation, and promotion will be merit-based.

Think back to the earlier description of Bentham's Panopticon, and the distanced, disembodied supervision of people and their behaviour: it is apparent that this model of objective observation and organisational structuring was a precursor to bureaucratic design. Ironically, for many of us our job security and sense of safety at work are dependent on the dispassionate operation of the bureaucracy, because as employees we seek clearly established policies and rules to protect us from individual prejudice.

Linkage
In Chapter 5 we discuss the expanding workforce in the health and human services, and the coupling of this with increasing organisational and professional regulations and qualification requirements.

REFLECTION EXERCISE

Reflect on your own workplace context. Do you prefer to have a position description, clear lines of command and clarity of expectation? Does it increase your sense of job security and workplace safety to know who your supervisor is, what your rights and entitlements are, and that there are policies and procedures for guiding conduct within the organisation?

This is an ideal point to meet the first of our practitioners, whose insights as managers and leaders in organisations will help ground the ideas we are discussing. Marie Feeley shares aspects of her work and some of the challenges she faced as a middle manager in a large bureaucracy. Marie's description illustrates the point made above; that the principles of bureaucratic management are strongly embedded in present working conditions in the health and human services. As you read Marie's reflections, consider the features of bureaucratic management that are evident and how these shape her experience within the organisation.

PRACTITIONER PROFILE 1.1

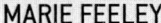

MARIE FEELEY

SENIOR PRACTITIONER, SPECIALIST SERVICES, BEHAVIOUR SUPPORT SERVICES

Position

This would be perceived as a middle management role. Major responsibilities include the coordination, operation and development of a direct service provision program; this may be at a primary, secondary and/or tertiary level. The role also requires the clinical and operational supervision of seven practitioners.

A secondary service provision, or consultation, may involve, for example, supporting a staff group through reflective practice sessions that might resemble a 'group supervision' model. A tertiary service provision may involve the development and delivery of 'educational' programs to a tertiary institution, for example, TAFE, university students, etc.

A typical day

Might involve two supervision sessions with program practitioners, and attendance at a case planning meeting where issues will be related to criminal offending behaviours and/or child protection issues, human rights violations, etc. A day may also include time spent responding to colleagues through direct contact or via phone/email, preparation of documents, reading of documents sent for input and feedback, project planning and development.

Challenges

- Marking items off my 'to do' list.
- Sitting within a large open workspace amongst many workers where, in my perception, consistent poor practice is evident that is outside my jurisdiction. How much or how little of this do I address directly? It is a challenge to get support to address this.
- Finding a private space for confidential professional conversations, by telephone and in person.
- Working in a large government bureaucracy with all the processes that this may suggest.
- Extensive travel, within a rural region as well as regular travel to a major city and metropolitan areas.
- Finding time for thinking and reflecting by myself.
- Time for lunch.

Lessons learnt

- There is sometimes extensive and unsurpassable distance between concrete and conceptual thinking.
- Realisation of what I am able to do, and what I am not.
- How to say 'no'.
- The value of clinical supervision.
- I cannot say that I regret any of my learnings; I learnt when I needed to, and when I was ready to.

Necessary skills and qualities

- A liking of people generally.
- Authenticity.
- Critical thinking skills.
- Conceptual thinking that can access concrete thinking.
- Awareness of one's own values, beliefs and prejudices as much as possible. However, there are many prejudices one is not aware of until 'they hit one in the face' so to speak.
- Tolerance.
- Empathy.
- Courtesy, time to listen and hear.
- Courage to speak.
- Courage in hearing other varied perspectives.
- Ability to accept constructive criticism.

Human relations management theory

The rise of the psychological sciences from the mid-nineteenth century focused attention on the reasons behind worker behaviour. With the drive to increase productivity and profit, there was interest in understanding what motivated and demotivated organisational employees. Studies were conducted on the affect of various factors within the organisational environment, such as the arrangement of workspaces, rewards and incentives, and the assignment of meaningful tasks. Behavioural management theories developed in the early 1900s were mainly based on empirical evidence and experiment, and they sat in contrast to the scientific management approach, which saw people as components of a production machine (Bartol et al., 2011; Ginsberg, 2008). A predominant behavioural theory approach is **human relations management**.

Early behavioural theorists linked with the burgeoning of human relations management are Elton Mayo (1880–1949) and Mary Parker Follett (1868–1933). While these two behaviourists share similar views regarding the importance of group work and relationships between management and workers, their perspectives diverge significantly.

Elton Mayo was an Australian organisational theorist who began his academic career at the University of Queensland before moving to the USA, where he became a professor at Harvard in 1926 (Clegg et al., 2011). Mayo analysed a series of three experimental studies that were conducted for the Western Electric Company in Chicago between 1927 and 1933, known as the Hawthorne studies (Bartol et al., 2011; Gray et al., 2010). These experiments involved observing the behaviour of factory workers when changes were made to their working environments. The research found that productivity increases were not necessarily dependent on environmental factors, such as changes to lighting and workspaces (Lewis et al., 2012), rather workers becoming more motivated and productive was linked with social factors, such as

Human relations management
Human relations management theory asserts that the psychosocial needs of workers must be addressed in order to maximise their performance. It was developed in reaction to the scientific management principles of Taylorism.

identification with an informal work group within the overall organisational structure and the increased sense of value and belonging that this created. This phenomenon became known as the Hawthorne effect (Clegg et al., 2011). But this explanation was not the end of the story.

These conclusions of the Hawthorne studies were criticised because it was later realised that the changes observed in workers' behaviours were in reality linked with their involvement in a research experiment, rather than changes in management practice strategies. Even so, the underlying principle that social factors influence worker motivation endures in contemporary management approaches. The most significant of these is that workers in an organisation perform better when there is a healthy group dynamic and when they receive positive attention from their supervisors (Ozanne & Rose, 2013).

The primary benefit of the Hawthorne experiments has been the redirection of attention away from bureaucratic and scientific management approaches toward the importance of fostering teamwork and meaningful, respectful relationships in organisations. However, it needs to be remembered, although these studies helped establish that motivation is not solely governed by economic reward or fear of punishment, the ultimate aim of Mayo and his colleagues was to maximise profit within a business environment. Their methods also still subscribed to the idea that organisational hierarchy and managerial control were necessary (Childs, 1995, cited in Lewis et al., 2012).

Mary Parker Follett, in contrast, promoted radical ideas about organisational management that are evident today in **participatory management** approaches. She was a social work manager for 25 years before turning her attention to the business sector during the early twentieth century.

Follett argued for group autonomy, and the benefits of communication and power-sharing across all levels of the organisation; utilising power 'with' rather than power 'over' subordinates (Bartol et al., 2011; Follett, 1951; Ginsberg, 2008).

The ideas of Mary Parker Follett and Elton Mayo founded the human relations approach to management, and drew attention to organisations as social environments comprised of human beings, the benefits of encouraging collaboration and cooperation, and the need for supervisors and managers to practise people skills (Bartol et al., 2011; Coulshed et al., 2006). At this time, in the early twentieth century, psychological and sociological theorising promoted reconsideration of the relationship between the individual and society, new understandings about the way people behave in relation to their environment, and the importance of meeting physical and emotional needs.

Abraham Maslow (1908–70) is well known to students in health and human services courses for his theory on human need and human nature, commonly referred to as Maslow's hierarchy of needs. Maslow argued that throughout the life course human beings are driven by the will and necessity to satisfy a series of needs. These progress through five stages: physiological (food, warmth and shelter), safety and security (absence of threats and violence), social (relationships with others), esteem (sense of self-worth),

Participatory management
A management approach that encourages consultation and genuine participation in organisational decision-making across all levels.

Linkage
The concept of participatory approaches to management is a theme that we revisit often throughout this text.

and ultimately a happy and fulfilled life (self-actualisation). Significantly, Maslow claimed that people must have their needs satisfied at each level before progressing to the next. In other words, if a person does not have adequate food, warmth and shelter, they cannot begin to feel safe; if they do not feel safe, they cannot develop functional social relationships; if they are not socially connected, they are not able to feel good about themselves; and if they have a negative self-image, they will not be able to reach their potential and feel satisfied and fulfilled with their life (Clegg et al., 2011).

An understanding of the needs that drive human behaviour strengthened the case against scientific management approaches. Maslow's conceptual framework encourages organisations to recognise that workers have basic human needs that must be met (Bartol et al., 2011; Gray et al., 2010). Today these principles are woven into theorising about effective approaches to health and human services management. This is quite possibly because they provide not only a common-sense model for explaining human motivation and why some people struggle to achieve, but also a level of certainty about how people's needs and associated issues can be addressed.

Douglas McGregor (1906–64) is another humanist psychologist, whose ideas shaped modern management theory, and with whom you may already be familiar. McGregor was concerned with the way managers viewed workers, developing the iconic notion of **Theory X and Theory Y management types**. These oppositional categories classify managers according to their view of human nature.

Theory X managers see people as self-interested, work-avoiding and unwilling to take responsibility. Therefore, the appropriate management style is to be highly directive and authoritarian; lines of accountability need to be clear. People are considered to be organisational resources that are expendable, like all resources, which do not contribute to profit (Clegg et al., 2011; Lewis et al., 2012).

Theory Y managers have a more positive view of human nature. They believe that people like to work and to take responsibility, that they are capable of working autonomously, have creative ability, and are independently aspiring towards self-actualisation (Bartol et al., 2011; Lewis et al., 2012). Management from this perspective assumes worker autonomy and capacity for self-management, and focuses on building worker self-esteem and career development. Delegating responsibility and shared leadership are encouraged. People are valued for their contribution to the organisation, and redundancy is not considered a desirable means of cost cutting (Clegg et al., 2011).

Even though these polarised extremes of management style are in many ways caricatures, the image illustrates the continuity in the influence of scientific management at the Theory X end of the scale, and the trend towards a human relations and participatory approach in the Theory Y orientation. It is reassuring that support for management approaches that adopt a positive view of workers, value the social dimensions of the workplace, foster individual potential and encourage participatory approaches continue into the present.

Rensis Likert (1903–81) was an American organisational psychologist who developed the **Likert scale**, a psychometric measure that is still used in surveys and questionnaires for measuring people's beliefs or feelings about a particular issue or factor. In the 1960s,

Theory X and Theory Y management types
Theory X managers assume workers are fundamentally lazy, only motivated by financial reward, and in need of constant supervision. Theory Y managers believe workers are self-motivated, can be left unsupervised and ultimately strive for self-actualisation in work.

Likert scale
A survey tool that measures opinions about a particular issue. Respondents are provided with a defined range of options, usually five (for example: strongly disagree, disagree, neutral, agree and strongly agree). These are then collated and analysed.

he also developed a framework for classifying organisations according to four types—or systems—of management. These range from highly controlling and disempowering for employees, to genuinely participative (Lewis et al., 2012). The table below outlines and compares the elements that define each system.

TABLE 1.1 Likert's management systems

SYSTEM 1: EXPLOITATIVE AUTHORITATIVE	SYSTEM 2: BENEVOLENT AUTHORITATIVE	SYSTEM 3: CONSULTATIVE	SYSTEM 4: PARTICIPATIVE
Power concentrated at top in hands of a few	Power concentrated at top in hands of a few	Power concentrated at top	Distributed power
Distrust of subordinates	Condescending trust in subordinates	More trust in employees	Complete trust in employees
Punishment to achieve compliance	Punishment and reward	Rewards with some punishment	Rewards and responsibility
Hierarchical decision-making	Limited and highly controlled participation in decision-making	Participation increases at higher levels Employees at bottom consulted, but do not make final decisions	Participation in decision-making across all organisational levels
Top-down communication	Top-down communication	Upwards and downwards communication (more downwards)	Communication in all directions
Employees alienated from organisational goals	Employees alienated from organisational goals	Less alienation	Engagement across all levels in goal formation
Low worker morale	Low to medium morale Competition between workers	Higher levels of morale Employee input, but final decisions made by top level management	Highest levels of morale Widespread responsibility Highest productivity

Source: adapted from Lewis et al., 2012, p.87; Tyson, 1998, p.96

Likert advocated for a System 4 approach: participative management. This involves the organisational structure incorporating group decision-making, and team leaders and managers acting as 'linking-pins' between work groups and other management levels (Coulshed et al., 2006).

Community sector organisations tend towards management approaches that are heavily informed by human relations principles. This includes:

* Valuing the people who work in the organisation.
* Attention to workers' needs.
* Encouraging informal groups and teamwork.
* Fostering multi-directional communication.
* Distributed leadership and participatory decision-making.

You will find that these concepts recur regularly throughout the chapters to follow. However, as encouraging as it is to engage with these ideas about management and to appreciate their fit with the values that underpin health and human service organisations, it is also important to be mindful of criticisms that have arisen regarding human relations ideas.

Coulshed et al. (2006) warn that these theories emerged from studies in the business sector. Despite the contributions of the humanities and social sciences, which illuminated valuing workers as people, and attending to needs and aspirations, their overriding intent is to maximise organisational profits. Therefore, the application of the human relations model in organisations has been oriented towards understanding people and their motivations in order to control and direct their behaviour so that the goals of the organisation can be achieved, rather than to better understand and nurture workers themselves. Coulshed et al. (2006, p.42) observe that: 'It is almost as if aspects of people's humanity are being understood only to be used against them, so as to turn them into more compliant workers'. Furthermore, they claim that this focus on the individual detracts from a critique of organisations as entities and of the quality and appropriateness of the services provided. Coulshed et al. observe that knowledge can be used to engage people in behaviours and practices which ultimately result in their own exploitation is supported by the view of power discussed earlier—that it is most effective when people are willing participants.

Of course, the trajectory of development in management approaches did not stop here. Up to this point, we have considered some of the features and progression of classical, scientific and human relations management. It is worth pausing to reflect that community sector organisations did not follow the same management path as business sector organisations. For the social welfare professional, management was considered a necessary evil, but not their real work. Different conceptualisations of the organisation as an entity contributed to the adoption of other management approaches, and many social and community sector organisations engaged with alternative models, such as collectives and community-based management (Lewis et al., 2012).

We hope it is now clearly evident that management and management theory has a lengthy history of concern with resolving the problem of getting people to do things within an organisational framework. As we saw in the profile provided by Marie Feeley, and will continue to observe in further practitioners' accounts, contemporary management approaches have not dispensed with this body of knowledge and its strategies and approaches. As management and organisational theory moved towards the twenty-first century, the relationships of organisations with their wider contexts, as well as the worlds contained within their boundaries, was brought into focus by the biological sciences.

Systems theory

While Likert identified four management 'systems' within organisations, other theorists were beginning to study organisations as open systems, with a two-way flow of interaction involving people, technologies and other systems. **Ecological systems theory**, which endures as a popular model in social work and human services practice,

Linkage
We discuss some of the alternative organisational formations adopted by community sector organisations later in this chapter and again in Chapter 3, when we explore organisational culture.

Ecological systems theory
Proposes that understanding human development and behaviour requires looking at the person in the context of the interrelated systems within their environment.

was developed by Urie Bronfenbrenner in the late 1970s. The ecological model seeks to make sense of the interactions between the person and their environment, which is understood as composed of other people and other systems (Morgan, 2006). Political, social, technological, legislative and economic factors in an organisation's environment are recognised as influencing human behaviour, as well as organisational practices and potential (Coulshed et al., 2006, p.43).

In the systems schema, organisations are understood as having internal components, or sub-systems, that dynamically interact with one another (the intra-organisational), as well as external relationships (inter-organisational) that are mediated by flows into and out of the organisation across permeable boundaries (see Figure 1.1). These exchanges between the internal and external domains of the organisation are constantly influencing and affecting both environments and the animate and inanimate elements within them. If we understand power as a form of relational energy, these flows can be seen as evidence of the actions of power.

Linkage
In Chapter 6 we revisit these concepts when looking at methods for analysing the organisational environment in the course of strategic planning.

FIGURE 1.1 Basic ecological system

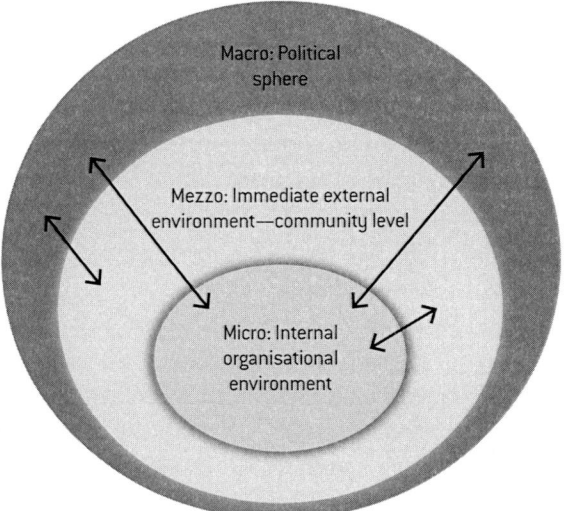

This concept of the organisation as a system redirects attention from structures toward processes. It also recognises forces beyond the control of management that act on the organisation itself, those employed within it and the people to whom services are provided. An important characteristic of an open system is the ability to exceed its component parts—to produce greater outcomes than are achievable by its individual elements. A common example is working towards the attainment of organisational goals, or resourcing and establishing a new program. You may recall Mary Parker Follett's observation that groups are more productive and effective than individuals working alone. This is described as synergy by ecological systems theorists (Bartol et al., 2011), and refers to the interaction of two or more entities that results in a greater outcome than is achievable by the individual components.

As a way of conceptualising organisations, the systems perspective fits more comfortably with health and human services than the business sector. This is because of the need in the former to be responsive to the multiple variables influencing the lives of clients, the heightened vulnerability of organisations to the socio-political environment, and because of recognition that health and human services are implicated in, and dependent on, networks (Lewis et al., 2012).

Constant tension exists between an organisation's aspiration to a sense of order and stability for internal functioning, and its externally driven need to adapt and change to remain viable. The capacity, willingness and necessity to engage in this dynamic varies across organisations and contexts, although it bears recognition that adaptive systems are more likely to survive and succeed (Page, 2011). Lewis and colleagues observe that 'most of the organisational theories that have emerged over the last half century operate under the assumption that all formal organisations are in fact open systems that respond to the environments around them' (Lewis et al., 2012, p.90).

Seeing organisations as complex, dynamic, open systems highlights the fluidity of the organisational environment; in which change is an inevitable feature of a normal order, rather than evidence of disorder. This notion that organisations are in a constant state of change and adaptation—an essential part of which is the constant flow and action of power—is critical for studying management in health and human services. We will return to this concept as we explore strategies for addressing the challenges presented to managers and leaders by the realities of the contemporary practice climate.

Contingency theory

Contingency theories build on the systems theory perspective by acknowledging that organisations must be responsive to fluctuations and changes in their internal and external environments to enable them to be effective and fulfil their purpose (Lewis et al., 2012). In short, contingency theory argues that organisations change their structures and management approaches to adapt to the unavoidable contingencies of the working environment (Clegg et al., 2011; Lewis et al., 2012).

In 1958 Joan Woodward (1916–71) observed that technologies directly impacted various components of the organisational environment, including lines of authority, and policy, rules and procedures. Subsequently, Burns and Stalker (1961) classified organisational structures as either mechanistic or organic.

Mechanistic organisations adhere to classical, scientific management principles; they are highly formalised, 'machine-like' and hierarchical. **Organic organisations**, on the other hand, are flexible, informal, 'biological' and flat structured. Where the environment is stable and certainty is high, organisations are more likely to be mechanistic. Where the environment is turbulent and uncertain, the greater need for adaptability results in more organic organisational structures (Ozanne & Rose, 2013). Contingency theory argues that neither is better than the other, rather it is context that determines what is appropriate; organisations are not stable entities, so they can adjust as required.

Mechanistic organisations
Organisations, often large, with a hierarchical structure, rigid rules, procedures and lines of accountability, and centralised decision-making.

Organic organisations
In many ways the antithesis of the mechanistic organisation, these are often small and flat structured, with open communication, and flexible decision-making processes to support emergent developments.

These ideas are particularly pertinent in the organisations that we studied in our case study research. Managers described needing to balance and maintain multiple relationships, and hold everything together, while also changing and adapting according to shifts in their environment. The following practice example, from a training and vocational enterprises manager, illustrates this.

PRACTICE EXAMPLE 1.1

The balancing act of managing within a system

The challenge for us as an organisation and as managers is balancing the government's requirements, the funders' requirements and the organisational requirements with what we believe is the best way to deliver services. Have you ever seen the Chinese balancing-plate act? Imagine, we've got government over here and we're trying to keep them happy, we've got the organisation over here and we're trying to keep them happy, we've got the media and the community over here and we're trying to keep them—oops, this one's starting to wobble, now that one is. So that's what it's like, trying to keep the plates in the air, but what matters most is how important has our work been. Not to the government, not to the funders, but to the person who's used it. So it's really about finding that balance.

Situational leadership
Situational leadership argues that to be effective, managers must select a style or strategy according to the presenting situation.

In terms of management approaches, contingency theory informs models such as **situational leadership.** Originally developed by Paul Hersey and Ken Blanchard, the situational leadership model is encapsulated in the popular management text *The One-Minute Manager* (Blanchard & Johnson, 1993). It argues that the most effective managers adapt their style to each situation. For example, novice workers require highly directive and controlling management styles, while experienced workers thrive on autonomy and responsibility, and so for them a laissez-faire approach is appropriate. Alternatively, an organisation dealing with mandated clients and highly risky public safety situations will require a more controlling and bureaucratic management approach than a community-based agency, which provides services to clients on a voluntary basis.

One example of organisations responding to contingencies in their environment has been the trajectory of the women's refuge movement. In the 1970s, with the rise in awareness about social problems facing women, such as domestic violence, women's refuges were established throughout Australia. As a resistance to and reaction against the disempowerment of women caused by patriarchal organisational and professional arrangements, women chose to establish feminist collectives. These were largely staffed by volunteer labour, they eschewed the notion of a leader or manager, and one criterion for appointment to a salaried position was *not* having a professional qualification. All paid staff were expected to contribute volunteer time and decisions were made collectively. However, increasing pressure from the governments that funded refuges, and the rise of economic rationalism, impelled these organic agencies to adopt managerial principles and move towards more mechanistic practices (Weeks, 1994).

Alternative approaches

Lewis and colleagues (2012) refer to non-bureaucratic organisations. These emerged as a critique of the unexamined use of power, and the lack of attention to the structural oppression that contributed to the marginalisation of particular individuals and groups. These alternative organisations were often small-scale, community-based, poorly funded, creative and experimental, and deeply committed to their clients and to social change. Disconcertingly, the majority have not survived the managerialist wave of the last decades; many have disappeared due to lack of funding or have been subsumed into larger auspicing agencies or clustered structures, like the present community health service model.

Coulshed et al. (2006) comment that the rate of change has become so fast and organisations so complex, that the management models developed in the nineteenth and twentieth centuries are no longer adequate. In the twenty-first century, health and human service organisations are implicated in a demanding and competitive environment that places more emphasis on management and leadership than ever before.

Emerging perspectives

As discussed at the outset of this chapter, and explored in more detail in Chapter 2, contemporary community services management is characterised by the ideology of managerialism imported from the business sector. In order to 'survive and thrive' and to be able to offer effective services to a wide range and significant number of people, health and human services have engaged, sometimes willingly and often reluctantly, with the discourse of scientific management and mechanistic processes. Policy-makers and funders, predominantly government, have instituted escalating levels of control through accreditation standards, and evaluation and accountability processes. Funding dollars must now be utilised *more efficiently* and achieve greater outcomes, and service delivery is being standardised towards predictable outcomes and *consistent* responses to clients. As we explore in the chapters to follow, not all of this is negative, and it is worth remaining mindful of Foucault's words:

> My point is not that everything is bad, but that everything is dangerous, which is not
> exactly the same as bad. If everything is dangerous, then we always have something to do.
> So my position leads not to apathy but to a hyper- and pessimistic activism. I think that the
> ethico-political choice we have to make every day is to determine which is the main danger.

Source: Foucault, 1983, pp.231–2

In discussing current management practice, Clegg and colleagues (Clegg et al., 2011) lament the lack of attention to contemporary management theory. They observe the 'fast track' mentality of management literature, trapped as it is within a culture of short time lines and pressure to succeed 'yesterday!' Scientific management principles are applied because they are expedient and achieve quick results, rather than because they are effective in the long term, well informed or just. Clegg et al. point to George Ritzer's concept of **McDonaldization** to describe contemporary approaches to business management.

McDonaldization
A concept that identifies four dominant mechanisms current in organisational management, based on fast-food industry principles: efficiency, calculability, predictability and control.

Ritzer identifies four dominant mechanisms that are based on fast-food industry principles. These are: efficiency—the smallest input for the largest gain; calculability—minimising production costs; predictability—standardising products so that the same service is delivered at all outlets; and control—regulating labour through machinery or, where people must provide the service, instituting rigid, prescriptive codes of conduct. The McDonaldization phenomenon has not only infiltrated the business sector but, according to Ritzer, this routinisation pervades contemporary life (Ritzer, 1993, cited in Clegg et al., 2011).

The consequences for the health and human services of this pervasive approach to managing organisations and everyday life take effect at a number of levels. At the dire extreme, management principles are imposed on organisations that contravene ethics of social justice, equity and the valuing of human (and all living) beings and the natural environment; placing the future well-being of people and communities at risk. On the other hand, increased accountability for public funding spending, the ability to provide immediate responses to increasingly complex client groups, and service system integration, impels the need to coordinate and standardise responses, and to find faster, more efficient ways of working. A critical issue for health and human services is identifying what these 'fast-food' approaches to organisational management do have to offer, while being alert and resistant to their pitfalls.

REFLECTION EXERCISE

Reflect on an organisation that you are familiar with. Have you seen any of the effects of McDonaldization taking place?

Into the future: Postmodern paradoxes

Lawler and Bilson (2010) also lament the popularity of simplified management models, commenting on the preference in social work management for approaches that promise concrete and pragmatic solutions in an increasingly unpredictable practice environment. They make the observation that many of these models are left wanting because they attempt to simplify complex theoretical ideas, and in so doing, depth of understanding, nuance and the importance of variable and unique contextual factors are overlooked. The paradox, they argue, is that the crushing demands in our ever more complex social world cannot be addressed with simple, one-size-fits-all solutions. And yet, time and resource limitations, and escalating external demands for responsiveness mean there is no time to engage with complicated theoretical frameworks, much less apply them to practice. Thus, organisational leaders are compelled to find quick fixes and 'simple' strategies, which can only offer inadequate, short-term solutions (Lawler & Bilson, 2010).

Somewhat ironically, one of the primary paradigm shifts in the transition from modernity to postmodernity was the rejection of the belief that one set of ideas could be found that would explain everything. Pluralism was embraced, and notions of hierarchy and elitism were disrupted. Postmodernism focused attention on how power operates within organisations in a web-like way, through discourses of 'expert' knowledge. Rather than a uni-directional flow from the top, power is understood as dispersed and diffuse, pervading all organisational levels. All of the people associated with an organisation— workers, clients and community members—are seen as constantly negotiating their position within, and in relation to, the organisation, through opposing interplays of power. At the same time, this constant tug and pull between demand to comply and resistance to compliance constructs the organisation and, in turn, this shapes and defines the workers' identities.

It can be a struggle to realise the implications of these ideas for health and human services management in a practical way. On one extreme, the values of the organisation and the professions that it supports are in danger of being undermined, and overridden by policy-makers and funders. On the other hand, these concepts lend support to the necessity for perpetual critical dialogue, the dismantling of hierarchical structures, the promotion of distributed leadership, the fostering of participatory practices, and the undoing of privilege in organisational relationships. Throughout this text, we encourage you to reflect on how to work with these paradoxes and challenges, as we explore the various dimensions of organisational management and practice in health and human services.

SUMMARY OF KEY ISSUES

In this chapter we traced the trajectory of the development of management into a specialised field from pre-classical to contemporary times. We considered some of the most influential thinkers arising from scientific and humanist schools of thought, and looked at how these two paradigms have contributed to knowledge about, and approaches to, management in the health and human services. We also reflected on various meanings and effects of power, and why—as managers and leaders—it is important to be aware of the way power operates, and how we can use this understanding productively, rather than oppressively. The intensifying complexity of the practice environment, the specialisation of management, and the need to find different ways of working effectively and successfully towards improved client outcomes, is impelling exploration of approaches and ideas capable of guiding us in new directions. This requires knowing what to select and retain from past practices, while fostering and engaging with new and emergent approaches. Next we look more closely at the factors that shape the practice environment.

PRACTICE ACTIVITIES

1 Management approaches
Identify whether elements of the management concepts listed below are evident in the organisation where you work, or one with which you are familiar. Specify the elements that you have observed.
1   Bureaucratic management
2   Human relations
3   McDonaldization
4   Panopticism
5   Participatory management
6   Scientific management/Taylorism

2 Organisational forms

Would you describe the organisation you have just analysed as mechanistic or organic? In what ways?

3 Managing now and into the future

List up to ten challenges that you see confronting management in health and human services as we move into the next decade. Identify strategies for addressing them.

FURTHER READING

The history of management theory

Bartol, K., Tein, M., Matthews, G., Sharma, B. & Scott-Ladd, B. (2011). 'Chapter 2: Pioneering Ideas in Management', in *Management. A Pacific Rim Focus*. Australia: McGraw-Hill, pp.36–57.

Clegg, S., Kornberger, M. & Pitsis, T. (2011). 'Chapter 12: Managing One Best Way?', in *Managing and Organizations. An Introduction to Theory and Practice* (3rd edn). London: Sage, pp.445–83.

Power

Foucault, M. (1992). 'The Subject and Power', in Dreyfus, H. L. & Rabinow, P.(eds), *Michel Foucault, Beyond Structuralism and Hermeneutics*, Chicago, University of Chicago Press, pp.208–28.

Lukes, S. (2005). 'Chapter 2: Power, Freedom and Reason', in *Power. A Radical Review* (2nd edn), Hampshire: Palgrave Macmillan, pp.60–107.

Tremain, S. (ed.), (2005). 'Foucault, Governmentality, and Critical Disability Theory. An Introduction', in *Foucault and the Government of Disability*, USA: The University of Michigan Press, pp.1–24.

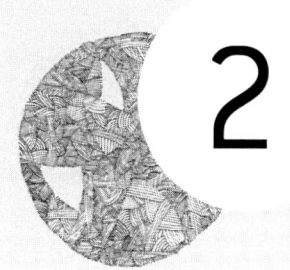

2

External Factors that Shape Health and Human Service Organisations

OVERVIEW

This chapter will:

- outline how health and human service organisations have changed in accordance with changes in the funding environment and in community expectations
- explore impacts of new public management and the role of government in the evolution of health and human service organisations
- discuss notions of equity and effectiveness and their relationship with resource distribution.

This chapter is about the origin of health and human service organisations in Australia, and major impacts on their structure and function.

KEY TERMS

Community Service Organisations (CSO)
equity
government-operated non-government
    organisations (GONGO)
horizontal equity
new public management (NPM)

not-for-profit (NFP) and non-government
    organisations (NGO)
policy stasis
quasi-autonomous non-government
    organisations (QANGO)
vertical equity

The origin and nature of health and human services in Australia

The values promoted in today's social services reflect their origins. Many were established because of community action to provide a service or advocate a cause. Historically, services received substantial social and practical support from religious groups, charities and philanthropists (Lyons, 2009, p.200). In many cases, this support has been maintained, while government also has a substantial role in supporting services.

Some services have become government-operated over time, while others are independent community organisations, typically described as **not-for-profit (NFP)** or **non-government organisations (NGO)**. These organisations may include voluntary as well as paid workers and funding comes from a range of sources. NFP/NGO are required to use any profit to advance the agency's purpose; any surplus must not be distributed to owners, members or any other individuals or groups (Commonwealth of Australia, 2001). The Australian Productivity Commission (2010) describes the NFP sector as one that includes organisations with a community orientation, which operate for altruistic or mutual benefit. In simple terms, NFP/NGO do not have shareholders, and all income is expended in the provision of services or used to improve the organisation (Black & Gruen, 2005).

Not-for-profit and non-government organisations
Organisations that do not have shareholders; all income is expended in the provision of services or used to improve the organisation.

Quasi-autonomous non-government organisations
Organisations that are semi-independent from government. They may have an independent board that includes government representatives.

Government-operated non-government organisations
Organisations that may be established by government but run separately, so the organisation maintains a level of independence and may qualify for government funding.

Community Service Organisations
Umbrella term covering a range of non-profit health and human service organisations that provide services to the community. Includes NGO, NFP, QANGO and GONGO.

REFLECTION EXERCISE

Identify an NGO in your area that has existed for a long time. What was the origin for its service and how has it changed?

Non-government organisations and independence from government

NGO must be understood in the context of a complex political environment, ongoing competition for funds, and changing discourses around social problems and the roles and importance of NGO in responding to these problems (Fisher, 1997). Substantial variations on the classic NGO have emerged, involving different funding arrangements, governance structures and levels of independence from government. For example, **quasi-autonomous non-government organisations (QANGO)** may involve an independent body that includes government representatives. **Government operated non-government organisations (GONGO)** may be established by government but run separately, so the organisation maintains a level of independence but may qualify for government funding schemes. The term **Community Service Organisations (CSO)** is often used to encompass NGO that offer programs funded from diverse sources. The practitioner profiled on the next page is the CEO of a regional not-for-profit organisation and she provides a valuable illustration of what is involved.

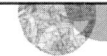

PRACTITIONER PROFILE 2.1

FIONA BOYLE

CHIEF EXECUTIVE OFFICER, GIPPSLAND CENTRE AGAINST SEXUAL ASSAULT (GCASA)

Position

My role involves oversight of all facets of the organisation from clinical practice, prevention and community education, finances, legal, HR and quality assurance. The role reports to a board that requires knowledge about governance. A critical function of the role is lobbying, both for the organisation and also on behalf of the community and clients we serve in respect to the issue of sexual assault.

Typical day

My workdays are varied and can involve anything from attending meetings and briefings, reporting to government, supervision of staff, preparing budgets and reviewing financial documents, and meeting with politicians, funders and key stakeholders.

Challenges

The greatest challenge of this particular role is related to the size of the organisation. Being a small rural organisation means that resources are limited and it is a challenge to work within these constraints. It is important to look for creative solutions to these challenges and this is sometimes difficult. It also means that there is an expectation to have knowledge across multiple areas because there are not the resources to employ specialist staff, for example, a quality HR or finance manager.

Skills and qualities

The most important skill is that of social intelligence. Relationships form the basis of all aspects of this role; with clients, staff, key stakeholders and funders. It is really helpful to have interpersonal skills that can promote team cohesiveness, assisting clients directly or through lobbying, forming and working in partnerships and attracting funds.

In addition, a sound understanding of the clinical processes, and the impact of sexual assault, needs to form a lens for everything that is worked towards and achieved. The vision and mission of the organisation needs to be fully understood and be consistent with personal values—this creates passion.

Lessons learnt

The greatest lesson I have learnt as CEO is that it takes time to really understand both the role and the organisation. There are relationships to be negotiated and this takes time. I was once told that it takes two years to be operating fully in a CEO role—at the time I did not think that was the case; I now do. The role can be performed on a much deeper level, with richer connections and understandings; this maturing approach has positive implications for the organisation.

Funding for services

Funding for health and human service organisations comes from many sources, including private foundations and bequests, client fees, and contributions from the corporate sector, in addition to government (local, state, territory, Commonwealth). We shall briefly look at non-government sources of funding before exploring government funding and associated expectations.

Non-government

In 2006–07, 9.5% of the income for non-profit organisations came from donations, sponsorship and fundraising. Almost all this income was for social services, which include youth and family welfare, childcare, the disabled and elderly (excluding high-care residential services), refugee and homeless assistance, emergency accommodation and shelters (Australian Bureau of Statistics, 2009). Further:

- In 2004, 13.4 million adult Australians donated $5.2 billion to non-profit organisations.
- A further $2 billion that year was provided by 10.5 million Australians who bought raffle tickets or attended charity auctions and similar events.
- In 2003–04, over half a million Australian businesses donated $3 billion to non-profit organisations.

Source: Commonwealth Department of Families, Housing, Community Services and Indigenous Affairs, in Lyons, 2009

Religious-based associations (for example, Uniting Care, Salvation Army) have maintained their commitment to community well-being throughout a long history of service provision. They provide financial support for organisations and specific projects; these organisations deliver services that are funded through government and non-government sources.

Many organisations in Britain and the USA benefit from a long and generous tradition of philanthropy. Large foundations have been established, with the imprimatur to improve social circumstances in the community—possibly connected with particular causes, but often in a more general sense. Australia does not have the same history of benefaction; in 2006–07 only 10% of the income for NFP was from philanthropy (Australian Productivity Commission, 2010).

There are some substantial philanthropic organisations in Australia, for example, the Ian Potter Foundation, which is described in Case example 2.1. Other examples include the Melbourne Community Foundation and the Sidney Myer Fund.

CASE EXAMPLE 2.1

The Ian Potter Foundation: A philanthropic organisation in Australia

The Ian Potter Foundation was established in the 1960s and since that time it has provided more than $30 million to organisations. It allocates grants in the area of community well-being that seek to alleviate disadvantage and generate well-being. Projects are selected based on the capacity of the host organisation (for example, they must have a proven track record) and the innovative nature of project ideas in seeking to tackle entrenched problems. For example, in South Australia the Adelaide Day Centre for Homeless Persons received support to ease the transition from homelessness into housing. Another example, the Adults Surviving Sexual Abuse organisation in New South Wales, received financial support to provide a telephone helpline and information service. The foundation's website has further information on the projects they fund: www.ianpotter.org.au.

Government

Government departments allocate funds for specific service areas and administer schemes designed to boost organisational capacity. Government money that is designated for public works helps fund building improvements and equipment purchases.

Over time, the amount of government support for community service organisations has increased to around one third of all funds received (Australian Bureau of Statistics, 2009). There is considerable discussion about whether this reliance on government funding has meant a change in the values of organisations, as their philosophy and objectives may be impacted by government priorities (Donovan & Jackson, 1991).

In addition, governments have become increasingly concerned about the benefits obtained from their investment in services. Quality assurance systems have been introduced to promote a level of uniformity in program operations that is consistent with good practice (Johnson-Abdelmalik, 2011). An evaluation and monitoring framework has been developed for the identification of inputs, outputs and outcomes that define service functions and effectiveness (Australian Productivity Commission, 2010). If you would like to read more about this, the Productivity Commission's report is included in the reading list for this chapter.

In response to government pressure and the drive for increased efficiencies and effectiveness, organisations have adopted more business-oriented management practices. There is potential benefit in the articulation of project activities and expectations, and efficiencies in administrative functions, while a continued commitment to organisational values remains important. However, values may change as organisations strive to compete within a complex funding environment.

In particular, the contractual environment brings a level of insecurity to organisations, partly as services are typically under-funded and budgets do not fully account for infrastructure costs (for example, clinical supervision or operational management) or sustainability measures (for example, staff development and succession planning). The long-term under-investment in management capability among community service organisations (Houlbrook, 2011) and the escalating demand for services means that those doing good work may not be well placed to effectively document and report on their successes. The health and human services manager thus faces substantial and competing challenges.

New public management and the role of government

In this section we consider the introduction of managerialism in the health and human services, and subsequent changes in these organisations.

The consequences of managerialism

Since the late 1980s the management of human service organisations has become increasingly aligned with management in the business sector. Government interest in cost containment

Linkage
Different approaches to management are explained in Chapter 1.

and the size of the public sector have meant that policies seeking to control and contain service operations are attractive (Willis et al., 2005).

Principles of the marketplace have been applied to public institutions, with the assumption that services will become more efficient if subject to challenges faced by the private sector (particularly competition), applying market principles to working conditions, and introducing performance management strategies (Willis et al., 2005). While these new forces have driven funding and reporting models, the exact nature of their implementation has been left to the sector—posing challenges but also opportunities regarding how organisations will function into the future.

The introduction of managerialism to the human services sector was perceived by many social and welfare workers as an unwarranted and unethical imposition that threatened to undermine the very nature and culture of practice (Hughes & Wearing, 2013). Hasenfeld (2010, p.2) argues that, coinciding with the establishment of managerialism, the human services as a field of practice and organisationally has translated from 'an institutional logic of care and equal access to an institutional logic of the new market and personal responsibility'.

This shift, of health and human service organisations being held accountable to their funding sources, has produced a range of challenges. Though resistance to now-entrenched managerialist techniques was ultimately moot, it was successfully asserted that distinct boundaries between the business and human services sectors needed to be acknowledged and retained. A trend during the 1990s towards the appointment of top-level managers with generic, business-oriented experience and qualifications, but no professional background in social work or welfare practice, intensified this imperative. At the same time, social welfare and social work educators worked to increase management content in undergraduate programs, and introduce postgraduate courses in relevant areas (for example, social work and human services administration) in an effort to address the evident qualification and skill gap in the professional workforce (Donovan & Jackson, 1991; Jones & May, 1992; Patti, 2003).

The differences between public sector and business organisations at that time could be seen at all levels, from direct practice to upper management. Drawing on a range of sources, Donovan and Jackson (1991) identified features that make human service organisations unique:

- Meeting socially recognised needs is the reason for their existence.
- Access to services is controlled by the providers and not the consumers of services (Martin, 1985, cited in Donovan & Jackson, 1991, p.220).
- Practices and behaviours are ideologically driven and characterised by conflicting demands and multiple expectations (Sarri & Hasenfeld, 1978, cited in Donovan & Jackson, 1991, p.19).
- A key function is to operationalise social policy through program delivery.
- External and internal environments are characterised by complexity and uncertainty (Donovan & Jackson, 1991, pp.18–20 & p.357)

While the overall direction of grants and incentive require that clinicians increase the delivery of services, they do not directly demand changes to the way work is organised, nor to clinical decision-making (Willis et al., 2005). However, when time is short and staff are underqualified (as a consequence of funding regimes), there is a flow-on effect to everyday practice.

Despite assertions that unique features in health and human service sectors make it difficult to anticipate and accurately measure program performance or truly reflect client outcomes, the benefit in trying to enhance efficiency and effectiveness has been recognised. This support for a re-orientation of the management of organisations is firmly grounded in the imperative to demonstrate benefits for clients, and acknowledgment of the need for organisations to be better managed in order to improve service provision comes from several sources: Donovan and Jackson (1991), Hasenfeld (2010), Jones and May (1992) and Patti (2003).

In the early 1990s, the profound paradigm shift that managerialism represented was described by Jones and May (1992, p.387), who urged workers to 'understand that managerialism is not a set of unquestionable techniques, but rather a political programme and campaign to bring about far-reaching changes in human service organisations'. Of course, service users have a right to expect quality services. To this end, workers are encouraged to commandeer managerialist principles for the benefit of clients by extending the criteria of efficiency and effectiveness to include equity, excellence and expansion (Jones & May, 1992, p.399).

> **Linkage**
> Understandings of equity and effectiveness are explored later in this chapter.

The fundamental distinction between management in the human services and administration in the business sector was in the professional values that underpin social work and welfare practice. The managerialist regime posed a threat to the retention and upholding of the moral codes and values that underpin health and human services practice, and this concern remains relevant today. However, the moral commitment to improve outcomes for clients impels workers and organisations towards providing high quality, equitable, efficient and effective services to all who need them. This application of managerialism in the public sector is referred to as **new public management (NPM)**.

> **New public management**
> Major reform of the public sector toward a market-oriented model: services need to be responsive to citizens and politicians, and to demonstrate desired outcomes within an efficient organisational framework.

The changing role of government

The exercise of neo-liberal ideology through the institution of managerialist and economic rationalist principles over the past three decades has profoundly changed management and practice in health and human services (Jones & May, 1992; Laming et al., 2011). Arguably the most significant macro-level change to take place began with governments adopting the now clichéd principle of 'steering not rowing' (Osborne & Gaebler, 1992).

This backing away of government from the welfare state, to play the role of funder, direction setter and regulator, but not the deliverer of public sector services, was implemented by the sale of government assets to private enterprises, and the introduction of a competitive funding environment (Willis et al., 2005). Health and human service organisations, which were previously not-for-profit or cost neutral, could now include private enterprises, all vying for government support through competitive tendering processes. This has meant substantial changes in the services that exist and the manners in which they operate.

A significant consequence of new public management has been the detrimental impact on small community-based organisations, many of which have found it impossible to survive as stand-alone agencies (Hughes & Wearing, 2013). From an initial period of competition, mistrust and divisiveness, many organisations learnt to work together to increase their marketability and pool resources. A raft of amalgamations resulted in the formation of larger organisations. These new arrangements necessitated a management approach that could transform, position and sustain organisations in a competitive climate modelled on the business sector (Hughes et al., 2007). Managerialist technologies are now commonplace in health and human services practice. They include:

- strategic, business and operational plans
- statistical reporting on program activities and client outcomes
- measurements of efficiency and effectiveness
- quality assurance frameworks
- accountability to clients.

In addition, some organisations have adopted a corporate identity, with catchy slogans, specially designed logos and staff uniforms. But managerialism is not just about administration or corporate image. It is informed by a transformational discourse that privileges the right to manage, positions the manager as a heroic leader, and promotes organisational obligations to engage in change while not simply achieving, but exceeding, performance targets. In other words, 'doing more, better, with less, by doing things differently' (Harris et al., 2004, pp.20–1).

In the 21st century, structural boundaries that once seemed firmly established have been blurred; for example, public and private domains, left and right wing politics, and gender and sexual identity. This does not of course mean that all borders have entirely broken down, or that new ones have not formed. Despite reductions in the delineation between business and community sector organisations, with both engaging in delivering services that previously would have been considered outside core business, fundamental differences have been retained. The distinction is not associated with the work or the environments within which the work takes place, but aligned with the goals and values that drive the work of health and human services.

Health and human service organisations continue to be defined by their focus on work that seeks to improve people's circumstances; for their own and society's benefit (Hasenfeld, 2010). Services aim to improve people's social and economic circumstances and enable access to specialist interventions that remedy or reduce negative impacts from physical and mental health problems. Empowered individuals take charge of their lives and work toward personal goals. Lewis et al. (2012, p.2) observe that while 'people working in unity to achieve common goals' constitutes an organisation, the shared focus on primary goals that seek to improve community and individual well-being ultimately distinguishes public health and human services, and this shapes the way they are managed.

Before we continue this exploration of the external factors impacting health and human services, it is useful to read the practitioner profile following. Simon Ruth provides a sophisticated account of the mechanisms involved in managing a large program that is part of a community health service. Key aspects of his role include contributing to management across different parts of the organisation, working with the community to enhance services, and being cognisant of changes at government level that may impact the operating environment.

PRACTITIONER PROFILE 2.2

SIMON RUTH

DIRECTOR—COMPLEX SERVICES, PENINSULA COMMUNITY HEALTH

Position

My position as Director—Complex Services, within the organisation is a middle management role. I am responsible for approximately a third of the programs of the community health service, which equates to roughly $10 million worth of funding. I am also site manager for one large site and four smaller sites. My program streams include alcohol and drug programs, Indigenous health, youth services, aged care programs, homelessness services, family violence programs, health promotion, post-acute care and access. In several of these areas, I am the senior person within the health service and represent the health service on these matters. I have three direct reports. I chair several internal committees, including several community advisory groups.

Typical day

A typical day involves attending meetings, writing reports and submissions, responding to queries both internal and external, examining reporting data and managing staff matters.

There is a range of meetings, both internal and external. External meetings are with a range of key stakeholders including funders, other service providers, members of the public, researchers, and consumers who want to discuss the service they received. Some of these meetings are for information sharing and gathering; others are to discuss organisational performance. Some meetings are in order to lobby for change. Meetings with consumers and the public may be to address complaints or they may be to hear ideas. Our community advisory groups are a forum for two-way communication with our community. These meetings allow the attendees to raise ideas with the health service about how it could be improved and also provide an avenue for the health service to seek advice on current or planned service provision.

Internal meetings involve meetings where management issues and processes are discussed and confirmed. Other internal meetings may occur with other parts of the health service to plan for projects or joint work to address common issues, such as looking at ways that alcohol and drug services can support other parts of the health service.

At my level, there is less day-to-day management of staff and programs, although this does still occur, and more oversight of systems, such as quality control, service improvement and data reporting. I work with managers and others to ensure that key performance indicators are met. There are certain areas, such as 'Closing the Gap' for Aboriginal and Torres Strait Islander consumers, that sit in my program stream but have a mandate to effect change across the entire health service.

As the lead person in the health service in certain areas such as alcohol and drug services, I attend many external meetings with funders, policy makers and other service providers. Both local government areas that fall into our catchment have keen interests in the issue and I meet

(*continued*)

with them regularly. I have been on the board of the state's peak body for alcohol and drug services for the last eight years, spending five years as president, and I attend meetings with funders representing the peak body as well.

Challenges

The biggest challenge I face is time. Is it quicker to complete an urgent project myself or teach someone else to do it? Teaching someone else to complete something will pay off in the long run but often in a time-poor environment it is easier and faster to do it yourself. Having the time to progress side projects, to adequately support staff, to complete the range of tasks expected and to maintain my own learning is a struggle. Working with more senior staff that have even less time creates further pressure, as there can be little opportunity to progress requests.

Managing in periods of significant change, such as government reform or periods of government downsizing, can be challenging as it can create insecurities for staff and organisations. With large numbers of public servants departing it can create instability in program support from government, particularly with the loss of corporate knowledge that goes along with this.

Funding

In the areas I currently manage, there are large-scale reform processes ahead and a tightening of the government belt. Reform processes can create instability and insecurities for staff and the broader sector. They can create a lot of work trying to settle people down and require a large number of meetings with stakeholders in planning and networking.

The biggest impact around tightening of the government purse has been the large-scale use of voluntary departure packages that has led to a significant decrease in the number of people in government that are available to continue to support funded services. It has also led to the loss of corporate knowledge and the stagnation of particular projects that are of a lower priority. In program areas where all, or most, staff have departed, activity can virtually cease.

All government funding is finite and there are many competing voices for it. Sometimes governments need to make tough decisions to meet their election promises, so you have to learn to take much of this in your stride.

Community engagement

Community engagement is incredibly important to the work we do. The organisation I work for has several different ways it engages the community. Every consumer is provided with information about their rights and responsibilities and is encouraged to make informed decisions about their own treatment. Additionally there is a Customer Relations Department where consumers can provide feedback to the service or have complaints resolved.

The organisation has a Community Advisory Committee (CAC) that is a sub-board committee. The CAC is attended by senior staff, board members and around 15 committee members. The committee members represent 15 Community Advisory Groups (CAGs). Each CAG focuses on a specific geographic community, program area or diversity group and is made up of community members with an interest in that area as well as staff and representatives of interested external organisations. The CAGs are invaluable in providing advice and support to the service around program and service development. This structure also allows the service to easily and quickly engage the local community on a range of issues. Without the support, and lobbying, of the CAGs many projects and new services would never have been conceived.

External to the organisation's official structures there are many opportunities to meet with individual community members, or self-help and social support groups, and these meetings are valuable opportunities to create partnerships and identify further gaps in service provision.

Management implications

The adequacy of funding has long been a concern for health and human services, and the emphasis on contracted programs has prompted changes in the way organisations 'do business'. These changes have significant implications for managers: contracting is often specific to projects and does not account for infrastructure costs; and funding contracts are often short-term and continuity is uncertain. As a consequence, there are advantages in having a range of funding sources so services can more easily compensate for the shortfall in individual contracts and acquire a pool of funds to support organisational planning and sustainability.

This context usually benefits larger agencies, as they have management and planning resources to promote their services, lobby potential funders, and develop sophisticated proposals. In addition, infrastructure expenses can be spread across programs. Arguably, larger agencies have better capacity to attract and retain talented staff in comparison with small organisations, as better salaries and benefits can be incorporated, along with a defined career path. The readings list at the end of this chapter includes an interesting case study that describes how a rural health service responded to changes in the service environment to ensure viability. An overarching framework was used to examine sustainability requirements in the areas of workforce; funding; governance, management and leadership; linkages; and infrastructure (Buykx et al., 2012).

Many health and human services have evolved to survive in an unpredictable financial environment, and have improved their business practices to account for requirements of funders, but they are responsible to a broad range of stakeholders, including clients and community members. These stakeholders may have different priorities and perspectives about what constitutes the 'core business' of the organisation, resulting in multiple and possibly competing demands. For example, program timelines and deliverables set out in funding contracts may not account for the actual time needed to establish new programs. There may be competing priorities based on business principles and those informed by client need. Management may decide that the organisation should invest in particular aspects of work that have appropriate funding levels and good continuity, while letting go of other services—perhaps involving uncertain financial arrangements and complex clients.

The practitioner profiled below is of someone who works in an Aboriginal organisation. You are encouraged to read the profile carefully to identify the skills particularly important for connectedness with the community.

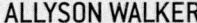

PRACTITIONER PROFILE 2.3

ALLYSON WALKER

MANAGER, SOCIAL AND COMMUNITY SERVICES, DANDENONG AND DISTRICT ABORIGINES CO-OPERATIVE

Position

I manage many different programs in the organisation, for example, 'Strengthening and Connecting Koori Young People' (Grades 4–6 boys), Youth Worker (12–25 years), Family Services (including emergency relief and food bank), 'Bringing Them Home' (first-, second- and third-generation stolen generations), and Mental Health Development and Outreach Workers.

I also provide supervision for all staff, attend meetings with funding bodies, the board and community members, and undertake casework.

Typical day

- Catching up with staff—I have an open door policy where they will pop in any time to discuss a case or run something by me
- Chatting with community members if they pop in for a yarn or would prefer to meet with me rather than another staff member
- Attending meetings and returning or making phone calls
- Sorting out issues if they arise
- Communication with community, staff and government

Challenges

- Time to complete admin work with people popping in and out of the office
- Case advice and direction then and there
- Sorting out disagreements
- Having a huge portfolio and generally keeping on top of it all
- Lack of support and understanding of the social and community services programs from the hierarchy

Lessons learnt

- Need to look after yourself so you can be an effective manager
- Need for support, someone to offload on; a need for outside supervision
- Can't have the door open all the time, sometimes you need to shut the door to get administrative tasks done
- Effective policy, processes and forms help make the job easier

Skills and qualities

- You need to be someone who is approachable both to staff and community members
- Good listener, let them tell their story—sometimes that's all they need
- Follow through with actions and don't make promises that you can't keep
- Value your staff, their expertise is unique; if you value and support your staff they will give their all to the community and their position

- Overall knowledge of your area so you can advise in the right direction
- Counselling; you will often be in a situation where you need to sort out disputes
- The ability to communicate with many different groups: government, directors, community members, youth, children, elders, community partners, etc. This includes written communication, through reports, email or letters, and the ability to speak publicly at meetings and give presentations
- Qualifications in social work, community development or welfare

To recapitulate, operating in an era of managerialism has been reflected in organisational developments that include:
- Amalgamating smaller services into larger, multi-program and possibly multi-site organisations.
- Adopting business management principles ranging from detailed financial planning to careful alignment of the workforce according to project needs.
- Developing a corporate layer in the organisation that demonstrates management infrastructure and acumen.
- Establishing partnerships across organisations that provide similar or complementary services.
- Building and maintaining the organisation's profile among potential or existing funders, potential partners and members of the community.
- The moderation of advocacy activities so as not to offend funders.

There is also evidence of a more corporate style of management in some organisations, which involves:
- Larger, more professionalised boards of directors.
- A focus on risk management with regard to financial and programmatic decision-making.
- Limited investment in management infrastructure.
- A workforce that may be required to work across roles, with some casual and contract-based positions. (Smith, 2010).

Managing with less

Operating within the NPM framework and a tight fiscal environment may require management strategies such as those outlined in Table 2.1 overleaf. When reading through the table, you may find it useful to think about an organisation that you are familiar with, and whether these strategies (and the associated benefits, risks and consequences) apply. You may also identify other strategies, benefits and risks that are not shown here.

At best, these strategies resemble management approaches that guide the wise investment of resources while accommodating funding constraints. At worst, an over-reaction to budgetary issues (short-term funding, future uncertainty) will see organisations reduce their capacity and lose considerable resources (staff, facilities) that are not easily replaced. Rather than operate from a business model using a risk-averse approach and an annual funding cycle, managers need to understand the level of risk they can accommodate in a funding environment where opportunities are likely to arise

Linkage
Funding and budget approaches are explored further in Chapter 8.

without a great deal of notice. Past performance is important for this and budgetary approaches that account for soft funding, multiple funding schemes, and policy cycles will assist.

TABLE 2.1 Management strategies to allow for a reduction in funding

STRATEGY	EXAMPLE	POSSIBLE BENEFITS	POSSIBLE RISKS AND CONSEQUENCES
Downscaling resources	Reduction in norms regarding work-related travel or catering (e.g., fewer pool cars, chocolate biscuits not cream cakes!)	• Reduced cost	• Insufficient resources to undertake work • Staff dissatisfaction and resentment
Contingency budgets	Defining the staff profile in the context of no growth (e.g., core positions plus contracted roles)	• Low risk; no financial commitment to unfunded positions	• Staff self-interest impacting decision-making processes • Limited capacity to take on new opportunities
Recruitment freeze	Staff vacancies are not filled, unless absolutely necessary	• Savings	• Increased workload for remaining staff • Reduced capacity to undertake tasks likely to bring in new work (e.g., networking, promoting organisation, preparing funding bids)
Reorientation of services	Review programs to identify principal areas and those that may need to be dissolved	• Freeing up resources • Savings	• Insufficient understanding of subliminal benefits from individual services may translate to the loss of valuable programs
Change in staff roles	Reallocating duties and reducing non-core staff activities	• Refocusing on organisational priorities	• Reduction in staff skills • Staff dissatisfaction
Top-down approach	The use of more directives and less advice/information for communicating the direction of the organisation	• Management control	• Reduced staff motivation and loss of allegiance to organisation • Development of subcultures with conflicting values

Forces that impact government funding

With this understanding of the roles of government and organisations in the NPM environment, we turn now to factors that impact decisions about which projects are funded. The determination of priorities and the process of policy change are described.

Limited resources

When considering challenges in the allocation of government funds for social services, it is important to note that funds are limited and that there are many possible inclusions under the banner of health and human services. At the macro level, what is best for the public should guide decisions about what is funded. Public attitudes about the importance of particular social concerns (for example, homelessness, domestic violence, teenage pregnancy) are pivotal given the community orientation of services and the political impetus to demonstrate responsiveness to community concerns.

In reality, the continuation of government funding for contracted services is often the product of **policy stasis**. That is, contracts are rolled over and government support remains essentially the same for long periods of time. Major changes in established government funding regimes generally occur in a climate of policy reform. This is often brought about by a change in government, a striving to reduce expenditure, and possibly fresh perspectives involving new initiatives or organisations that appear best placed to deliver effective care.

Policy stasis
The continued application of an existing policy, which may persist despite external factors indicating that the policy needs amendment.

Policy development and the distribution of government funds

The distribution of 'new' government funds for services (or adjustments involving existing funds) is the product of policy change. However, this process is not straightforward. Factors with varying importance that can affect this include public opinion, political imperative, existing evidence, and the capacity to implement change (Edwards et al., 2001; Bowen & Zwi, 2005). In simple terms, stages in policy development and resultant funding for services involve the process illustrated in the following figure (Edwards et al., 2001).

FIGURE 2.1 The process of policy development

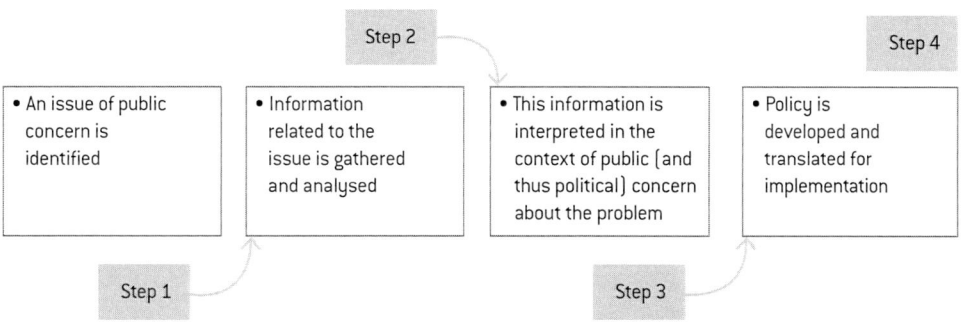

Each step in this process is explained below.

Step 1. Examples include a new viral infection, elevated rates of youth homelessness, or family breakdown. Alternatively, initiatives from other locations (for example, a successful program on parenting skills for young single parents) may be disseminated and prompt public interest and policy action.

Step 2. This may involve the use of data already gathered (for example, population statistics, service evaluations, literature and policy reviews) and include gathering new information via consultation and research. The exact nature of the issue will be clarified and available options for its remediation will be outlined.

Step 3. Is the issue likely to cause major problems for the public? Is there a known and feasible remedy? What level of political caché (community concern) is involved if action is or isn't taken to address the issue?

Step 4. This includes consideration of the cost, timeliness, effectiveness and review of proposed interventions.

There is considerable variation in how this process unfolds—the time involved and thoroughness of investigation—according to characteristics of the specific issue. For example, recent policy (and legislative) changes regarding plain packaging for cigarettes are the product of a long and exhaustive process that has been informed by evidence on harms from nicotine and the effects of packaging, and faced challenges from powerful industry lobbyists. In another example, pilot programs involving clients on substitution pharmacotherapy in residential rehabilitation are being undertaken to test the effectiveness of this approach. This will provide evidence for a possible change in policy regarding this service type (Step 2, shown above) and, depending on impacts at Step 3, policy development and implementation (Step 4) may eventuate.

REFLECTION EXERCISE

Think about a recent policy development that has impacted your work or your personal life, for example new initiatives targeting social concerns or strategies to improve education. Were there any markers of policy development in the media? What has driven the change?

Equity and effectiveness

Having explored challenges of the funding environment and management implications, in this section we consider who 'should' have access to health and human services in the context of increasing demand for care and limited public resources. We explore what is meant by **equity** and its relationship to, and understandings of, program efficiency and effectiveness.

Equity
An important concept that impacts on the configuration of services according to fundamental views regarding equality, ethics and efficiency in health care.

With reference to health, Black and Gruen (2005, p.74) explain that resource allocation should be guided by three goals:

- *Equity*, which they explain as access to care by those in need.
- *Allocative efficiency*, where resources are invested in services that are likely to be successful rather than services that are likely to provide low return.
- *Technical efficiency*, where the combination and nature of expenditure on equipment and staff resources is optimal for the initiative being funded.

Equity

Equity is difficult to define and there is no single 'correct' explanation. It depends on value judgments about access to care and equal rights, as well as the relative emphasis placed on different aspects of health and human services (Mooney, 2003). This is best illustrated by the importance placed on equal access to services versus the efficiency of services—their performance on agreed measures of output. For example, a prevention-oriented intervention that targets the entire population may produce a moderate risk reduction. Using the same resources to support fewer people at high risk may bring greater dividends. This latter approach is *unequal*, in that health and human services resources are not evenly distributed across the population. However, the distribution of resources may be *equitable* given the higher levels of need among the high-risk group. It reflects allocative efficiency in terms of a good return on the investment made.

This brings us to two major aspects of equity. **Horizontal equity** is about equal treatment of people in similar circumstances. **Vertical equity** is concerned with unequal treatment that varies because of the different levels of need in the population—the unequal status of potential clients (Mooney, 2003). By enabling people's access to services according to their level of need, we may expect substantial improvements in their health and well-being (Harris et al., 2004).

Linkage
As you may appreciate, values are critical to decisions about equity; we explore this area further in the next chapter.

Horizontal equity
The equal provision of services among people with equal levels of need.

Vertical equity
The unequal provision of services among people according to their unequal levels of need.

REFLECTION EXERCISE

Equity in health care may be defined differently across locations, as beliefs and judgments about differential access impact the allocation of resources in relation to need. As noted above, horizontal and vertical equity represent views about providing equal services for equal need versus unequal services based on unequal need. How is equity defined in your organisation? Identify some examples of service access that illustrate this understanding of equity.

Effectiveness

The drive for increased effectiveness, or at least the capacity to demonstrate positive outcomes, means we need to understand what is being sought from services and how this may be measured. This is not straightforward in health and human services as gains at client level may be incremental and service delivery improvements may take some time to be realised. It is important that everyone (from management to staff and clients) understands and agrees on the purpose, activities and desired outcomes of each program.

Tolbert and Hall (2009) define organisational effectiveness in three ways:

- *System-resource approach*: where the long-term survival of the organisation is the key goal. This is the consequence of performance across many projects, some of which may not be operating at optimum level at any given point in time.
- *Client-satisfaction approach:* individuals attached to the organisation feel their goals are being met and they continue to contribute to the organisation, ensuring its survival.
- *Stakeholder approach:* involving the understanding of what various stakeholders to the organisation seek to achieve and their relative importance in terms of conceptualisations of organisational effectiveness.

For government (a major stakeholder) it is important to know what they are purchasing and that it works. For organisations, adapting principles of business management alongside the definition and measurement of 'what matters' to the organisation (and funders) is critical. Clients need programs that are responsive to their concerns; utilising strategies that are effective, and drawing on service and system networks to maximise resource availability. Management will benefit from understanding how separate components contribute to the whole; how individual program performance is consolidated to show organisational effectiveness. Staff will be able to direct their energies to activities matched to agreed objectives. Clients will better understand the potential gains from program participation.

Linkage
In Chapter 7 we describe two collaborative evaluations of community services.

As you can appreciate, this context means it is important to define the target group for health and human service organisations and tailor interventions and expectations accordingly. Subsequently, services need to examine the extent to which characteristics of their client group match that of the target group and gather information on their achievements against desired outcomes. Evaluation is a useful tool for services and we revisit this area later in the text.

SUMMARY OF KEY ISSUES

Health and human services evolved as a result of community action to address social problems, and public opinion continues to be an important driver of investment in these areas. A substantial proportion of funding for non-government organisations is from various levels of government and the era of new public management has seen government take the position of 'steering not rowing' the orientation and function of services. Limited resources, increasing demand and competing priorities all impact on the distribution of funding. Different views on equity and effectiveness impact decisions about what areas should be funded and to what effect.

PRACTICE ACTIVITIES

1 New public management

Approach a senior manager in your workplace or another organisation that you are connected with and ask them whether there have been any changes in the philosophy of management and what this meant in relation to the values upheld by the organisation.

2 Non-profit and profit-oriented organisations

Make a list of the organisations that you access in a day, for example, the supermarket, public transport, an educational institution, or your local community health service. Divide the list into organisations that are primarily profit making, those that are primarily about providing a service to people to improve their well-being, and those that combine these approaches. Now think about whether you encountered any managers while you were there. How did you know they were in a management position? What distinguished them (or not) from other people who work there? When you were engaging with the organisation did you think of yourself as a customer, client or service user? How did this affect the way you interacted with the people who worked there? Does managerialism help to explain your perceptions?

3 Effectiveness

Think about how effectiveness is described in the commercial sector; for example, involving a media outlet or insurance company. How does this contrast with understandings of effectiveness in health and human services?

4 Policy development

Identify a 'new' policy in your area of work or study and map out the process of development using the stages that are described in Figure 2.1. Adjust these stages according to the nature of the policy development process you have identified. What stages were prominent in this process of policy development?

FURTHER READING

Contribution of the NFP sector

Australian Productivity Commission (2010). *Contribution of the Not-For-Profit Sector*, Research Report, Canberra: Australian Government.

Indigenous health organisations in Australia

Baeza, J. I., & Lewis, J. M. (2010). 'Indigenous Health Organizations in Australia: Connections and Capacity', *International Journal of Health Services*, *40*, pp.719–42.

Rural health services

Buykx, P., Humphreys, J. S., Tham, R., Kinsman, L., Wakerman, J., Asaid, A. & Tuohey, K. (2012). 'How do Small Rural Primary Health Care Services Sustain Themselves in a Constantly Changing Health System Environment?', *BMC Health Services Research*, *12*(81). Retrieved from www.biomedcentral.com/1472-6963/12/81

3

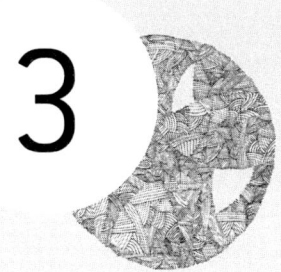

Organisational Culture and Operation

OVERVIEW

This chapter will:

- describe organisational culture and its relationship with staff well-being
- explain the multiple sets of ethical obligations encountered by managers
- outline diversity and discrimination in organisations, and management strategies against discrimination and for diversity
- describe organisational policies and explore their development and implementation.

In this chapter we explore the inner environment of the organisation, focusing on mechanisms that shape its culture and approach to practice. Processes in support of diversity and equal opportunity are outlined, and the nature and role of policy development and implementation are explained.

KEY TERMS

corporate culture	organisational culture
discrimination	organisational ethics
diversity management	organisational policies
managerial ethics	professional code of ethical conduct
operative culture	values
organisational climate	

Organisational culture
Understanding organisational culture

Organisational culture is a somewhat elusive concept, often referred to in academic literature and workplace conversations, but difficult to define and fully understand. It involves a system of shared meaning, developed and maintained by a group in response to external conditions and the need for internal cohesion (Robbins et al., 2004; Schein, 1990).

The culture in an organisation conveys a sense of identity for members and facilitates their commitment to a common purpose. It can enhance the stability of social aspects of the work environment and help to make sense of decisions and operations that guide and shape staff behaviour (Smircich, 1983). Organisational culture thus represents the accumulated learning of a group and the integration of this learning into a common understanding that shapes how an organisation works.

This common understanding is partly about the purpose of the organisation and also about how the organisation operates from day to day. The purpose, or core business, of the organisation will determine people's commitment to tasks and events; the amount of energy they are prepared to contribute and the priority they give to one thing over another. How the organisation operates is about common practices that are largely unquestioned, except in a time of change. Examples include operating hours and mechanisms for communication, in addition to the level of responsiveness to clients that is implicit in how work is organised. It is important to recognise that organisational culture is not about whether employees *like* their workplace, it is about *features* of the work environment (Robbins et al., 2004) and their translation into how the organisation functions.

Manning (2003) explains that each organisation has its own 'mini-society', which may include particular terms and patterns of interaction, as well as regular rituals and topics of conversation. A number of factors provide a foundation for the culture that develops in an organisation:

- The scope for innovation and risk-taking.
- The use of shared problem-solving.
- Management expectations about the quality and speed required to complete one's work.
- The relative emphasis placed on outcomes as well as the processes involved in realising these aspirations.
- The presence and importance of working in teams.
- The norms about staff interactions, including basic courtesies as well as efforts to support new staff and those experiencing difficulties.
- Management attitudes toward change and growth.

The strength and stability of the culture in an organisation depends on characteristics of the staff; their foundation, stability, longevity and shared experience (Schein, 1990). For example, having a common interest may instil ownership of and loyalty toward the existing culture. Where staff turnover is high, the culture may be subject to change as values and beliefs are no longer reinforced and new workers bring their own perspectives on how the organisation works. When there is a clear sense of purpose that is reinforced

Organisational culture
A system of shared meaning that distinguishes the organisation from other workplaces. This culture is evident in the policies, practices, attitudes and rituals of the organisation.

by external conditions and internal achievements, the organisation's culture is generally well supported and stable.

The practitioner profile below is of the CEO of a small non-government organisation. It highlights the importance of a healthy organisational culture.

PRACTITIONER PROFILE 3.1

GEOFF SOMA

CHIEF EXECUTIVE OFFICER, WESTERN REGION ALCOHOL AND DRUG CENTRE (WRAD)

Position

My overall responsibility is for operations, employing 21 staff. We provide a drug and alcohol program as well as a medical service. Funding is split into state, commonwealth and fee-for-services. The role covers HR, marketing and profile, media, finance, fundraising, contracting with various departments and developing strategic relationships and directions.

Typical day

- Administration tasks including correspondence, telephone calls, emails and internet
- Meetings with management staff, finance staff and medical staff
- Submissions and application writing
- Budget control, fundraising, internet banking
- External meetings: local, regional, metropolitan
- Media contact
- Preparing presentations and briefings and progress reports
- Reading background and relevant documents
- Planning and review

Challenges

- Maintaining morale
- Juggling meeting attendance
- Funding pressures
- Keeping up to date with information
- Managing stress levels
- Communicating adequate information to others
- Dealing with ongoing reforms
- Maintaining the required quality and standards
- Juggling roles
- Managing deadlines
- Being responsible for other people

Skills and qualities

Qualification in health-related field (nursing is a good starting point); finance skills; media and marketing skills; good communication skills; problem solving skills; a sense of humour; passion, commitment and energy.

Lessons learnt

- Think before you act
- The value of listening and including people
- Being able to admit to mistakes
- How you behave and what you project will be remembered by others
- Management requires a significant amount of people and practical skills
- Understanding financial areas and knowing the business is essential
- Being productive with political issues
- To ask for help
- Patience
- Respect is something that you earn
- Encouragement and praise are valued
- How to handle the media
- How to manage difficult people
- Each situation has its own solution and requires flexible strategies
- Do not procrastinate
- Celebrate achievements
- 'Act your age and not your rage'

Managing organisational culture

Where possible I stop, reflect, consider and act. In some circumstances urgency can threaten this approach and then it becomes very much management on the run until things slow down and get back to plan. Time out is important and of course I try not to overact and can usually get back on track eventually.

Clear leadership, direction and modelling have been important in providing some stability and confidence within the organisation. Recognising people's strengths and including them have been vital. I have tried to communicate on many levels across the organisation and involve staff in strategic direction but also have taken charge and made hard decisions when required.

Teasing out staff strengths and tapping into individual creativity have supported the organisational culture. Providing rewards both financial and through praise has also been essential. I try to identify and address conflict as quickly as possible. Celebrating achievements and history together have helped people feel part of the organisation. Providing structure, creating some excitement and being able to meet challenges and move forward as an organisation have helped.

REFLECTION EXERCISE

Look again at the final section of the practitioner profile and consider the strategies that Geoff Soma has identified to manage organisational culture. Does Geoff mention items that you have found important? Is there anything you would add?

As you may appreciate, organisational culture is fundamental to worker satisfaction and performance. When leadership is lacking and there is a misuse of power by those in management roles, the ramifications can be widespread and difficult to rectify. Geoff Soma's comments on organisational culture reflect the importance of 'leadership, direction and modelling', in addition to ongoing communication, shared decision-making and valuing staff.

Many of the structural elements in an organisation shape the health of the workplace. For example, having a 'clear purpose, appropriate culture, specified tasks, distinct roles, suitable leadership, relevant members, and adequate resources' is important (Mickan & Rodger 2000, p.202). These aspects of organisational culture build trust, cohesion and motivation. In turn, this reduces the scope for decision-making based on self-interest, while countering the impact of external pressures that may undermine organisational effectiveness.

We explore many of the structural elements impacting organisational well-being throughout this text from a constructive perspective, but it is also useful to reflect on what may occur when the culture is considered to be problematic. The second practice activity at the end of this chapter provides a thought-provoking example of the importance of organisational culture.

Developing and maintaining organisational culture

Establishing a new organisation is a unique opportunity to shape culture. Three factors are critical in this process: the selection of employees; the training and socialisation of these employees; and the role models provided by senior staff (Robbins et al., 2004).

Linkage
Processes for staff recruitment and support are described in Chapter 5.

Organisational culture is a learnt phenomenon and two models have been put forward to explain how this learning occurs. The first model is about the creation of behavioural norms while the second model focuses on identifying with leaders (Schein, 1990).

In the first model, the way that staff respond to a highly charged situation communicates their shared expectations and establishes group norms for future operations. For example, a staff member may highlight an error made by a leader and suggest that it needs to be rectified. If the leader responds by acknowledging the mistake and affirming the behaviour of the staff member before discussing ways to remedy the situation, then other members of the staff group learn it is okay to identify mistakes and important to focus on problem-solving. Conversely, if the leader attacks the staff member for her comments and the other staff members remain quiet, then the hidden message is that the leader should not be openly criticised. This set of experiences becomes a common understanding of how to operate in similar situations.

The second model involves leaders modelling the assumptions and values they promote (Schein, 1990), and staff perceptions of appropriate behaviour. Examples range from working hours—in moderation or without limits—to the emphasis placed on timely and open communication with staff.

A number of mechanisms assist in the creation and maintenance of organisational culture, according to Schein (1990, p.115):

- What leaders pay attention to, measure, and control
- How leaders react to critical incidents and crises

- Deliberate role modelling and coaching
- Operational criteria for assigning rewards and status
- Operational criteria for recruitment, promotion and retirement

Over time, the culture that has been developed becomes self-sustaining. Staff with the 'right' values and assumptions are recruited, and existing staff are encouraged and rewarded on the basis of their demonstrated alignment with the culture. There are formal and informal indoctrination processes, both for new staff and to maintain and reinforce existing norms among current staff. Policies promote and reinforce behaviour that is consistent with the preferred culture, and staff who are not comfortable with the culture may be encouraged, or feel compelled, to leave. While maintaining the desired culture is important to guide staff according to a shared vision and purpose, having a reflective approach is essential for organisational renewal and adaptation to changes in the external environment.

Linkage
We explore organisational change and analysis of the external environment in Chapters 6 and 9.

Symbols of organisational culture

By now, you may have developed an appreciation about the complexity in trying to describe the culture in an organisation. A good place to start is by examining formal documents and statements. Examples include mission statements, strategic plans and standards. Profiles of senior staff and the major achievements that are highlighted by the organisation may also be useful. Most organisations have a website that contains significant statements and information on key policies and people, as well as other illustrations of organisational culture. Table 3.1 outlines some of these features.

TABLE 3.1 Elements of websites that may reflect aspects of organisational culture

FEATURE	ELEMENTS
Home page	The slogan A brief description of core business Photographs and other images Client and partner testimonials Information on legal status (e.g., not-for-profit, area health service)
What we stand for	Vision Mission Principles Values Strategic goals
Our history	Origin of the organisation Major developments
Key people	Brief biographies of managers and board members
External links	Partner agencies
Visual layout	Logo/s Colours Structure Text size and font

Less formal, but equally important, symbols and activities help to define and maintain the culture of an organisation. Popular accounts of the organisation's beginnings, and stories about significant staff, events and programs are shared with new staff and recounted during meetings and social gatherings. Ceremonies that celebrate events and achievements consistent with the culture of the organisation occur as part of the daily routine or through staff initiatives. Physical elements, ranging from awards and noticeboards to the layout of furniture and working arrangements, display 'what matters' to the organisation (Jones & May, 1992).

Corporate and operative cultures

Corporate culture
The official culture of the organisation that is represented in formal elements that are promoted through documents, websites and displays.

Operative culture
The actual culture of the organisation that is evident in staff behaviour and physical aspects of the work environment.

The official culture of organisations, espoused in policy documents and on display in reception and on the web, may be incongruous with elements that you have observed. For example, there may be statements about valuing excellence and striving to make a difference in people's lives, while staff behaviour reflects an entrenched way of operating that is more about 'business as usual'. Jones and May (1992) distinguish between two aspects of organisational culture: official and operative. The official culture is designed to represent the organisation to external stakeholders. These overt representations that promote the preferred culture of the workplace are sometimes referred to as the **corporate culture**. In contrast, the **operative culture** is closer to what you may have observed in organisations; involving the meaning that is *actually* given to behaviours in, and features of, the workplace. Some elements of the operative culture are covert, in that they are not officially displayed or sanctioned.

Subcultures

Most large organisations have a dominant culture and several subcultures. These subcultures arise from the particular roles and experiences that define groups and departments in the organisation. For example, the clinical services group in a health service will prioritise clinical practices and responsiveness to clients, while the information technology department is likely to focus on maintaining efficient operations by attending to equipment, software, licences and so on. Ideally each group will have a common understanding of the organisation's purpose, though they may develop a particular set of values according to their role in contributing to organisational effectiveness.

The physical separation of work units, in different buildings or geographical locations, may also contribute to the development of subcultures in an organisation. Daily work patterns and characteristics of the external environment are likely to vary across these locations. In addition, there may be different access to basic resources— ranging from management and administrative support to the ease with which in-house training and social events can be attended. Building on this discussion, the list of readings for this chapter includes a paper by Wilcoxson and Millett (2000) on multiple group identities in the organisational setting and implications for management. You may find this interesting.

The dominant culture in an organisation supports consistency in staff behaviour, based on common goals and understandings. However, if an organisation has many subcultures but a weak or poorly supported dominant culture then groups may operate in different ways and focus on different objectives. There is also a risk that divided loyalties will develop across groups with diverse areas of activity and professional orientations. Examples include professional groups that have contrasting values (for example, business, social work, medicine, psychology), contrasting social and ethnic orientations (for example, class, culture, sexuality), and different occupational groupings (for example, union employees, management, paraprofessionals and professionals) (Manning, 2003). The strength of the values underpinning the dominant organisational culture will determine the extent to which these divided loyalties can be reconciled. With general agreement about the nature and purpose of the organisation, different subcultures can be layered upon this foundation.

Benefits of, and challenges to, a healthy organisational culture

While the benefits of a strong organisational culture are apparent, negative aspects may also exist. Employing individuals who are closely aligned with the existing culture will add to the homogeneity of members—reducing opportunities for diversity and innovation that arise from contrasting professional backgrounds, experience, cultural heritage and so on. An organisation with a strong and static culture may find it difficult to be responsive to a dynamic external environment.

In addition, there is a natural tendency to stagnation and decay in organisations. An ongoing cycle of review is important to refresh the energy and sense of purpose held by staff, board members and others in the organisation. This enables entrenched routines and decision-making processes that may be focused on preserving a person's position and influence to be challenged, and enables teams to focus on what is best for advancing the purpose of the organisation. Complacency about what is important and achievable may be challenged by perspectives from new staff, who contribute their own expectations and novel views on what is possible (Brody, 2005).

Managers can guard against natural decline in a number of ways. Taking the time to document your concerns and possible solutions is an important step toward renewal. It may be useful to discuss your thoughts with others in the organisation, or involve an external colleague or mentor in deciding what needs to change and how. The most challenging issues may not be resolved, but there is scope to balance their impact with affirming activities and achievements.

At a personal level, changing your routine or your approach to regular tasks may be of benefit. Taking on a new assignment may encourage new ways of operating, and renewed enthusiasm for the work. In terms of managing others, valuing staff work and taking interest in their general well-being is critical to staff motivation and dedication. Sharing information about individual and team successes engenders a competitive environment that can support staff motivation and commitment. This needs to be balanced by the recognition that failures are learning opportunities (Brody, 2005).

Organisational culture and organisational climate

Before moving on from organisational culture, it is important to consider what is meant by the related concept of **organisational climate**. There are two ways of thinking about organisational climate: how it is defined and how it is measured.

The organisational climate refers to a shared understanding among staff about how the workplace affects them (Hemmelgarn, 2010). Staff develop an understanding of this climate by examining how the organisation deals with what is personally important to them. The alignment between core values and views on appropriate and just organisational practices are involved.

There is a long history of research in this area and a range of surveys and other tools have been developed to measure organisational climate. Areas that are often examined include role clarity and reporting structures, worker satisfaction and challenge, peer support, and feeling valued. Organisational climate can also be considered using information on staff turnover and sick leave, staff commitment and service achievements. It is in the best interests of managers to strive for a positive organisational climate given that productivity and performance are both influenced by the workplace environment. Weinbach and Taylor (2011, pp.92–9) outline some workplace characteristics that contribute toward a positive organisational climate:

- Team affiliation and cooperation toward shared goals
- Mutual respect and confidence
- Role clarity
- Advocacy for staff
- Autonomy and independence at all levels
- Good communication

Values

We move now to consider the importance of **values** in guiding the culture of an organisation. As we have been discussing, particular values are intrinsic to health and human services. These values are fundamental components of the area and refer to perspectives and behaviours that are esteemed and prized by all involved with an organisation (Jones & May, 1992; Donovan & Jackson, 1991). The Ethics Resource Center (May 2009) has an extensive list of values that are often cited by organisations. Examples include:

- Altruism, involving the unselfish concern for the welfare of others.
- Community, which is about sharing, being involved, and having fellowship with others.
- Justice, which is concerned with conforming to what is right in terms of actions and attitudes.

The strategic framework for Parenting WA, which is part of the Western Australian Department of Communities (Government of Western Australia Department of Communities, 2010), provides a further example. Consultations with staff led to the identification of the following values:

1   Respect for families, communities, colleagues and cultures.
2   Partnership approach to working with families, practitioners and agencies.

3   Supportive relationships are established and nurtured.

4   Inclusive approach to culturally diverse and Indigenous families.

5   Advocacy for individuals, communities and sound practice.

6   Responsiveness to the needs of families and communities.

7   Strengths-based focus as the foundation for practice.

These values are described as foundational to Parenting WA, guiding business processes and articulating the philosophy that is reflected in how staff approach their work.

As we considered earlier in the chapter, there are both overt and covert values in an organisation; values which are put forward to represent positive and desirable attributes of the workplace and those not formally celebrated but important in guiding staff behaviour. This is a reflection of the corporate and operative cultures in place. For example, an organisation may promote values of acceptance and charity toward others while operating within systems that exclude those most in need of an accepting and responsive approach to service delivery. Similarly, equality may be officially promoted while, at the same time, males dominate in senior roles. It is important for staff and managers to consider the level of consistency between what is meant to matter in the organisation and what really matters. This understanding will assist in determining the motivation for management decisions and staff behaviour.

The example below is a description of a relatively new organisation, which provides a range of services. As you read through the case example, think about the nature of the organisational culture and climate, and note the values that are upheld.

CASE EXAMPLE 3.1

An NGO for clients with mild to moderate mental health conditions (part one)

This organisation provides a range of programs for people experiencing disability and mental illness in combination with social disadvantage. The programs include disability support, mental health outreach, acquired brain injury, mental health care coordination, intensive home-based outreach, and service development.

Values of the organisation are excellence, integrity, equity, respect and honesty. The offices do not have a corporate feel, but retain the comfortable atmosphere of a community-based service; well worn and unpretentious. This seems like an effective engagement strategy—a more clinical environment may be alienating and stressful for the client group.

Enthusiasm for the work, a commitment to social justice and a 'can do anything' attitude contribute to positivity and pride among staff. Creativity and passion are fostered and highly valued.

The organisation is governed by a board, which takes responsibility for the corporate plan. The CEO and executive team have developed the operational plan. They are constantly reflecting on the business they are doing and how they can do it better, creating the systems, policies and processes to move forward but without being deterministic and limiting the scope to take on new opportunities. This involves 'trying to find a balance so that we don't lose that creativity and that innovation aspect. We found that we still have to have some kind of base to ensure that we can spring forward in a positive direction'.

Linkage
Further discussion on the place of values in organisational planning, design and function is included in Chapter 6.

Ethics in the organisation

Having described components of organisational culture and the importance of values, our focus shifts now to ethics in the organisational setting, with a particular focus on management. Ethics is concerned with values, principles and rules that guide behaviour. It refers to what is regarded as right and beneficial for individuals and for society, shaping expectations regarding daily conduct and the obligations and duties we owe one another. The strength of these views is influenced by the level of homogeneity in the social group and the negative consequences resulting from individual transgression. When this understanding of ethics is applied to **organisational ethics**, it focuses on rules of conduct in relation to internal and external stakeholders, board members, clients and the broader community (Pettinger, 2004).

> **Organisational ethics**
> Principles and rules of behaviour established to uphold the values of an organisation.

The ethical stance of an organisation promotes crucial values and reinforces preferred behaviours and approaches to decision-making. Staff who are committed to the ethical perspective bring fresh energy to the workplace and maintain motivation. This constitutes a unique force that enables organisations to strive for ambitious goals even when client circumstances and external conditions are complex and challenging (Manning, 2003).

Multiple sets of ethical obligations

> **Managerial ethics**
> Obligations and duties regarding internal and external stakeholders, board members, clients and the broader community.

Managerial ethics involves multiple sets of ethical obligations that are linked to different elements of the organisation. These elements include the work environment, client group and the broader community, as well as structures and processes that underpin organisational culture and effectiveness. Ideally, these multiple sets of ethical obligations coalesce for the benefit of all stakeholders—including managers. This is not always the case, though, and sometimes managers must make difficult choices that involve weighing up the relative priority attached to different responses to an ethical dilemma.

Workplace conditions

As a manager, you are ethically obliged to ensure the internal environment is appropriate for staff. Associated duties and ways of operating to achieve this include:

- The provision of a structured schedule of salary payments, superannuation and career advancement.
- Attention to the physical quality and resourcing of the work environment.
- Clarity in expectations attached to staff positions.
- Practical supports for staff development.
- Clarity and effectiveness in communication mechanisms within and across groups and departments.
- Respect for religious or other rituals, beliefs and considerations among staff.
- Recognition of staff contributions, achievements and efforts.

Source: Pettinger, 2004

Ethical practice

Robbins et al. (2004) report on a number of strategies managers can use to promote ethical practices among staff.

1   *Select employees with high ethical standards*, using a recruitment process designed to identify the value system of applicants and their compatibility with values upheld by the organisation. New staff can uphold and strengthen the ethics of the organisation or challenge established principles. Managers can use the recruitment process to explain the ethics of the organisation and associated expectations of staff.

2   *Develop organisational policies* that state the ethical rules employees are expected to follow. These policies may refer to various codes that are developed by and for professional groups. The codes are useful as long as organisations are aware of their content, and staff reflect on how consistent their practice is with the principles and values in the guidelines.

3   *Lead by example.* Management should provide visible role models who set a benchmark for defining appropriate workplace behaviour. This is more important than what is said or included in formal documents. Ethically questionable practices (for example, preferential treatment to colleagues who are personal friends, or other forms of favouritism) send a strong message to employees that these practices are acceptable, and that there is a difference between behaviour that is formally sanctioned and that which occurs in practice. There may be ongoing effects on staff morale, due to feelings of mistrust and uncertainty about what really matters. Staff commitment to the organisation's stated mission may be compromised as a result.

4   *Be clear on the expectations and goals of positions.* Employees will benefit from understanding how their work contributes to organisational success. With unrealistic goals or role ambiguity there is a risk that staff will feel that 'anything goes', or that they must modify their behaviour to survive in the dysfunctional environment. Having clear and realistic goals provides strong motivation for staff, which translates into ethical behaviour that is aligned with the purpose of the organisation.

5   *Provide ethics training.* Some training programs explore ethical codes and dilemmas in the workplace, thereby highlighting the organisation's commitment to ethical practice that is consistent with the values and principles that have been formally adopted.

Organisational viability

Another obligation for the manager is about ensuring the organisation is financially viable. Managers may experience ethical conflict when there is a need to make decisions based on business principles that do not align with the needs of staff, clients or other stakeholders (Finkelman, 2006; Weinbach & Taylor, 2011). A common example is the short-term nature of program funding in health and human services and the need to wind down programs toward the end of their funded period. This may occur in the context of increased demand for care, as clients are aware of and engaged with the program, and might involve making staff redundant irrespective of the quality and effectiveness of their work.

Linkage
Decision-making structures are further explored in Chapter 4, when we look at management, leadership and governance.

A more complex example involves management decisions about the relative merit of programs when resources (funding or staff) are limited. Which client group takes precedence? How will decisions impact the organisation now and into the future? These management dilemmas require unpopular decisions that may challenge the ethical stance of the organisation. They may separate the manager from clinicians as business-oriented principles compete with those underpinning the services being provided. Attention to decision-making structures and an awareness of useful styles of decision-making in health and human service organisations are critical supports for managers in these situations.

Professional codes

Many workers in health and human service organisations are members of one or more professional associations for those with particular qualifications. These associations generally have a **professional code of ethical conduct**, which provides principles and rules for practice that represent visible, coherent and enforceable guidelines (Manning, 2003).

Professional code of ethical conduct
An official guide to the values and standards of a professional group.

One example is the *Code of Ethics* for the Australian Association of Social Workers (AASW), which identifies three core values: respect for persons; social justice; and professional integrity. The AASW expands on each value by providing a definition and listing general and specific objectives. For example, the value 'respect for persons' is about believing each one of us has inherent worth and a right to well-being, self-fulfilment and self-determination. There are three objectives linked to this value: fostering individual well-being, and recognising and respecting group identity and interdependence (Australian Association of Social Workers, 2010).

In another example, the *Code of Ethics* for the Australian Community Workers Association (ACWA) aims to provide practice standards for professionals in the sector. Members of ACWA are bound by the code, which promotes desired values, attitudes, knowledge and skills (Australian Community Workers Association, 2012). Other examples include codes developed by the Australasian Psychological Society and the Australian College of Nursing.

Membership of a professional association brings a level of prestige and identity to employees. The ethical code of the association is also a substantial resource for individuals and employers, communicating expectations regarding appropriate conduct that reach beyond organisational boundaries. As with all tools of this nature, it is important that professional codes of ethics are not just window dressing. Members should be familiar with the codes and apply them in daily practice (Berglund, 2012). Similarly, managers need to support the professional nature of their workforce.

REFLECTION EXERCISE

Obtain a copy of the *Code of Ethics* for your profession, or one that is relevant to the area you are studying. How is the document structured? What are the key principles? Is the code a useful guide to appropriate behaviour in the workplace?

Diversity and discrimination

Another area important to the culture of an organisation is the value placed on diversity, and associated efforts to counter discrimination. Our exploration of this area is about the effort of organisations to be inclusive of various characteristics among potential recruits and existing staff. These characteristics include culture, religion, sexual orientation and the like. After this, we explore discrimination against women.

Diversity

In recent years, managing diversity has emerged as an important issue for organisations. A review of literature in the area illustrates that diversity has a positive impact on organisational performance. Put simply, diversity is good for staff, the organisation and its clients (Mor Barak & Travis, 2010).

There are a number of reasons why **diversity management** is important:

- Organisations that aim to be inclusive will strive to have a staff profile that reflects characteristics of the community, thereby appealing to a diverse client base.
- Having a diverse staff group fosters innovation and creativity, which is important to refresh and renew the culture of an organisation.
- Subtle forms of discrimination can be countered by heterogeneity in the staff group, as members have different norms and cultural nuances that impact how they operate.
- Legislative frameworks promote understanding of diversity in the client population.
- Staff diversity gives organisations a competitive edge, something unique to offer community members and funders.

Michàlle Mor Barak and Dnika Travis examined research on the link between diversity management and organisational performance and identified implications for human service management. Their work, which is included in the reading list for this chapter, provides an interesting description of diversity issues and the organisational responses that have emerged.

Diversity management
Actions designed to support an inclusive approach to employment and to foster awareness and acceptance of various backgrounds of staff.

Linkage
We revisit the importance of diversity in Chapter 10 when looking at community engagement.

The legislative framework

The Diversity Council of Australia (DCA) is an independent, not-for-profit advisor to organisations. It provides a range of resources to support organisations in the development of processes that counter discrimination. Particular groups include those defined by gender, cultural diversity, disability, age (older people), Aboriginal and Torres Strait Islander status, being lesbian, gay, bisexual or transgender, and religion. The DCA notes that employers have a legal responsibility to take 'reasonable steps' to prevent harassment and discrimination in the workplace (Diversity Council of Australia, 2012).

The legislative framework for workplace diversity and equal opportunity in Australia includes a number of acts and related documents. An outline of Commonwealth legislation, from the Human Rights and Equal Opportunity Commission and Diversity Council of Australia, is shown on the next page. The web includes considerable information on each act and its purpose (for example: www.dca.org.au; www.humanrights.gov.au; www.wgea.gov.au).

1   The *Australian Human Rights Commission Act (1986)* is the statute for the Australian Human Rights Commission, a national institution that is funded by, but operates independently of, the Australian Government. Grounds for arguing the existence of discrimination in employment may involve race, colour, sex, religion, political opinion, national extraction, social origin, age, medical record, criminal record, marital status, impairment, disability, nationality, sexual preference, or trade union activity.

2   The *Age Discrimination Act (2004)* aims to protect both younger and older Australians from discrimination.

3   The *Disability Discrimination Act (1992)* makes it unlawful for an employer to discriminate against a person on the grounds of disability.

4   The *Racial Discrimination Act (1975)* makes it unlawful to discriminate in employment on the grounds or race, colour or national or ethnic origin.

5   The *Sex Discrimination Act (1984)* addresses grounds of discrimination based on sex, marital status, pregnancy and family responsibility.

6   The *Workplace Gender Equality Act (2012)* is designed to promote and improve gender equality outcomes for women and men.

7   The *Fair Work Act and National Employment Standards (2009)* provides a legislative framework for workplace relations and includes a set of ten basic entitlements. While these documents are at national level, there are also state and territory laws.

Discrimination

Effective managers support diversity in their workforce as a simple extension of the broader community. Australia has a strong multicultural population. The 2011 census showed that around one quarter of its population was born overseas and a further fifth had at least one overseas-born parent (Australian Bureau of Statistics, 2012).

Another issue related to diversity in the workplace (and at different levels of operation) is gender. Just over half the people in Australia are women, whose rates of workforce participation are gradually increasing (in 2010–11 79.4% of males and 65.3% of females aged 20–74 years were in work; Australian Bureau of Statistics, 2012); however, women are under-represented in senior leadership and management roles.

Interestingly, Aboriginal and Torres Strait Islander peoples are well represented in some areas of the health and human services. For example, a 2007 survey of the community-managed housing and support workforce in Victoria showed that 2.2% of respondents identified as being of Aboriginal or Torres Strait Islander origin, compared with 0.6% of the state's population (KPMG, 2007, p.12).

Discrimination in the workplace involves disadvantaging someone because of their race, colour, sex, sexual preference, age, physical or mental disability, marital status, family or carer's responsibilities, pregnancy, religion, political opinion, national extraction, or social origin (Australian Government, Fair Work Ombudsman, 2013, p.218). It may be reflected in recruitment processes and approaches to staff promotion, and the failure to recognise different cultural and religious beliefs among staff and

Discrimination
Disadvantaging a person because of their personal characteristics or situation, which can include race, sex, sexual preference, age, physical or mental disability, family responsibilities or political opinion.

other stakeholders. Inappropriate behaviour, including harassment based on gender or sexual orientation, may be inadvertently condoned by an organisation when there is limited attention to awareness raising and communication about appropriate staff conduct.

Insufficient access to necessary information has the most direct negative impact on people's capacity to perform their management functions. Managers need good information, available in a timely fashion, to undertake sound planning and decision-making. The denial of this information may be deliberate and designed to hinder someone's ability to function as a manager. It may also stem from a paternalistic perspective, where mid-level managers are 'spared' from exposure to information that others decide they do not need. A common problem stems from social structures within and across organisations, like the 'boys' club', where valuable information is shared during informal engagements such as a regular social gathering after work or other recreational activities (Weinbach & Taylor, 2011).

These discriminatory practices disadvantage women and others who have been the subject of negative stereotyping in the broader community. People from cultural or religious minorities may experience these barriers to effective management and succession within the organisation. In many situations, the behaviours are not discussed and they are certainly not formalised in policy documents. This is part of the insidious and ongoing nature of the problem. For the organisation, it means the full capacity of staff is not realised and there is a risk that talented staff will leave.

Equal opportunity

Women have always been over-represented in health and human service organisations, partly because these roles are consistent with traditional understandings of women as carers. Discriminatory practices such as salary inequality and limited access to promotions have impacted women across all areas of the job market. The Victorian Equal Opportunity and Human Rights Commission (2011b) has developed resources to assist organisations in developing policies and creating an equal opportunity workplace. It provides an introduction to relevant legislation and an overview of equal opportunity in practice. An outline of its policy template is shown in Table 3.2 overleaf.

The commission has also developed a complaint procedure checklist that focuses on the scope of the issue and the options available to the person making a complaint. In addition to the complaints process, it covers possible outcomes and the storage of documents related to the complaint (Victorian Equal Opportunity and Human Rights Commission, 2011a).

REFLECTION EXERCISE

Think of an organisation that you know well in terms of staff diversity (for example, ethnicity, male/female mix, gender balance at different levels). Have you identified any areas of concern? What has contributed to this situation and how would you go about changing things for the better?

TABLE 3.2 Policy outline: Workplace equal opportunity

POLICY ELEMENT	WHAT THIS COVERS
Scope	• Who the policy applies to • What work situations are covered • Interactions between what parties
Aims	• Organisational commitment to policy • Requirements of staff • Benefit of policy
Staff rights and responsibilities	• Staff entitlements and requirements • Managers and supervisors' additional responsibilities
Unacceptable workplace conduct—discrimination, bullying, sexual harassment, racial and religious vilification, victimisation, gossip	• List of relevant legislation • Definition and explanation of terms
Merit	• Organisational commitment to recruitment based on merit
Resolving issues	• Direction to relevant complaint resolution policy and procedure document, or contacts for advice and support, or action on their behalf
Equal opportunity contact officers	• Definition and role of EO contact officers
Employee assistance program	• Definition and staff entitlements
Other relevant policies	• Reference to associated policies (e.g., flexible work arrangements, enterprise bargaining agreement)
More information	• Contact details for queries regarding the policy
Review details	• Policy date and review schedule

Source: Victorian Equal Opportunity and Human Rights Commission, 2011b, p.205

Management strategies against discrimination and for diversity

Managers can guard against negative stereotyping and discrimination at an individual level through reflective practice and, at an organisational level, by including strategies such as staff audits and affirmative action. They can actively promote diversity in the workplace using several strategies:

• Identify and monitor the number of women and minorities in the organisation.
• Develop guidelines and goals to support the promotion of competent women and minorities.
• Establish policies that mean the workplace is 'family friendly', for example involving support for maternity leave, flexible work hours and job sharing.
• Establish diversity awareness teams.

- Take part in training that encourages you to examine and reflect on your assumptions and expectations regarding minority groups and women.
- Survey staff to obtain information on perceived discrimination and its impact.
- Assign a mentor to work with promising female staff and those from a minority background, to support their success and advancement in the organisation.

Source: Brody, 2005

There are a number of challenges for all staff in countering institutionalised discrimination:

- *Recognise* the differences between masculine and feminine styles of management and take what is best from each.
- *Understand* that we are dealing with how men and women have been socialised, so their behaviours may be interpreted as perfectly natural and beyond change.
- *Accept* that substantial difference exists within as well as across social divisions, for example sex and sexual identity, culture and class. Don't simplify the power struggles and identity concerns that may be involved (Coulshed et al., 2006).

Despite these substantial challenges, as a manager you are obliged to operate according to values and codes that are consistent with fostering and recognising staff potential. In addition, both you and your organisation stand to benefit from the realisation of this potential.

Policies in the organisation

The final section of this chapter is about how the culture, values, ethical perspectives and support for diversity in an organisation relate to organisational policies. Figure 3.1 shows the flow of information and influence between various components of the framework for organisational culture, climate and policy development.

FIGURE 3.1 A framework on information and influence for organisational culture, organisational climate and policy development

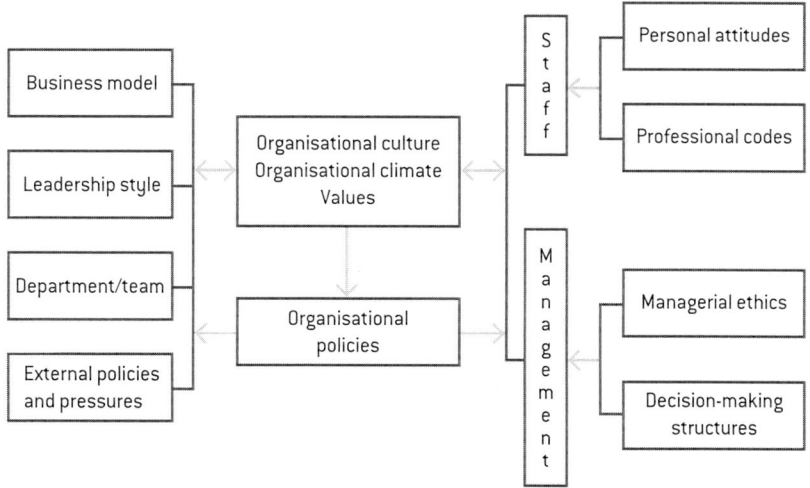

Understanding organisational policies

Organisational policies
General statements intended to communicate expectations and guide staff behaviour.

Organisational policies are general statements that communicate expectations to staff. They are designed to guide staff decision-making and behaviour in accordance with the organisation's mission and objectives. These documents support consistency across cases and time, and provide transparency for managers and other employees regarding the rationale behind decisions and actions. In contrast, procedures provide step-by-step instructions on policy implementation (Weinbach & Taylor, 2011).

Policies sometimes address different levels of the organisation. For example, a policy on annual leave applies to everyone while a policy on needle-stick injuries may be relevant only for staff and management working in medical services. Policies are generally rather abstract, being concerned with the principles and standards of operations (Finkelman, 2006). Put simply, policies address the 'what' and 'why' of organisational operations and they form the basis for procedural documents that address the 'how' and 'when' of organisational operations—the application of general perspectives to daily practice.

Developing policies

Linkage
Policies are often reviewed in the context of formal accreditation, which is explored in Chapter 8.

Policy formation involves basic tenets of good planning along with a reflective approach that allows for personal views to be identified, challenged and resolved. Each of us brings our own interests, wants and needs to the workplace, resulting in multiple sets of interests and political affiliations. A good planning process includes scope for different perspectives to be considered and resolved. The aim of the process is to produce a relevant, accurate and recognised document that assists staff in making decisions and understanding the context for decisions made by others in the organisation.

Some basic questions to consider in organising the process of policy formation include:

- Who should be involved (for example, what roles, levels of seniority, representation of particular interest groups)?
- When should consultation occur (for example, formative work developed by senior staff or tailored working groups, general consultation based on a draft document)?
- What information is required to ensure the policy is relevant to legislative, sector and professional contexts for the organisation's work?
- How can the policy formation process and the final product be effectively communicated to staff?
- What strategies will reinforce to staff that the policy is integral to how the organisation operates?
- What structures are required to ensure the policy remains relevant (for example, scheduled reviews)?

You may wish to read further about policy development in community services. The Victorian Council of Social Services (2007) has worked with the Victoria Law Foundation to develop resources for the management groups of community service organisations. They have produced a manual describing what policies and procedures are, why they are necessary and how to develop them. This manual is included in the readings list at the end of the chapter.

Implementing policies

It is critical that policies and procedures are communicated regularly to staff so they understand the significance of these documents and use them on a regular basis. Policies are communicated through formal and informal mechanisms. Documents may be available via the organisation's intranet and in printed form, and new or revised policies are generally highlighted. Policy details are communicated via staff memos and attached to job descriptions. They are also the subject of informal discussions among staff, and raised at staff meetings when the need arises.

In the case example below, we revisit the NGO described earlier in the chapter, focusing on the process for policy development. This case study is a useful reminder that the process of policy development may not go according to plan.

CASE EXAMPLE 3.2

An NGO for clients with mild to moderate mental health conditions (part two)

The organisation has grown quickly, from a small community service to an organisation with more than 100 staff who operate from three sites. This rapid growth has meant that planning, policies and procedures have not always received due attention. As this is a highly community-oriented and practice-focused organisation, resources have been directed towards clients and programs, rather than governance and administration.

The management structure is described as 'a transparent, collaborative, open hierarchy', driven by the energy and vision of those who established the organisation. The organisation has reached the stage where the establishment of more formal practices and processes is well overdue. The major challenge for the organisation is consolidation and order. The manager explained that, 'if we're going to be effective and successful in the future we actually have to have good grounding, policies and procedures, and ensure that those things [for] future planning are embedded in the organisation'.

As a consequence, management has funded a dedicated role to attend to policies and planning. It was explained that, 'we are finally going to be creating a new position (director of service development) and it will be their role to document and draft all these policies, procedures, and these types of things and do research and development'.

Monitoring decisions in support of policy relevance

In day-to-day operations, decisions may be made in an ad hoc manner, without reference to formal policies. The significance of these actions may not be immediately apparent, but there is a risk of setting a precedent regarding appropriate responses to specific elements of a situation and in relation to the salience of policies in decision-making (Donovan & Jackson, 1991).

It is important that managers review and reflect on these circumstances to avoid behaviours that contradict stated policies. This self-awareness involves developing an understanding of why particular decisions are made and applying what has been learnt to other situations (Donovan & Jackson, 1991). Regular policy reviews should include consideration of these experiences and the recognition of decisions that need to be amended. Weinbach and Taylor (2011) suggest that when a policy is no longer a useful shortcut to decision-making then it needs to be reviewed, perhaps through the provision of a more general document. Alternatively, case examples may augment a policy by illustrating the range and complexity of the decision-making process.

Within any organisation there is potential for negativity and stress among staff, particularly when management and leadership are lacking. For example, where goals are not shared and decision-making processes are not communicated then employees may pursue their own interests without regard to the goals of the organisation or the welfare of colleagues. The formalisation of processes and participation in decision-making and policy review assist with staff communication and shared motivation (Aryee et al., 2004).

SUMMARY OF KEY ISSUES

Organisational culture is a system of shared meaning that is a powerful determinant of staff well-being and service effectiveness. It is a learnt phenomenon that is shaped by corporate and operative mechanisms. In large and diverse organisations, subcultures may develop.

Managers face multiple sets of ethical obligations. They are ethically obliged to ensure the organisation provides an adequate work environment and that it is financially viable. Broader obligations refer to appropriate service provision for the target client group and making a positive contribution to the wider community.

Efforts to counter discrimination and support diversity are underpinned by a legislative framework. Attention to recruitment processes and approaches to staff promotion are important, in order to guard against systemic discrimination. Despite long-standing strategies for equal opportunity, women remain under-represented in management roles. The process of policy development is seldom straightforward and often results from the coalescence of will, information and planning.

PRACTICE ACTIVITIES

1   Exploring organisational culture

One way to learn about the culture in an organisation is to explore formal and informal mechanisms that promote and reinforce the culture. You may wish to undertake this exercise to explore the notion of organisational culture from an applied perspective. Start by selecting an organisation that you are connected with, as an employee or student, for example. Visit the website and note some formal elements of the organisation. Try to identify statements, phrases, words and possibly characteristics of staff that reflect the organisational culture. Next, visit the organisation and look for further information. These questions may assist you:

- What items are valued in the workplace? This may include awards or plaques that are on display, things that are given priority on noticeboards or in newsletters, and items placed strategically on desks or shelves.

- What is the physical arrangement of the workplace? Is it open plan? Are there offices? What is the proximity of workspaces? Do you get the sense that people desire privacy or welcome the opportunity to socialise with their colleagues?
- Observe the nature of interactions between people. Do staff act in a positive way toward each other? Is there much communication (formal and informal)? How are problems solved? What are the decision-making processes?

Finally, think about what you would tell a friend who was considering a position in the organisation. How would you describe the organisational culture? What are the good things and what concerns you?

2   A toxic culture?

The reference below gives a dramatic account of problems attributed to the poor organisational culture in a Canberra hospital. Read the sections about the hospital and consider the aspects of organisational culture described and the purported consequences of the toxic culture, the level of bias in the comments made, and external factors that may have affected the hospital's performance.

Debates of the Legislative Assembly for the Australian Capital Territory. Daily Hansard. Edited proof transcript, 22 August 2012. www.regnet.anu.edu.au/sites/default/files/Debates%20 Educ%20right.pdf Accessed 5 September 2013

3   Legislative requirements

Select one of the Acts listed in this chapter, preferably in an area relevant to your interests or your area of work. Use the web to explore requirements of the Act and how it has been interpreted in organisational settings. Identify three or more key messages to include in organisational policies, to support practice that is consistent with the legislation you have reviewed.

4   Exploring policies

You may be interested in exploring a policy example from your workplace or another institution. Consider these aspects of the policy to decide on its usefulness:
- the date the policy was created
- the purpose of the policy
- the timeline for review
- the person or position responsible for the policy
- the links to procedural documents.

FURTHER READING

Organisational culture

Wilcoxson, L. & Millett, B. (2000). 'The Management of Organisational Culture', *Australian Journal of Management & Organisational Behaviour*, *3*(2), pp.91–9.

A review of organisational culture

Carson, E., Chung, D. & Day, A. (2009). 'Evaluating Contracted Domestic Violence Programs', *Standardisation and Organisational Culture. Evaluation Journal of Australasia*, *9*, pp.10–19.

Diversity

Mor Barak, M. E. & Travis, D. J. (2010). 'Diversity and Organizational Performance', in
　　Hasenfeld,　Y. (ed), *Human Services As Complex Organizations* (2nd edn), USA: Sage,
　　pp.341–78.

Policy development in the community sector

Victorian Council of Social Services (2007). *Policies and Procedures: A Guide for Community
　　Management Groups*, Melbourne: Victoria Law Foundation & Victorian Council of Social
　　Services.

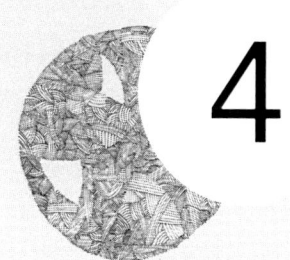

Management, Leadership and Governance

4

OVERVIEW

This chapter will:

- define and discuss management, leadership and governance in health and human service organisations
- critically explore the inter-relationships and differences between management, leadership and governance
- identify and describe key functions, roles, tasks, skills and responsibilities of management in health and human services.

This chapter describes key aspects of management, leadership and governance in health and human service organisations. It emphasises the importance of developing management and leadership skills from the moment a new worker enters the field, to enhance their own practice, address issues and challenges, and contribute to successful outcomes for clients and the organisation.

KEY TERMS

governance	management role
leadership	management skills
management	management tasks
management functions	

Fundamentals of management, leadership and governance

In this chapter we discuss the three fundamental components involved in the administration and leadership of health and human service organisations: management, leadership and governance. These concepts do not reflect an inflexible reality. Rather, as we have seen, they emerge from a wide variety of organisational contexts that exist within a constantly shifting socio-political environment. These three key intra-organisational arenas are structured in a dynamic relationship, and the way each is enacted varies considerably across organisational contexts. Their meaning is constantly being revised, resulting in a diversity of definitions (Donovan & Jackson, 1991; Weinbach & Taylor, 2011). In spite of these discrepancies, the combination of management, leadership and governance constitutes an essential sub-structure for the facilitation of necessary organisational processes. When this relationship is effective, and power and authority are employed productively rather than oppressively, the work of the organisation gets done, the needs of clients and staff are met, professional values are upheld, there is direction and accountability to stakeholders and, perhaps most importantly, the organisation flourishes. We will explore some of these complexities, while at the same time aiming for clarity in terms of their separate elements and purposes.

Intersections

The intersections between management, leadership and governance are illustrated in Figure 4.1 below. We offer this simple depiction as a starting point for building a more nuanced appreciation of the way these arenas overlap and, at the same time, retain substantial distinctions. While it is tempting to conform to the typical hierarchical arrangement of most organisational charts, which place governance above both

FIGURE 4.1 Relationship between management, leadership and governance within the organisation

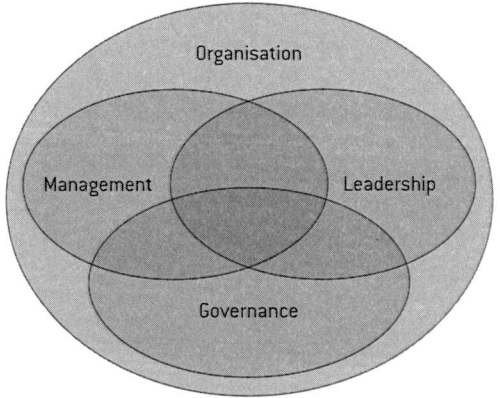

management and leadership, we see governance as supporting management and leadership, providing a foundation for the overall organisational structure. The degrees of interaction, the overlap in functions, and differences between these domains are, of course, dependent on specific organisational context. You will no doubt have your own image, based on your organisational experience, of how these arenas fit together, and therefore you may wish to develop and work with your own representation.

Management

Management in health and human service organisations is often primarily focused on maintenance and administration, with the purpose of achieving 'the healthy functioning of the organisation' (Hughes & Wearing, 2013, p.17). J. P. Kotter (2011b) argues that management is concerned with creating order and consistency, so that organisations can cope with the complexity of the present. Management activities involve organising people, systems and resources, supporting and supervising workers, forming and maintaining strategic alliances, communicating with stakeholders, making decisions, monitoring progress, problem-solving, evaluating results, revising plans to improve future outcomes and ensuring that the organisation remains committed to its professional value base and ethical obligations (Anheier, 2005; Lewis et al., 2012; Pine & Healy, 2007).

Being a manager involves synthesising specific skills, knowledge and attributes to perform a role that is designed to conduct these various core functions. The ultimate purpose of management in the health and human services is to ensure an efficiently run organisation (Pine & Healy, 2007) that delivers effective services, which facilitate positive change in people's lives (Lewis et al., 2012). In today's organisational environment the successful enactment of all of these management functions requires that they are dispersed across levels and shared by a range of people—from base-grade workers to chief executive officers.

Management
Involves purposeful planning, organising people, systems and resources, supporting and supervising workers, communicating with stakeholders, making decisions, monitoring progress, evaluating results and revising plans to improve future outcomes.

Linkage
We return to management functions, roles, tasks and skills in greater detail later in this chapter.

Leadership

Leadership involves having a vision for future directions, seeking new opportunities and providing a sense of purpose for an organisation, as well as guiding, motivating and enabling people to achieve shared goals (Hudson, 2009; Hughes & Wearing, 2013). Leadership requires the passion to embrace change and the skills to bring it about. In health and human service organisations leadership should not be driven by the imperative to increase profits, but instead by a commitment to maximising individual and community well-being and the pursuit of a just and equitable society.

The trend of the escalating pace of change and the importance of bringing staff 'on board' has seen leadership being treated as synonymous with management (Carlopio, Andrewartha & Armstrong, 2001). But it is also stridently argued that, although related, leadership is very different from management (Kotter, 2011b). Kotter makes the point

Leadership
Different from management, leadership involves seeing future directions, seeking opportunities and providing a sense of purpose, as well as guiding and motivating people to achieve goals.

that while managing and leading involve similar tasks, such as deciding what needs to be done, ensuring people are able to carry out their work, and establishing networks and strategic alliances, these are achieved in different ways. Managers plan and organise resources while leaders align and inspire people and set directions. Pine and Healy (2007) succinctly identify the difference by explaining that management is about efficiency, while leadership is about effectiveness.

Although leadership and leading are often positioned as functions of management, it is our view that the role of leaders and the practice of leadership differ from that of manager and management processes in some significant ways. We suggest that while it is possible to manage well without being a leader, it is not possible to lead well without also having management competence. That said, it does need to be recognised that the separation of management and leadership functions, tasks and skills is not always formalised in the separation of the roles of manager and leader. As Jackson and Donovan (1999) observe, the smaller the organisation, the more likely that a manager will be expected to lead, and that all workers will be required to participate in managing and leading. We continue to unpack these similarities, differences and intersections in this and further chapters.

Governance

Governance

Governance is not about day-to-day management, but about *overseeing* the management of an organisation; providing guidance to ensure an organisation has good management and leadership and that it honours its values.

The concept of **governance** as a system for directing and controlling organisations originates in the world of corporate business. Governance in the not-for-profit and public sectors, on the other hand, is about aligning an organisation's purpose and vision with its activities and performance (Anheier, 2005, pp.230–1).

Governance is about providing guidance, 'insight, wisdom and good judgement' (Hudson, 2009, p.54). It involves ensuring an organisation has efficient management and effective leadership, that values are honoured and that strategic goals are achieved. Governing bodies are responsible for financial viability, making sure plans are current and appropriate, that the concerns of stakeholders are heard and interests addressed, and that effective monitoring and quality improvement processes are in place. In brief, governance is ensuring that an organisation stays true to its course.

Caution and clear boundaries are required to ensure governance does not become entangled with management. It is important to be mindful that the governing body is not responsible for the day-to-day management of the internal operations of the organisation, but it is responsible for managing the organisation as an entity. It is critical for very clear distinctions to be maintained between management within the organisation, and the governance of the organisation overall.

This confusion is often exacerbated in the community sector by the way the governance body is named; frequently being referred to as the committee of *management*, or board of *management*. Mackay (1991, p.13) cautions that the governance body (however named) 'needs to adopt an attitude of trust and confidence in their staff so that staff can "get on with the job at hand" in a spirit of goodwill and confidence, without unnecessary interference or intimidation'. In actuality, the function of governance is more closely aligned with leadership. At the same time, it is essential to recognise the intersections that exist between all three of these administrative domains.

The practice example below raises some issues about the need to honour and recognise the distinctions, and attend to the intersections between management, leadership and governance. It will be helpful to reflect on this scenario as you read the rest of the chapter. The example describes the work of the manager of employment and training programs in a large clustered service community health centre. The structure, diversity and size, and the change and growth in the organisation over the past twenty-five years are outlined and, importantly, the manager describes his role and what it involves.

PRACTICE EXAMPLE   4.1

Managing in a community health centre

The organisation is set up with six different service streams; they range from our finance or corporate service area, mental health, disabilities, primary healthcare or allied health services—that's the dentistry and the podiatry and those sorts of things. Then we've got the counselling folk and then there's us, which is the employment service and training area. We sit within the employment services and training departments. We've now got 700 staff members across the organisation. We used to just work mainly in the one region, way back in the early days, and I'm talking about twenty/twenty-five years ago. We've since expanded to have services across the state, and now there's further plans for expansion interstate.

Essentially my role is providing for the training needs of the organisation, but also developing it as a financially viable service area; that is, we still need to seek external contracts of work to make it something that will take us through into the future and provide subsidised training for our internal staff. So what that means is we use the external environment to offset some of the costs of training for our internal constituents.

Then, in the other half of my role I am responsible for developing little business ventures. So for clients, some people with disability or long-term unemployment, what I do is go out there, set up little business enterprises, have clients come through our training and perhaps learn some skills—for example, horticulture, that sort of stuff. They then go on to working in a nursery, which we purchased about twelve-and-a-half months ago now. The idea was that it would provide the training as well as the experience for clients so that they can go on to the open labour market.

Management levels

As in many other organisational types, management positions are commonly structured across three levels in health and human services:

1   frontline managers: team leaders, coordinators
2   middle managers: program managers, division managers
3   top-level managers: executives, directors.

Linkage
The DHS restructure is considered more fully in Chapter 9 when we explore organisational change.

You will remember from Chapter 2 that some organisational structures are more complicated and hierarchical than others. Often this relates to their size, with smaller agencies having flatter structures and therefore fewer management layers. In these organisations, the middle management layer is often absent. In large organisations this tier can be an early target in restructures and workforce rationalisations. For example, the Department of Human Services (DHS) in Victoria, which represents one of this Australian state's largest government bureaucracies, recently underwent a significant restructure, which involved reducing middle management positions and increasing frontline workers.

Management tasks
Specific activities relating to management in an organisational setting. Although often seen as the work of managers, all workers are required to perform management tasks to some degree.

Of course, as we have noted, managing as one of many organisational practices is not exclusive to 'management' positions. All workers carry out **management tasks** to varying degrees. New workers must be able to manage their workloads and prioritise tasks, they need to make decisions, plan, and participate in meetings. If they want to bring about change, developing the skill of managing 'up' is essential, and to do this, understanding is required about 'what managers do and why they do it' (Weinbach, 2007, p.13). There is also a trend towards creating management teams comprised of workers from all organisational levels, which are assigned responsibility for making significant organisational decisions (Weinbach & Taylor, 2011)—keep this in mind while you read about levels of management in the next sections. That said, despite distributing and sharing management functions across the organisation, managers by name (those in the three tiers of management we identified above) have added responsibilities towards other staff and the organisation, and they spend a greater percentage of their time on management tasks than other workers.

Frontline managers

Managers at the frontline, who are closest to practice, are frequently identified as team leaders, supervisors or coordinators. These managers may have recent direct practice experience and they require more knowledge specific to the practice area than managers at higher levels (Hughes & Wearing, 2013). This is because they must support and supervise staff who are providing services to clients. Sometimes these managers are actively engaged in service delivery, for example, house supervisors in residential settings.

Leadership in some form is important and, like management, it is required in workers across all organisational levels (Coulshed et al., 2006; McDonald et al., 2011). However, there is less expectation that a frontline manager will carry formal leadership responsibilities commensurate with executive, organisational and strategic planning levels. On the other hand, team leaders or small work group coordinators are usually expected to show leadership and exercise initiative within their team as a component of their supervisory role. In the following profile, Vanessa Bleier talks about the variety in her dual role as team and project manager. Vanessa's position involves frontline as well as program management duties.

PRACTITIONER PROFILE 4.1

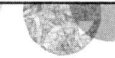

VANESSA BLEIER

TEAM MANAGER AND PROJECT MANAGER, YOORALLA, GIPPSLAND

Current position

I currently hold two roles, Team Manager of staff, providing information, planning and case management, and Project Manager. Essentially the role is to support the programs (supporting best practice and adherence to organisational policies and procedures), and the staff who work within these programs at an operational and professional level, to ensure that all are working towards maximising opportunities and outcomes for clients.

A typical day

In a typical day I work across many different levels, including day-to-day interactions with staff, formal and informal supervision, consultations with staff dealing with complex client issues, discussion regarding funding and budgets, application of legislation to program guidelines and ensuring staff comprehension of guidelines. I may at times attend network meetings or client case meetings, and my role in these circumstances is to act on behalf of the client, as well as the agency in their support of the client. Sometimes incidents occur and there is a significant amount of follow-up that needs to be put in place, such as debriefing, problem solving. Most of my day-to-day space tends to be toward planning and being proactive, and trying to ensure things do not get to a critical level.

Challenges

Managing competing priorities and often having to multi-task, across varying types of programs and client needs. The tyranny of distance—often having to manage quite critical situations remotely can be complex. Getting familiar with the use of technology and long drives is a key to success. Also trying to plan for the unexpected, by being proactive with routine work. Building room and delegating the routine work is essential to being able to respond to crisis more effectively, although this formula is challenged quite regularly.

Lessons learnt

- You cannot please all of the people all of the time.
- Client outcomes are the priority, as this seems to allow all things to fall into place with a flow-on effect.
- Keep your staff happy, and trust them.
- Be available to them always.
- Be willing to let go of broken processes; if it is not working, throw it out and try something else, as sometimes we try to salvage too much.
- Always look for the 'WHY?' If you cannot find the 'why?' go deeper and keep looking, because this is where you will find the thing that needs changing, and this is regardless of the issue.
- Understanding that crisis is never a single and isolated issue.

(continued)

Skills and qualities

Being able to communicate effectively, and accommodate and adapt to different communication styles; to utilise or be open to the use of technology; to learn to delegate (something I am not exactly good at). The ability to cope with competing priorities and demands, and still stay relatively sane. Being approachable, regarding the needs of others, and your own needs. Understanding budgets and finance, and their application, is essential.

Supporting staff, formally and informally

Formal strategies include the use of formalised supervision in a one-on-one and team environment, and training and development opportunities.

Informal strategies include having an open door policy; asking staff at least daily how they are going and what is working well; never walking past a negative comment without asking about it or offering a solution; clearly communicating expectations.

Middle-level managers

Managers at program or 'middle' level supervise team leaders and ensure that specific areas of service delivery are meeting goals and targets. Middle managers are also often responsible for particular areas of work or programs. Recent direct service-delivery experience and strong professional knowledge are still regarded as highly important. In many but not all health and human service organisations, these positions engage in some level of direct service delivery, although this is generally less than frontline managers. As with team leaders and frontline managers, program and middle managers are commonly expected to show leadership qualities and to be leaders within their work teams. At the middle management level it is also particularly important to exercise leadership by 'managing up'. This involves engaging the attention of the next line manager, such as the CEO, and advocating on behalf of the work teams or programs for which the manager has responsibility. Middle managers often belong to an executive team, which brings middle and senior management together.

Top-level managers

The executive team is responsible for liaising between the executive level and frontline staff, providing support and advice to the CEO or director. The executive group undertakes leadership roles in strategic planning, as well as making decisions about internal organisational policy and procedures.

No matter what type of structure, or how widely management and leadership tasks are distributed and performed through teams, it would be exceptional to find an organisation that does not have a person located at the top executive level, as either the chief executive officer (CEO) or director. This person is ultimately responsible for the whole organisation, including staff and services. It is their role to ensure that programs are in accordance with the strategic plan and that quality services are delivered within budget.

REFLECTION EXERCISE

Refer back to Practice example 4.1. How many management tiers and how many managers do you think might be necessary in a service that employs 700 staff, has six separate service streams and operates across numerous sites? What type of organisational structure do you believe would be the most appropriate?

Executive level managers rarely engage in direct service delivery, and according to managerialist principles, do not need to have knowledge and experience associated with service delivery in the profession. In reality, with the current trend towards service clustering and amalgamations, they are likely to sit across a range of professional areas. For example, the CEO of a community health service is potentially responsible for health, primary care and social services; with staff teams comprised of nurses, doctors, social workers, counsellors, health promotion and community development workers.

The balance between leadership and management shifts significantly at the executive level and many CEOs find the bulk of their workload is taken up with leadership activity. In publicly funded community service organisations, the CEO acts as the conduit between the organisation and its employees, and the board of governance. As a member of the board, the CEO also has governance responsibilities.

We have described a simplified three-level schema; it is worth being mindful that there are many variations to these three broad management levels. The following profile provided by Jenny Smith, the CEO of the Council to Homeless Persons (CHP), offers insight into the diverse role expectations and skill requirements of someone sitting in the 'top' position in a peak body.

Linkage
For further information on the Council to Homeless Persons, see www.chp.org.au

PRACTITIONER PROFILE 4.2

JENNY SMITH

CEO, COUNCIL TO HOMELESS PERSONS

Position

The Council to Homeless Persons is the peak body for the specialist homelessness sector in Victoria. Jenny has over twenty years of experience in leadership and management in the public sector. She has worked at policy, management and service delivery levels in health, mental health, community health, within government and now the community sector. Jenny is a social worker and family therapist and has completed Masters degrees in social work as well as public policy and management. Jenny is also a graduate of the Australian Institute of Company Directors and a board director of St Mary's House of Welcome and the Victorian Mental Health Carers Network.

The specialist homelessness service sector in Victoria comprises around 150 organisations providing more than 500 programs, with key approaches including the provision of case management, transitional housing and brokerage. CHP works to end homelessness through leadership in policy, advocacy, capacity building and consumer participation. CHP is a company limited by guarantee and has a small staff of around ten people. As Chief Executive Officer Jenny is responsible to a board of twelve directors for the strategic and operational management of the organisation.

(continued)

A typical day

The CEO of a peak body is a wonderful all-round role. Such a small organisation has little infrastructure and so most days include some hands-on running of the organisation, addressing issues including staffing, finance, quality assurance, governance and administration. Most days also include liaison with a range of stakeholders drawn from: government ministers and their offices, government departments, specialist homelessness services providers, consumers and other peak bodies. The foci of discussion ranges across national and state social service and homelessness policies, strategic considerations about how best to influence government decision-making, how to maximise positive relationships between various stakeholders, public presentations and media interviews. On the organisational home-front, daily considerations include prioritising the work to be done, seeking additional resources, keeping expenditure within budget, making sure the organisation remains accredited, recruitment and retention of staff, the relationships between staff, and maintaining the office premises and equipment in good condition.

Challenges

The most important role for a peak body is to represent the sector in a way that is influential in improving outcomes for consumers. Like most peak bodies in Australia, CHP is funded by (state) government. There is a genuine challenge in finding the best way to go about assertively influencing the government that funds you. So the best approach is to establish and maintain good working relationships with the diverse stakeholders across policy and practice. Politicians, public servants, service providers, members, consumers, businesses and philanthropic bodies usually look at social issues including homelessness from slightly different perspectives. It is important to engage constructively with all stakeholders and maintain those relationships through times when differences become difficult.

Lessons learnt

Too many important things to begin to list! However, some key thoughts:

* Diplomacy and integrity are vital to maintain at all times.
* The motivations of employees vary enormously, and you will make fewer mistakes if you assume that staff enthusiasms are not the same as your own.
* Both you and the organisation are rarely in a steady and stable state. It's wise to assume you are either moving forward or slipping back.
* It's important to have sound research and policy development processes. However, include in your plan the assumption that good outcomes are most likely to be associated with political influence and good timing.

Skills and qualities

* A genuine enjoyment of working with and in partnership with a wide range of other people.
* A capacity to cope well with ambiguity and uncertainty and to keep your sights on long-term goals, while enjoying small wins and shrugging off losses.
* A capacity to plan and act strategically while remaining actively engaged with the day-to-day and necessary detail.
* A capacity to manage conflict with a view to constructive outcomes for all involved.
* A capacity to work with people in groups, and to be able to write and speak well.
* A thick skin!

Skills, experience and qualifications

The work of the CEO is to manage and lead the organisation itself, and therefore expertise and knowledge in management become imperative. At the same time, in health and human service organisations there is generally an expectation that the CEO has a qualification relevant to a field of practice pertinent to the organisation, and at least some experience in direct service delivery.

Qualifications across the health and human services sectors vary widely: professions include medical doctors, dentists and nurses, counsellors, social workers, welfare and community development workers, psychologists, specialist support staff, housing workers, the list goes on and on. Some of these positions involve years of university study, others require undergraduate degrees, diplomas and certificates. Due to the introduction of accreditation standards, many workers across the sector now have some form of minimum qualification.

It is encouraging that, although still limited and contained to upper levels, qualifications in management are beginning to rise. In our own research we found that managers' qualifications and experience increased with the level of their position (Berends & Crinall, forthcoming). In an online survey, respondents were asked to identify their level of management, years of experience in the field and type of qualification. The respondents included twelve who were executive level managers, and eight who were program managers. Sixteen had more than ten years' experience in the sector, twenty-three had tertiary qualifications in a related field of study, and nine had management qualifications. Nine of the twelve executive level managers had ten or more years' experience in the sector, and seven had management qualifications. Amongst the program managers, four had ten or more years' experience in the sector, and two had management qualifications. This is summarised in Figure 4.2 below.

Linkage
We continue this discussion on qualifications held by the health and human services workforce in Chapter 5, highlighting the diversity that exists and the limited number of staff with management training.

FIGURE 4.2 Experience and management qualifications of executive and program managers

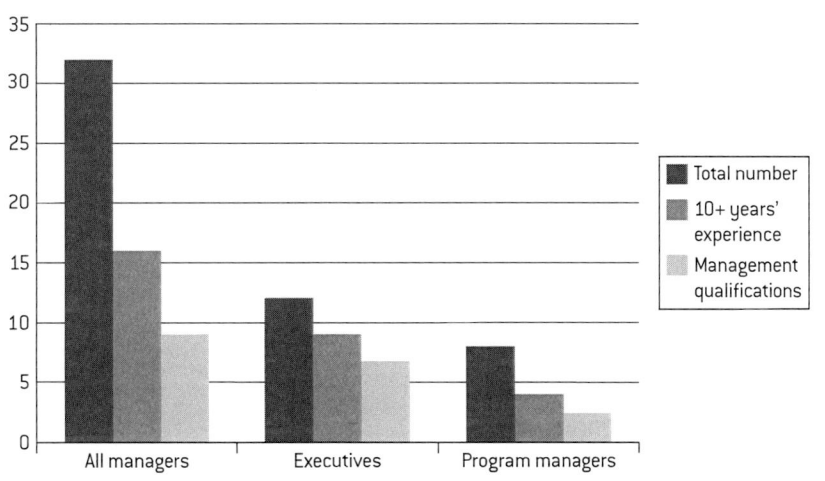

Responsibilities

We have been suggesting that employees at all levels in a health and human service organisation are required to perform management and leadership roles to varying degrees. But what does managing and leading in health and human services entail? We have acknowledged that managing in these services is complex and, as the practitioner profiles indicate, considerable self-care and level headedness is required to avoid a manager's role becoming overwhelming. Pinning down what is actually required of managers in human service organisations can be a frustrating and elusive task, and this is why these organisations are high on the list of 'the most difficult to manage' (Drucker, 2006, cited in Menefee, 2009, p.101). For this reason alone it is important to identify and clarify our expectations of managers and leaders. This is especially so if health and human services are to retain their value base, while also 'surviving and thriving' in a climate of competition, escalating demands and increasing complexity. The following core management responsibilities are included in the literature on health and human services management.

TABLE 4.1 Core management responsibilities

TASKS	ACTIVITIES
Planning	Goal setting and decision-making
Organising/designing	Coordinating work to be done; identifying, allocating and arranging tasks and resources
Leading and facilitating	Influencing others to achieve goals; enabling staff
Supervising	Supporting, motivating and resourcing staff and teams
Managing human resources	Recruiting and selecting staff; staff training and performance development
Managing finances	Planning budgets and controlling financial expenditure
Monitoring and evaluating	Tracking progress on program and organisational performance; determining achievement of program and service delivery outcomes
Communicating	Written and verbal communication in a variety of modes: face-to-face, digital, paper-based in a range of formats, presentations, reports, memos, information exchange, chairing meetings, etc.
Forecasting	Anticipating and identifying future directions and emergent trends; risk management
Boundary spanning	Building and maintaining networks and relationships outside the organisation
Policy administration	Developing, implementing and complying with organisational policies, as well as overseeing the translation of social policy into practice
Advocating	Presenting to major stakeholders on behalf of staff, client groups (at the macro level) and organisation
Team building	Ensuring functional teams and a safe, healthy, dynamic, supportive work environment
Problem-solving	Making decisions; finding appropriate resolutions to various issues

Source: Donovan & Jackson, 1991, p.13; Lewis et al., 2012, pp.8–9; Menefee, 2009, pp.103–7

We find it helpful to organise these areas of management responsibility into four broad categories: functions, tasks, roles and skills. Before discussing these in detail, you may wish to complete the following activity.

REFLECTION EXERCISE

Locate some recent advertisements for management positions in health and human services. If possible, acquire the position descriptions. Take note of the roles and responsibilities that are listed in the ads and position descriptions.

Our own scan of advertised positions in the health and human services sector revealed the following mix of requirements:

TABLE 4.2 Applicant requirements for health and human services management positions

QUALIFICATIONS	EXPERIENCE	SKILLS	QUALITIES	AREAS OF RESPONSIBILITY
• Graduate or post-graduate • Relevant to area of practice	• Financial management • Relevant to area of practice • In managing complexity • Staff support • Staffing • Administration	• Leadership • Relationship building • Ability to improve client outcomes • Crisis resolution • Maintenance of community partnerships • Exceptional communication skills • Ability to balance priorities • Exceptional problem-solving skills	• Positive attitude • High motivation • Strong core values • Team approach • Creativity • Innovation • Passion	• Stakeholder engagement • Operational management • Service development • Program establishment • Leadership

Power and authority

A particularly important responsibility for those in management and leadership positions is the ethical use of power and authority. This requires critical self-awareness and insight into the different forms that they take, and an appreciation of their complex operation through interpersonal relationships, and organisational structure and culture.

The privileges afforded by their positions authorise managers and leaders to exercise many forms of influence. Depending on the circumstances, supervisory and leadership roles carry varying capacity to enact power *over* others, power *with* others and power *for* others. As representatives of their organisation, leaders are expected to enable others to achieve their own and the organisation's goals, and to act in the best interests of the stakeholders, communities and society that the organisation serves and to which it is accountable.

The degrees and forms of power that a manager is able to exercise are also dependent on the organisation's structure and function: whether it is a collective or a bureaucracy, whether clients are voluntary or mandated, whether the practice philosophy is oriented towards advocacy and support, or care and protection. Leadership style also determines how individuals utilise power in their relationships with their peers, their superiors and those they supervise. Managers are also required to moderate the interplay of power between workers.

The inter-relationships between leadership, power and authority are complex. Leadership involves using power productively to motivate and inspire others towards a desired goal. Authority is the sanctioning of the right to use particular forms of power. As acknowledged in Chapter 1, power is both entity (something that is held and used) and action (a force or drive that operates through having the freedom to act and make choices). It is the *capacity* and *ability* to influence others, and it is the *actions* and *processes* that take place within all relationships; particularly where shifts between one state and another are involved. This form of power sits at the centre of bringing about change.

The ability to influence others often causes dilemmas for health and human services managers, who are guided by policy and practice codes that resist the idea of controlling others or exercising power over them. Professional ethics, practice and personal philosophies, and our own value systems mean that we are comfortable acting as mentors. But we are often not so keen to make evaluative judgments of others, or to exercise influence to the point that we are seen to be *making* someone do something when they might be reluctant or resistant (which is, in fact, a very effective use of power by the resistor). That said, a manager occupies a privileged position, and is able to access and exercise forms of power that those in subordinate positions cannot. Therefore, it is important to recognise this capacity, and to employ it fairly, justly and effectively, according to the philosophy and values of the human service organisation, while at the same time, reconciled with one's own personal and professional values (Lewis et al., 2012, pp.154–5).

The many different types and sources of power include:
- exploitative (of others)
- manipulative (over others)
- competitive (against others)
- nutrient (for others)
- integrative (with others)
- coercive (punishing others)
- legitimate or positional (gained through privilege)
- expert (gained through knowledge)
- informational (gained through access to valuable information)
- reward (capacity to evaluate and provide incentives)
- referent (gained from personal relationships)

- connection (gained through contacts with influential people)
- productive (the will to change and achieve)
- oppressive (gained through the will to control)
- resistant (refusing to be influenced by another's power).

Source: Hughes & Wearing, 2013; Lewis et al., 2012

All of these types of power can be useful, depending on the situation and the amount of control that is called for in relation to others. For those in management and leadership positions, power derives from various sources: personal capabilities, such as qualifications and expertise; relationships, where power flows upwards from followers; and from the manager's position in the organisation, which affords control over rewards and resources, with power mainly flowing horizontally and downwards. Challenges for the manager are, firstly, to develop critical insight into their own use of power, secondly to be clear about their sanctioned authority to exercise influence, and thirdly to develop their skills in determining the most appropriate and productive form of power for a given situation. Although a difficult concept for many in the health and human services, workers, managers and leaders cannot perform the functions of their roles without exercising power. It is *how* power is exercised that determines the value of its affects and effects. It is the responsibility of those in authority to be self-critically aware of their own use of power, trying to ensure that power is deployed productively—increasing freedom and opportunity—rather than in limiting, exploitative and oppressive ways.

REFLECTION EXERCISE

Reflect on the forms of power listed.

1 What forms of power are evident in your workplace?
2 Which do you use to achieve management tasks?
3 Can you think of a situation where it may be appropriate for a leader to use manipulative power? When and why?

Functions

Functions are processes that authorise particular roles and establish their purpose in an organisational context. The identification and definition of a set of functions determines which tasks will be performed and which skills are required. In this way, they play a fundamental role in shaping the flow of power, and how and by whom it can be exercised towards achieving productive ends. The core functions listed in generic management literature have been described as 'limited and somewhat overlapping' (Weinbach, 2007, p.7). Although there are numerous variations, the four most commonly identified are:

- planning
- organising
- leading
- controlling.

Source: Bartol et al., 2011, p.6

In literature specific to health and human services management, this list tends to be more expansive. For example, Lewis et al. identify seven key functions in human services management: these are represented in Figure 4.3.

FIGURE 4.3 Management functions

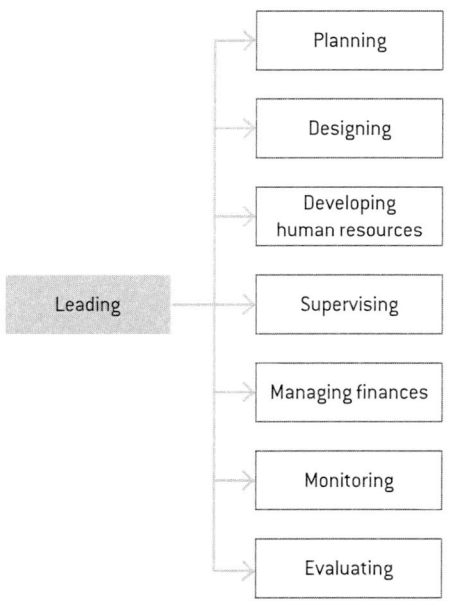

Source: adapted from Lewis et al., 2012, pp.8–9

As this diagram indicates, Lewis et al. consider leadership to be 'the force that binds together and energizes' the seven functions (2012, p.8). Other authors include 'coordinating, marketing, consulting, liaising with external stakeholders' (Anheier, 2005, p.245) and staffing (Weinbach, 2007, p.73).

REFLECTION EXERCISE

Think for a moment about management in your own organisational context. What do you believe are the essential management functions? Create your own list.

Management functions
The fundamental management processes. These establish the purpose of a management role and circumscribe management tasks, roles and skills.

Management functions

Management functions relate to the day-to-day administration of an organisation, and are variously applied across management levels. From our own review of literature, and consultations with health and human services managers, we identified a list of twelve core functions:

1   planning
2   organising

3   developing
4   communicating
5   facilitating
6   influencing
7   monitoring
8   evaluating
9   decision-making
10 resourcing
11 supervising
12 problem-solving.

Each function is briefly outlined below and these concepts are interwoven throughout the text. It is worth restating that these functions overlap to some degree. Separating and organising them into a number of discrete processes is simply a method that helps make sense of the complex work of managing (Weinbach & Taylor, 2011). Remember too that functions are dynamic; adapting and changing according to socio-political context, culture and time.

Management with leadership

You may have noticed that we have not included leadership as a management function. This is because, as explained earlier, we believe it is possible to perform a **management role** successfully, without being a leader. That said, we also recognise that many of these functions do involve drawing on leadership skills, and of course, at the upper levels of management in today's organisations, leadership is essential.

Much of the health and human services literature blurs management and leadership when discussing functions, roles and tasks, and then discusses leadership in terms of style, quality, dimensions and characteristics (McDonald et al., 2011). We appreciate that the topics of management and leadership and their interrelationship has become complex and confusing. In a quest for clarity and to maintain some distinction, we address management, leadership and governance functions separately, while continuing to acknowledge and promote their interconnectedness.

Management role
A formally or informally defined position that has responsibility for performing a management function.

Linkage
These management functions are described in Box 4.1

BOX 4.1

Management functions

Planning is a multi-layered process involving forecasting, setting organisational policies, establishing the overall direction for the organisation, setting goals and identifying appropriate programs.

Organising involves arranging systems, processes, resources and people, so that plans and work can be monitored and successfully carried out. It involves making decisions about including and excluding.

Developing refers to building the capacity and potential of the organisation and the people associated with it. It refers to growing and fostering potential.

(continued)

Communicating requires effectively conveying information through a variety of spoken and written media and methods within, and external to, the organisation. Effective communication is essential for organisational success.

Facilitating involves mentoring staff and ensuring that organisational processes and culture are enabling, so that programs and work can be carried out effectively. Facilitating is also about appropriately sharing management and leadership tasks and responsibilities.

Influencing is about causing things to happen. It entails leading, affecting and shaping the organisation and its work. Influencing also entails team-building.

Monitoring is the process of continuously checking and tracking how the organisation, staff and programs are performing.

Evaluating requires judging, measuring, interpreting and analysing the value of programs, policies, processes and practices occurring within the organisation.

Decision-making involves deciding what needs to be done and how it will happen, and then delegating tasks and responsibilities to the appropriate team or person. Essentially, decision-making is about selecting an option from a range of alternatives.

Resourcing is about supplying. It relates to ensuring that adequate fiscal, human and knowledge resources are provided for the organisation and staff to efficiently and effectively carry out the services it has undertaken to deliver.

Supervising in health and human services is about administering and overseeing the work of others; it also relates to supporting staff to achieve their performance goals and targets. It involves assisting people to work towards the attainment of their own career aspirations.

Problem-solving involves identifying issues, gathering and processing information, and finding a solution. This function also relates to arbitrating and mediating when parties cannot resolve disputes and complaints.

Leadership functions

As stated earlier, the purpose of leadership is to guide and provide organisations and workers with vision and purpose. Leadership processes involve exercising significant influence to bring about change, risk-taking, working with possibilities and building potential, while management functions are largely about exercising influence to ensure efficiency and survival. Within an organisation there is ideally a dynamic but balanced relationship between leadership and management, and it is preferable, but not always possible or necessary, for this to be present in the one person (Kotter, 2011b).

Many leadership functions can be conceived as extensions, or perhaps enhancements, of management functions. Kotter (2011b) explains that while managers are engaged in planning processes, they work within strategic planning frameworks, setting goals and future targets, detailing the objectives for attaining these goals and allocating resources. Leaders, on the other hand, are involved in planning for change—creating visions and taking calculated risks that inform future planning. Gardner explains that leaders are 'expected to enthuse and inspire staff to work well' (Gardner, 2006, p.143). She also emphasises the importance of leadership being dispersed across all positions in an organisation.

We see leadership functions as necessarily incorporating all of the above management functions, because in order for leadership to be successfully translated into organisational processes and practice, a leader must have proficient **management skills**. Leadership is the creative edge of management; it is where the art of management is realised. In addition to the management functions listed above, we include the following essential functions of leadership: having vision, changing, inspiring and connecting.

Management skills
The ability and capacity to carry out tasks and functions pertaining to a management role.

BOX 4.2

Functions of leadership, in addition to management functions

Having vision requires seeing future potential, seeking opportunities and creating new directions for moving forward positively. It is about realising new solutions for old problems.

Changing involves guiding the organisation, individual staff and work teams into and through unfamiliar terrain and new directions.

Inspiring refers to enthusing and motivating people and extending them beyond their comfort zone.

Connecting is about establishing new relationships, building partnerships and aligning people and work groups. It also refers to ensuring that professional values lead and guide organisational decision-making and practice.

Although perplexing at times, it is not overly difficult to appreciate the relationship between the functions of management and leadership within an organisational setting. There is a large body of literature devoted to exploring this topic. Some key sources are included in the further reading section at the end of the chapter (and in references throughout the chapter). Governance functions, on the other hand, are rarely discussed as if they belong in the same arena. Before looking at the functions associated with governance, take a moment to consider Jodie Martin's list of tasks associated with her role as CEO of the Gippsland Women's Health Service (GWHS).

PRACTITIONER PROFILE 4.3

JODIE MARTIN

CEO, GIPPSLAND WOMEN'S HEALTH SERVICE

Current role

My role is to provide organisational leadership and operational management of GWHS. This involves:

- Oversight for the implementation of GWHS strategic directions and policy and procedures.
- Managing the resources of the organisation to deliver on strategic and operational priorities, continuous improvement processes and externally funded projects.
- Managing external relationships, including with key policy makers and service provider organisations.
- Providing leadership of internal organisational values and culture, staff and governance processes.

(continued)

Typical day

Given the small size of our organisation, my role is quite varied. A typical day involves a mixture of:

- Supervision/oversight of staff including dealing with HR matters
- Responding to emails
- Attending and/or chairing meetings—across the region and in the city (executive, network, partnership, departmental meetings)
- Reporting to the GWHS Board: CEO report, finance reports
- Responding to media enquiries
- Financial management.

Governance functions

Earlier we described governance as one of the three fundamental components underpinning management and leadership. We also emphasised the importance of maintaining the distinction between the functions of the board of management (or governing body) and management and leadership roles within the organisation. According to Hudson (2009, p.60), 'boards play specific roles in the delivery of certain organisational functions.' In comparison with management and leadership, governance functions are more circumscribed; they are linked with very specific purposes.

But, as with management and leadership, the functions attached to governance align and overlap. Hudson (2009) identifies these functions as: strategic planning, managing corporate performance, policy-making, managing risk and compliance. We replace 'corporate' with 'organisational' in our list, which is detailed in Box 4.3.

BOX 4.3

Governance functions

Strategic planning includes ensuring that the organisation has a current and appropriate process for developing the strategic plan, confirming the planning process, challenging key elements of the proposed plan and approving the final plan.

Managing organisational performance involves holding the management of the organisation accountable, praising achievements and challenging poor performance.

Policy-making involves assisting in developing policies, where appropriate, approving policies when they are developed, and ensuring that policies and procedures are in place and regularly reviewed. It is not the board's role to implement policies.

Managing risk is a key responsibility of a governance board. This involves identifying major risks and those responsible for their management, estimating their likelihood and potential impact, defining actions for addressing the risk, and reporting on recommendations for any further actions.

Compliance requires boards to take responsibility for ensuring that an organisation is compliant with regulatory requirements.

Source: adapted from Hudson, 2009, pp.60–2

As these functions and processes make evident, the governance body has a watching brief. It exists to ensure that the organisation has fulfilled the necessary requirements for efficient and effective functioning, but it is not responsible for actually carrying out that work.

REFLECTION EXERCISE

Spend a few moments reviewing the functions of management, leadership and governance. Reflect on how they overlap and where they diverge.

Review the practitioner profiles and consider how each person describes their role as a manager and leader.

What role might the board of governance have in the initiatives described in Practice example 4.1?

Tasks

While functions establish the processes and actions that are required of managers, leaders and governing bodies, these become meaningful when they are attached to tasks and directed towards outcomes. In other words, actions need to be purposeful. Tasks are perhaps best identified by the answer to the question, *What is required to be done?* The task list for managing, leading and governing an organisation will vary according to the type of services offered, its size, location and context. Specific tasks are defined by the functions that drive them. Table 4.3 provides an example of the relationship between management functions, processes and tasks. This is not a static or finite list; you will no doubt quickly identify missing components, as well as aspects that are less relevant in your own context.

TABLE 4.3 Management functions, processes and tasks

FUNCTION	ASSOCIATED PROCESSES	TASKS
Planning	Forecasting, setting, identifying, establishing	Strategic, operation and program planning, policy development, agenda setting
Organising	Arranging, including, excluding	Establishing systems, procedures and processes; arranging structures and areas of activity
Developing	Building, growing, fostering	Expanding programs and services; fostering staff development
Communicating	Conveying, informing	Writing memos, reports, and strategic documents; speaking with staff, chairing meetings; networking with external stakeholders; liaising between staff and board of management/governance
Facilitating	Mentoring, enabling, sharing	Enabling staff, identifying areas of strength, connecting people and teams
Influencing	Leading, affecting, shaping	Managing change, guiding organisation and staff in new directions

(continued)

TABLE 4.3 Management functions, processes and tasks (*continued*)

FUNCTION	ASSOCIATED PROCESSES	TASKS
Monitoring	Checking, tracking	Staff performance development; generating and gathering client data
Evaluating	Judging, measuring, interpreting, analysing	Interpreting and analysing data, preparing and responding to review and audit requirements
Decision-making	Deciding, delegating, selecting	Making choices about program development and resource distribution
Resourcing	Supplying, maintaining	Staffing and personnel issues; preparing and submitting tender documents; preparing and adhering to budgets
Supervising	Overseeing, supporting, administering	Meeting with staff; monitoring workloads
Problem-solving	Identifying, gathering, processing, finding, arbitrating, mediating	Working out the solution to problems; resolving conflict, responding to complaints

Roles

It is important to distinguish between management, leadership and governance as organisational functions and processes, and the people who carry out and perform the tasks associated with them. For example, being a manager may well be defined by doing management tasks; however, being a manager is also about adopting a particular identity within an organisational context. Furthermore, as we have emphasised, management and leadership tasks are not limited to people who have been formally appointed to management and leadership positions within the organisation (Coulshed et al., 2006; Gardner, 2006; McDonald et al., 2011).

As we propose, along with others, it is increasingly essential for workers at all organisational levels to engage in management and leadership activities to varying degrees and as appropriate (Gardner, 2006). However, many workers, particularly those in direct service delivery, find it difficult to put on a management or leadership 'hat', identify as a manager or leader, and take on the associated organisational responsibilities. This reluctance has been ascribed to the negative associations deriving from management as an administrative role involving the supervision of staff in a manner of power *over* them within a hierarchical structure (Aldgate et al., 2007; Coulshed et al., 2006; Patti, 2003; Weinbach & Taylor 2011). For others, it is related to the direction and focus of their work. Practitioners in direct service delivery are necessarily—and appropriately—primarily focused on facilitating change in their clients' lives, rather than directing their attention and energy at improving the performance of other staff or enhancing organisational survival and growth (Donovan & Jackson, 1991; Gardner, 2006; McDonald et al., 2011). Even so, frontline practitioners frequently draw on management and leadership skills with their clients, and in networking and liaising with other organisations in their task environment.

David Menefee (2009) aligns management roles with core competencies. Based on research that examined what managers actually do, rather than what they are 'supposed' to do, he identified these roles as: communicator; boundary spanner; futurist; organiser; resource administrator; evaluator; policy practitioner; advocate; supervisor; facilitator; and team–builder–leader (Coulshed et al., 2006; Hughes & Wearing, 2013).

Again, this list is by no means definitive; new roles arise along with new technologies, models and approaches. The roles of 'leader', 'futurist' and 'evaluator' are relatively recent, emerging along with the introduction of managerialist principles and the unfolding effects and requirements of the new public management regime in health and human services that we discussed in Chapter 2. Performing these tasks and roles is underpinned by the requirement for managers to have specific knowledge and skills. These too are interconnected with, and at the same time divisible from, core functions and processes.

Skills

Skills are the particular abilities that enable tasks and functions to be carried out. Menefee categorises skills into three main types: technical, conceptual and interpersonal (2009, p.103). We add perceptual skills to this list, elaborated in Box 4.4.

BOX 4.4

Management, leadership and governance skills

Technical skills involve being able to develop organisational plans and budgets, and to prepare funding, various reporting and evaluation documents. This requires experience, capacity and specialist knowledge (Lewis et al., 2012; Weinbach & Taylor, 2011).

Conceptual skills involve the ability to see the whole organisation and how its various components connect and interact (Bartol et al., 2011; Weinbach & Taylor, 2011). Weinbach and Taylor (2011) point out that conceptual skills also require an ability to accurately interpret and contextualise what is happening in the organisation. In leadership roles capacity for creativity and innovation is required.

Interpersonal skills refer to the ability to communicate effectively and respectfully with people at all levels in the organisation. Also referred to as 'human' or 'people' skills, these involve motivating and encouraging staff to perform their own duties well. For leaders this extends to being able to connect and align people, and to motivate and inspire.

Perceptual skills are particularly required in leaders and those in governance positions. These involve being able to see that which is not immediately obvious, and to form visions for new directions based on evidence and indicators that are not clearly defined.

Effective managers and leaders require competence in all of these skill sets, even though the importance varies at different levels. Top-level managers, such as directors and CEOs, must draw on conceptual and perceptual skills more often than frontline managers, who are more frequently required to utilise technical skills. Interpersonal skills, or people skills, are essential at all levels (Bartol et al., 2011).

REFLECTION EXERCISE

Review the descriptions by Jenny Smith (Practitioner profile 4.2) and Jodie Martin (Practitioner profile 4.3) of their tasks and responsibilities. List some of the skills that you believe might be required to competently perform their roles. Make a list of your own management and leadership skills.

The close alliance between the skills needed for direct practice, management and leadership is recognised by a number of authors. Coulshed et al. (2006, p.13) explain, 'many practitioner skills in social work are also managerial ones, and all social workers increasingly work to managerialist agendas, so the difference may be one of degree, rather than of kind'. Weinbach, too, asserts this alignment, and observes that 'management is an integral part of social work practice' (Weinbach, 2007, p.8). He further claims that, 'it is more similar to the other functions performed by social workers than it is dissimilar to them' (Weinbach, 2007, p.19).

Despite these observations, it is also important to be mindful that the skills and expertise required by a specialist practitioner diverge in significant ways from those necessary for efficient management. Hudson (2009, p.359) suggests that although managers often feel more comfortable when they are busy, and many believe that they can do a better job in a shorter time frame, managing is not about 'doing', it is about facilitating processes and others to deliver services and carry out tasks. A focus on this essential function of management is often difficult to sustain in work environments characterised by impossible time frames, demanding workloads, multi-tasking and the assignment of dual roles. Attentiveness to the organising, facilitating, influencing and initiating functions of management and leadership requires the development, in particular, of conceptual and interpersonal skills.

We have discussed the importance of health and human service managers possessing knowledge and experience relevant to the area of service delivery provided by their organisation, in tandem with knowledge about management. It is also important to recognise that capacity to perform a particular role varies widely across individuals. In the past, explanations for this variation have been ascribed to innate personal traits, environmental factors, learnt behaviours and access to training and education. Over recent decades there has been a rapid rise in popular literature about developing management and leadership skills. As an example, a search on the Amazon books website using the term 'management skills' generated 67,134 results, and 'leadership skills' elicited 35,015. This avalanche of texts on management and leadership skills delivers a strong message that contemporary culture not only places a strong emphasis on the capacity to manage and lead, but also on the ability we all have to learn these skills.

SUMMARY OF KEY ISSUES

This chapter unpacked the key functions, tasks, roles and responsibilities required in the management, leadership and governance of health and human services. It discussed the interrelatedness between these organisational domains and the distinctions between them; and emphasised the importance of encouraging workers across all organisational levels to develop leadership and management skills. We identified various forms and sources of power, and emphasised that effective management and leadership requires self-awareness, and skilful and responsible use of power and authority to achieve productive and positive outcomes. A key point throughout is the fundamental importance of ethical, competent and effective management, leadership and governance for organisational well-being. These messages are carried into the next chapter when discussing workforce support and development.

PRACTICE ACTIVITIES

1 Defining management, leadership and governance

Answer the following questions:
  a   What is meant by the terms management, leadership and governance?
  b   How are management, leadership and governance in the health and human services different from in the business sector?
  c   What key functions are performed in these organisational domains?
  d   What are the differences and similarities between management and leadership?

2 The role of the CEO

Imagine you are the CEO of a medium-size community service organisation. How would you begin your day? What might you expect to encounter in a typical working day?

3 Qualifications and experience

Think for a moment about your views regarding the professional qualifications and experience of managers. What do you believe is the correct mix of management practice and/or professional practice? Imagine that you are a member of the selection panel for the following positions in your organisation:
  • Frontline worker
  • Team leader or supervisor
  • Program manager
  • CEO.

  Using Table 4.4 overleaf, indicate the level of importance that you would place on qualifications and experience for positions at these four levels. When you have completed your selections, reflect on your choices. Was there a difference in your expectations of qualifications and experience across the four positions? If so, why do you think this was the case? If you were employing new staff for a business, such as a petrol station or restaurant, do you think you would have allocated the same importance to relevant qualifications and experience? If not, why not? You may like to share your responses with other students or colleagues and discuss any similarities or differences in their choices.

TABLE 4.4 Importance of qualifications across management levels

	NOT IMPORTANT	IMPORTANT	VERY IMPORTANT	ESSENTIAL
RELEVANT QUALIFICATIONS				
Frontline worker				
Team leader				
Program manager				
CEO				
RELEVANT PRACTICE EXPERIENCE				
Frontline worker				
Team leader				
Program manager				
CEO				
MANAGEMENT QUALIFICATIONS				
Frontline worker				
Team leader				
Program manager				
CEO				
MANAGEMENT EXPERIENCE				
Frontline worker				
Team leader				
Program manager				
CEO				

FURTHER READING

Leadership

Gray, I., Field, R. & Brown, K. (2010). *Effective Leadership, Management and Supervision in Health and Social Care*. Exeter: Learning Matters, Chapter 2, 'Self Awareness and Leadership' and Chapter 3, 'Developing your Leadership Style'.

Kotter, J. P. (2011b, originally published 1990). 'What Leaders Really Do', in H. B. Review (ed.), *On Leadership*, Boston, Massachussetts: Harvard Business Review Press, pp.37–56.

Management

Lewis, J. A., Packard, T. R. & Lewis, M. D. (2012). *Management of Human Service Programs* (5th edn). USA: Brooks/Cole Cengage Learning.

This is a classic human service management text. Chapter 1, 'Facing the Challenges of Management', is particularly relevant to much of the discussion here.

Menefee, D. (2009). 'What Human Services Managers Do and Why They Do It', in Patti, R. J. (ed.), *The Handbook of Human Services Management* (2nd edn), California, USA: Sage, pp.101–16.

Boards of governance

Mackay, K. (1991). *Community Management*, Melbourne, Australia: Victorian Council of Social Services & Victoria Law Foundation.

This plain-language manual was developed as a guide for management groups in community service organisations. Although it is over twenty years since this version was published, its common sense approach is enduring.

PART 2

PLANNING AND PRACTICE

The practice cases in this part are:

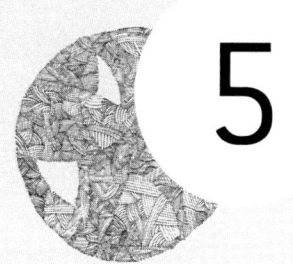

5

Workforce Support and Development

OVERVIEW

This chapter will:

- explore characteristics of the workforce in Australia's health and human service organisations, and associated challenges
- describe management processes for staff recruitment, development and review
- consider some of the factors that shape employment conditions.

This chapter is an overview of the health and human services workforce and the processes that support staff performance and well-being, and impact workplace functionality.

KEY TERMS

community services workforce
health workforce
human resource management
human services workforce
industrial organisation

performance appraisal
staff conditions
supervision
unions

Characteristics of the workforce

Working with people is central to health and human service delivery. Capable management requires a sound understanding of pressures on staff that arise from the nature of the work as well as from features of organisational and funding environments. In this section we explore characteristics of the workforce, such as age and gender, in addition to qualifications, and workplace arrangements. We describe trends in workforce demand and supply, and associated challenges, to illustrate some of the practical issues that may be encountered by managers.

'The workforce' in health and human services

The Australian Institute of Health and Welfare (AIHW) provides regular reports describing health and human service sectors, including information on the workforce. First, let us consider the size and nature of this workforce, to provide a foundation for related management considerations.

The workforce in health and human service organisations includes many industries and occupational groups. The AIHW describes this workforce in two domains, health services and community services. Both paid and voluntary positions are involved.

Health services

Health workforce
Comprises people employed in health occupations in health service industries. There are many types of occupations; major groups include nurses, medical professionals, allied health workers and social workers.

The **health workforce** is growing at a much faster rate than either population or workforce growth in other areas. Between 2003 and 2008 there was a 23% increase in the health workforce, which is almost double the increase across all Australian occupations (13%; Australian Institute of Health and Welfare, 2012b). Information from 2001 and 2006, in Table 5.1 below, shows that occupations involving nurses and medical

TABLE 5.1 Persons employed in health occupations: Australia, 2001 and 2006

OCCUPATION	2001	2006	CHANGE BETWEEN 2001 AND 2006 (%)
Medical practitioners	51,791	57,019	10.1
Medical imaging workers	8,170	10,477	28.2
Dental workers	25,876	29,624	14.5
Nursing workers	193,767	222,133	14.6
Pharmacists	13,925	15,339	10.2
Allied health workers	51,046	65,284	27.9
Complementary therapists	10,964	16,354	49.2
Other health workers	91,183	131,142	45.3
Total health workers	446,722	547,372	22.8

Source: adapted from Australian Institute of Health and Welfare (2009), ABS, Census of Population and Housing, 1996, 2001 and 2006, Table 2.1, p.5

practitioners are the most common, with substantial numbers in the categories of allied health and 'other health workers'. However, there has been considerable expansion in particular occupations, for example complementary therapists (49.2%) and medical imaging workers (28.2%).

More recent data reinforce this sense of growth and change in the workforce. In 2010 there were 766,800 workers in health, an increase of around one quarter from 606,900 in 2005. There has been a 50% increase in the number of social workers, psychologists and 'other health workers' during this period (Australian Institute of Health and Welfare, 2012a, p.496).

Human services

It is difficult to find an adequate definition for the **human services workforce**. Many of these professions overlap with professions in health services (for example, social work and psychology) and the area incorporates a vast collection of occupations; from advocacy, research and policy to residential care programs. However, human services is commonly recognised as a broad descriptor for professions that involve working with people and communities to improve their lives (Lewis et al., 2012). Healy and Lonne (2010) define the social work and human services workforce as:

> Those involved in practice with individuals, groups and communities to assess social needs and to intervene to promote quality of life through improving access to resources and services, or through the provision of social support or personal care services. This definition includes social welfare professionals, such as professionally qualified social workers, paraprofessionals, such as family support workers or youth workers, and intermediate support workers, such as workers providing personal care services to support people with disabilities to remain in their homes.

Human services workforce
A term used to describe the diverse field of workers employed across community and health services, sometimes referred to as 'the caring professions'.

Community services

The AIHW uses a separate classification for 'the community services industry', which also overlaps with human services. According to the AIHW, this industry involves residential aged care services and other residential care, childcare services, and other social assistance services (Australian Institute of Health and Welfare, 2012b, p.315). As of June 2009, more than half a million people (571,000) were employed in community services, and the majority (59%) were in NFP. One quarter (26%) were in for-profit organisations, and 15% were employed by government organisations (Australian Institute of Health and Welfare, 2012b).

As you may have recognised, the separation of workers into occupational categories and groups is somewhat arbitrary. 'Health' workers and 'human services' staff may be part of the same team, and 'community workers' may include staff that work across these areas. This diversity of professions and backgrounds among the workforce is generally regarded as a strength for organisations, as team members learn from each other and encounter fresh perspectives on client concerns and their remediation.

Our focus in this section has been on the provision of client services, but organisations cannot deliver services effectively without the support provided by

Linkage
Chapter 10 includes an exploration of teams, including interdisciplinary, multidisciplinary and transdisciplinary.

other staff. Administrative, financial and clerical roles are just some of the supports that maintain the required infrastructure.

Workforce characteristics and associated challenges

Table 5.2 summarises characteristics of community services and health services workers, which provide an indication of current and future challenges for management. We can see that workers are usually female and that a substantial proportion is aged 55 years or more. Workers have a range of qualifications and part-time work is common.

TABLE 5.2 Selected characteristics of the workforce in Australia's health services industries and community services industries

CHARACTERISTIC	COMMUNITY SERVICES	HEALTH SERVICES
Sex	The majority of workers are female (78%).	The majority of workers are female (76%; but there is considerable variation across professional groups).
Age	The most common age group is 26–45 years (43%) and 15% of the community services workforce is more than 55 years of age.	The average age is 42 and 19% of the health workforce is aged 55 years or more.
Place of birth	One in five workers were born outside Australia.	One in three workers were born outside Australia.
Part-time status	Part-time work is common (42%).	Part-time work is common (50% of females and 20% of males).
Rurality	There are fewer services in rural and remote locations.	Staff shortages are more acute in rural and remote areas.
Salary*	Workers earn less, on average, than people in other industries (i.e., averaging $982 per week, pro rata, in 2010).	There are too many different professions to make a general statement.
Qualifications	A diploma, certificate or equivalent qualification is the most commonly held qualification (43%), followed by a bachelor or higher degree (15%).	Graduation from a relevant university course is a requirement for some professions while others require a vocational training qualification.
Student populations	Increasing numbers are completing community-service-related university courses.	Increasing numbers are completing community-service-related university courses (37% increase from 2005 to 2010) and vocational education and training courses (42,879 students in 2010).

*In 2010 the average weekly salary was $1219 for all other industries (Australian Institute of Health and Welfare, 2011).

Source: based on material from the Australian Institute of Health and Welfare (2011); Australian Bureau of Statistics (2012), Australian Institute of Health and Welfare (2009)

Many of those in the **community services workforce** were born overseas, and this is even more the case in health services industries. The workers have a range of qualifications, with university degrees more common in health services industries. It is a time of change, in terms of tertiary education: university courses are in demand and student numbers are increasing. Salary rates for community services workers are lower than for other industries, while in health services, the breadth of occupations means it is difficult to generalise about salary rates.

Community services workforce
According to the Australian Institute of Health and Welfare the major services in this workforce involve residential aged care and other residential care, childcare, and other social support and assistance.

A broader understanding of the workforce

Our focus thus far has been on professional and paraprofessional staff who are employed to provide particular services—from dental care to nursing and aged care services to support for homeless youth. However, 'the workforce' in health and human service organisations includes other groups that provide a valuable and unique contribution.

Weinbach and Taylor (2011, p.179) identify two additional groups that are sometimes involved in health and human services. The first group involves paid staff with personal experience relevant to their role and the second group involves volunteers.

Those with personal experiences relevant to the area of work may have particular insights and skills that are useful for engaging with and providing an appropriate response to clients. For example, an Aboriginal hospital liaison officer may have links with the community, along with communication skills that foster people's trust in services and their willingness to engage in treatment. In another example, a peer worker may be well placed to build rapport with clients because of their own history of problems and progress (for example, in the case of youth homelessness or domestic violence) and their ability to operate in a non-judgmental and accepting manner.

Volunteers may include those with personal experiences and extend to those who are socially minded. These individuals offer their services without cost and their involvement is defined by organisational need matched to capacity. Volunteers had a substantial role in the establishment of community services and they continue to make a valuable contribution. You may wish to explore this area further: the readings list for this chapter includes a website that has useful information and resources for volunteer programs.

Summary

The general message from this information is that the health and human services workforce in Australia is growing and becoming more qualified. Also, while there is some variation, the workforce is ageing. With the increasing demand for services, key challenges for organisations and for government include attracting people into health and human services positions and retaining them in these roles. Having outlined trends in the workforce, we turn now to implications for policy, planning and practice.

Workforce demand and supply

The Productivity Commission is an independent research and advisory body, established to inform national policies on a range of economic, social and environmental issues.

In 2005, the commission did a review of Australia's health workforce that showed a substantial dissonance between demand and supply. The commission noted that:

- Australia is experiencing workforce shortages across a number of health professions despite a significant and growing reliance on overseas trained health workers. The shortages are even more acute in rural and remote areas and in certain special needs sectors.

- With developing technology, growing community expectations and population ageing, the demand for health workforce services will increase while the labour market will tighten. New models of care will also be required.

- Expenditure on health care is already 9.7% of GDP and is increasing. Even so, there will be a need to train more health workers. There will also be benefits in improving the retention and re-entry to the workforce of qualified health workers.

- It is critical to increase the efficiency and effectiveness of the available health workforce, and to improve its distribution.

Source: Australian Productivity Commission, 2006, p.xiv

Similarly, an analysis of welfare spending and service provision during 2008–09 shows that demand is considerable:

- Government spending increased an average of 5% (after adjusting for inflation) each year, over a ten-year period.
- Governments were the major funder for welfare services (73%), and 59% of services were provided by non-government community service organisations.
- The value of unpaid care was estimated at $68.4 billion, involving family members, neighbours and service volunteers.

Source: Australian Institute of Health and Welfare, 2011

Linkage
A set of standards
for health and
community services
is now in place, as
outlined in Chapter 8.

The Productivity Commission suggests a number of objectives for the health workforce (outlined in Box 5.1). These structures include regulatory groups, to guide and monitor service activities, and the introduction of standards for professions and organisations, to support effective service delivery.

BOX 5.1

Objectives for the health workforce

- Support local innovations, and objectively evaluate, facilitate and drive those of national significance through an advisory health workforce improvement agency.
- Promote more responsive health education and training arrangements through the creation of an independent advisory council; and a high-level taskforce to achieve greater transparency (and appropriate contestability) of funding for clinical training.
- Integrate the current profession-based accreditation of health education and training through an over-arching national accreditation board that could, initially at least, delegate functions to appropriate existing entities, based on their capacity to contribute to the objectives of the new accreditation regime.
- Provide for national registration standards for health professions and for the creation of a national registration board with supporting professional panels.
- Improve funding-related incentives for workforce change through the transparent assessment by an independent committee of proposals to extend MBS coverage beyond the medical profession; the

introduction of (discounted) MBS rebates for a wider range of delegated services; and addressing distortions in rebate relativities.

- Those living in outer metropolitan, rural and remote areas and in Indigenous communities, and others with special needs would benefit from these system-wide initiatives.

Source: Australian Productivity Commission, 2006

Having a capable workforce that matches community demand for health and human services will continue to be a major challenge for government and organisations (Armstrong et al., 2007). Three major strategies have been put forward to address this challenge (Fleming, 2008, p.10):

- Provide training for current and future staff.
- Bring in qualified workers from other countries.
- Encourage staff retention and re-entry.

Each strategy has its own complexities, as Fleming (2008, pp.126–7), explains:

- *Training* takes time and often requires curriculum development at tertiary level. Specialist courses may be offered as electives within health and social work degrees, or provided at postgraduate levels. Training opportunities for the existing workforce must be carefully designed and implemented to reach staff in need of advancing their qualifications.
- *Bringing in overseas staff* is a quick solution but it requires incentives, surveillance and support. Practitioners need to be convinced that moving to a new country will bring career and personal benefits, and they must be appropriately qualified. Ideally, support will be available to assist with their resettlement and integration.
- *Attracting qualified non-practitioners and retaining existing practitioners* seems like an obvious and practical approach, but sometimes factors outside the organisation's control are substantial barriers. Examples include staff remuneration, working conditions and career pathways, in addition to job satisfaction and lifestyle considerations.

Human services have limited capacity to offer positions that are attractive, well paid and have a logical career progression. This is also the case for some parts of health.

To understand this, it is important to note two factors. First, when positions are not defined through industrial agreements or recognised as formal professions there is limited foundation for staff to negotiate favourable employment conditions. For example, being an 'alcohol and drug worker' or 'housing support officer' does not carry the same professional clout as that attached to being a nurse or psychologist. Second, community service organisations are critically important to government because of their community orientation, independence *and* the fact that they tend to be cheaper to fund than government-owned services. There is something of a reliance on the goodwill of community-oriented workplaces (management and workers) to 'do more with less', without expecting conditions that are commensurate with the work they do.

The AIHW (2011) notes that the workplace in community sector organisations has been found wanting in terms of opportunities for career advancement and organisational capacity to provide professional, clearly structured work arrangements. For managers, this means pressure to maintain staff morale and maximise opportunities for career progression, while operating within considerable constraints. You may recall our exploration in Chapter 2 of external pressures and funding considerations. This is an important example of how these pressures impact organisational capacity.

REFLECTION EXERCISE

This may be a good point to pause and reflect on your own career pathway; what motivates you and whether there are clearly defined opportunities for career progression. What is the one thing you would change about your current position, in terms of conditions or opportunities for advancement? Is there anything you could do to support this change?

Our practitioner profile gives a soulful perspective on what is important and challenging at a regional service.

PRACTITIONER PROFILE 5.1

DARYL FITZGIBBON

CLINICAL MANAGER, WESTERN REGION ALCOHOL AND DRUG CENTRE (WRAD)

Position
The role aims to:
- promote good clinical practice across a broad range of services
- facilitate staff support and skill development
- provide counselling, consultancy and continuing care to clients with alcohol and drug problems
- assist with service linking with other related services.

Typical day
- Attend triage, clinical and staff meetings as required.
- Provide assessment of performance data.
- Provide assessments and reports to referring agencies as required.
- Consult and liaise with a range of individuals and agencies about alcohol and drug issues.
- Identify and implement adequate staff training initiatives.
- Assist with the development and updating of clinical guidelines.
- Identify and implement staff support mechanisms.
- Provide regular reports on the development of clinical services within the centre.
- Watch others grimace at some of the things I have to say.

Challenges
- Converting strategies into workable realities.
- Looking beyond jargon.

- Designing service documentation and data recognition systems that are compatible and collaborate in the same way our workers do.
- Training workers to a high standard and watching them leave.
- Educating other agencies and clients.
- Dealing with the 'noticeably nice' who nearly made a decision four years ago but didn't want to offend anybody.
- Windsock policies.

Skills and qualities

- At the end of the day it is *esprit de corps* loyalty to this unfashionable profession.
- You have to believe in what you do and work to continually improve at doing it.
- A clear understanding of your role to ensure we keep the main thing the main thing (alcohol and drug service provision).
- Learn to say no and mean it. You don't have to do anything, you just have to accept responsibility for not doing it.
- Genuineness.

Lessons learnt

- That the only people who make a profit working in alcohol and other drugs are printers and muffin makers.
- The evolution of the health system is somewhat akin to that of the fashion industry; styles and models re-emerge after years of being out of favour.
- People care is an inexact science.
- The saddest thing I have learnt is: that clients consistently pound the pavements to appointments that bring no result, relaying a story that was once an emotional plea from the heart but now seems pointless.
- Drugs and alcohol rob individuals of comfort and confidence. Ironically the quest for these qualities was the reason they took those substances in the first place. It's my comfort-theft theory (I don't expect any speaking engagements on the back of this mind-boggling revelation).

Supporting staff well-being and development

- I ensure they are well trained and not denied professional development opportunities.
- I protect my staff but I don't shelter them from responsibility.
- We have formal internal and external support mechanisms (personal support both internal and external).
- Internal clinical supervision.
- Open door policy with staff but professional boundaries and chain of command are adhered to.

Human resource management

Human resource management
Involves strategies for managing people to maintain a strong alignment between workforce characteristics and organisational goals. Areas include staff recruitment and development, staff welfare and workforce renewal.

Now that we have considered characteristics of the workforce in health and human services, we are well placed to consider daily activities involved in managing this essential resource. **Human resource management** is about strategies for managing people and addressing the alignment between workforce characteristics and organisational goals. It may be explained as involving four components:

1 *Acquiring workers*: including workforce planning, recruitment and selection, induction and initial training.
2 *Staff development*: involving professional development programs, supervision and career planning, as well as performance appraisal.
3 *Staff welfare*: attending to workplace conditions that influence people's motivation for work and their satisfaction with the workplace. Examples include salary and benefits, career opportunities and aspects of organisational culture.
4 *Workforce renewal*: including planning and replacing staff, and extending to processes such as retirement, retrenchment and resignation.

Source: adapted from Lansbury, 1982, cited in Donovan & Jackson, 1991, p.314

While some organisations have a separate unit for human resource management, others are too small to support this arrangement. In any case, many aspects of human resource management involve managers, including workforce planning, recruitment, induction and supervision, as well as staff development and appraisal.

Staff recruitment, selection and induction

The skills and commitment of staff are critical to organisational success. Brody (2005) notes the importance of having employees who are highly motivated and find intrinsic satisfaction in their work. Managers seek to retain the most capable staff in the long term and match qualities of the team with tasks at hand.

Salaries are the major expense in health and human service organisations, and employing new staff is a substantial financial commitment. When a position becomes vacant it is an opportunity to review the current needs of the organisation and the existing complement of staff. Given the uncertain nature of project funding, organisations may find it necessary to have a flexible workforce that includes casual positions and short-term contracts (Coulshed et al., 2006).

Questions for managers considering the need for recruitment include the following:
• Might current staff be deployed differently?
• What specific expertise would be most useful given current staff qualities and service demands?
• Is it better to employ new staff on a casual basis rather than on a contract?

Commencing the recruitment process

Once the decision to recruit has been approved, in the context of organisational need and budget capacity, selection processes can commence. These processes explore applicants' competence and their compatibility with the existing team and the organisation.

Initially, the position will be advertised and applicants will respond to a formal job description. Online advertising and recruitment systems are common and they streamline the process leading to short-listing. The job description typically has a set of selection criteria or essential qualities (or both), and you may ask applicants to provide a response to these items. This information can be useful as it provides a match between what you are seeking and what the applicant is able to offer; it may also filter out potential applicants who are not well suited to the position. Your first role as manager is to cull the set of applications and remove those not matched to your requirements.

Having developed a short-list of applicants, it is time to learn more about them.

Recruitment interviews

Interviews are useful for clarifying details in the job application, exploring some personal qualities of the applicant (for example, presentation and confidence), and explaining particular conditions of the position (for example, after hours work, working across sites). Importantly, interviews provide an opportunity to convey the values of the organisation and explore the attitudes of applicants.

An interview panel is generally convened, which includes management working in the same area as the position, and may involve someone from another part of the organisation. Depending on the position, it may be useful to include an external stakeholder to obtain an independent perspective on applicants. Gender representativeness and cultural diversity may be considered in decisions about the composition of the panel.

Brody (2005, pp.115–17) identifies eight categories of questions for recruitment interviews, which can be adapted according to characteristics of specific roles:

* the applicant's background relevant to the role
* areas of strength and weakness
* expectations of the position and alignment with career goals
* strategies for dealing with work pressure
* accomplishments
* analysis and decision-making
* approach to staff supervision
* cooperation and independence.

Box 5.2 is a generic interview schedule, which includes broad questions that are consistent with the categories put forward by Brody. Specific questions, based on key selection criteria for the role, may be added. The schedule may be formatted to include space for interviewer comments and a rating scale for each question, as well as an overall recommendation.

BOX 5.2

A generic interview schedule

1   What attracted you to this position?
2   Please describe your experience in a related area, highlighting a particular challenge and strategies you used to resolve this issue—along with the outcome and lessons learnt.
3   What do you see as the challenges of this role and how would you overcome them?
4   What are your key strengths and how would these strengths enable you to successfully undertake this position?
5   What strategies do you use to manage and support staff?
6   And what about working with peers and senior staff in the organisation and in other organisations; what is important?
7   What are your priorities for skills development?
8   How does this position fit with your career plans? Where would you like to be in five years' time?
9   Do you have any questions or further comments for the panel?

The schedule is a useful tool that guides the interview process and supports consistency across panel members, generating a set of information that can be used to further reduce the short-list and move toward selection.

Referees

Referees are another source of information that adds to what has been learnt from the written application and recruitment interview. Referee checks are generally undertaken on the final short-list of applicants, which is developed after the interviews. Having a set template, which includes a number of open and more-targeted questions, is useful. Strategies to get the most out of this aspect of the process include:

• Ensuring that the person doing the referee checks understands the requirements of the position.
• Ensuring that this person was involved in other aspects of the recruitment process (for example, short-listing and interviews).
• Including questions that address general staff performance, as well as questions specific to the role.

This is an opportunity to obtain insights from others' experience of working with the applicant regarding some of the more sensitive aspects of employment. Examples include validating their current role in terms of seniority and tasks, and exploring attributes such as their ability to work with others. The applicant's attitude to work and their efficiency, skills, and particular strengths and limitations should be explored. In addition, asking a referee whether they would re-hire the applicant if the opportunity arose and what is next for the applicant in terms of career development is useful to gain an understanding of the applicant's qualities, and how good the 'fit' is between them, other staff, and the role. While it may seem invasive to ask questions in these areas, as a manager you need to know the best and worst aspects of working with the applicant.

Selection

Now that you have information from the applications, interviews and referees you should be ready to select the successful applicant. On occasion, you may wish to hold a second interview to clarify uncertainties and fill gaps in the information already obtained.

Staff with oversight for the position usually guide the decision-making process regarding the successful applicant; ideally the final decision will reflect a consensus among panel members. It should be based on the competence and experience of the applicant in relation to requirements of the position *and* considered in terms of existing staff; who is best placed to complement the skills and qualities of the current group? Where senior positions are involved, the emphasis on potential contribution to part of or the entire organisation will also be considered. The final decision will be based on the skills, knowledge and compatibility of the preferred applicant in relation to current and projected needs of the organisation.

REFLECTION EXERCISE

Think back to a situation where you were applying for a position or involved in a recruitment process. What is your general recollection of the process? What was important for you and what would you do differently?

Induction

Activities to assist in settling a new employee into the organisation are sometimes overlooked, although this is critical to their sense of belonging and their capacity to understand and respond to requirements of the role. The introduction of quality assurance systems has seen more of a deliberate approach to induction, documented in policy and involving a set of orientation activities and the use of a 'buddy program' to support the new worker. As with all policies, this approach is only useful if translated into action. But managers will likely be busy with tasks they had set aside to allow time for recruitment, and juggling demands arising from the previously unfilled position. One option is to delegate aspects of induction to an established member of staff, so the new recruit can be given due attention. During supervision, managers can discuss and supplement these activities.

A common element of employment involves a three-month probationary or trial period, to see if the new staff member is performing adequately. It should soon become apparent if the anticipated fit between your new recruit and the position is a reality. Ongoing discussion with the new employee during this period is important, so they develop a good understanding of what is involved and how well they are doing in relation to your expectations as a manager.

Staff development and supervision

Linkage
Characteristics of staff are an important influence on organisational culture, as we explored in Chapter 3.

Staff welfare, ability and motivation are fundamental to organisational success and well-being. Having a structured approach to **supervision**, in addition to ongoing, informal contact, is essential. The most common form of supervision involves a regular meeting between an employee and their line manager. It is essentially a process whereby the supervisor and supervisee meet to achieve a number of common and different outcomes. Supervision will generally focus on three areas (Weinbach & Taylor, 2011):

1 Administration—is the supervisee able to do their job, at a pace and quality that is appropriate to their role?
2 Support—is the supervisee supported and encouraged in their work? Do they need emotional support because of stressors and challenges arising from the role?
3 Professional development—how can the supervisor best share information and provide guidance for skill and career development? Does the supervisee need access to mechanisms (for example, training) to improve their skills and knowledge base relevant to their role in the workplace? What areas of expertise are they developing and how can these be fostered?

Supervision
A process involving manager and employee, where the manager allocates and monitors work activities, provides support for work-related challenges, and fosters employee development through mentoring, advice and opportunities for skill development.

The supervisee will be seeking:
- Guidance on specific work activities; challenges, achievements, directions.
- Opportunity to share ideas and identify directions for their work.
- Information and support for professional development.

The common goal that unites the supervisor and supervisee is that they are trying, together, to provide the best possible service for their clients.

Supervision is particularly important in health and human service organisations because of the dynamic and challenging nature of the work. Staff may need to debrief on situations they have encountered—with clients or stakeholders, for example. This also applies to challenges arising from workload issues and skill deficits, which can be reviewed to identify possible remedies. Having a supportive and skilled forum to reflect on mistakes and successes is an opportunity for staff to explore what is needed for future practice, in an ongoing cycle of learning and improvement.

We are talking here about management supervision rather than clinical supervision, which involves discussion of therapeutic elements of work (for example, client cases, intervention types). Depending on the professional domain involved, staff may need supervisors with particular qualifications/registration (for example, in the field of psychology) so they can access clinical supervision that aligns with their philosophical and skill base. Some people seek clinical supervision outside their workplace, to access appropriately qualified supervisors and obtain a perspective from someone who is not connected with the organisation.

Brody has identified guidelines to enhance the supervisory relationship. As you read this list, it may be useful to think about examples from your experience that illustrate the points being made.

BOX 5.3

Ways to enhance the supervisory relationship

- Set and/or identify positive examples for others to follow.
- Take time to know staff.
- Give clear instructions.
- 'Sell' your requests; providing an explanation of potential benefits.
- Foster a collaborative spirit.
- Draw the line between supervision and therapy.
- Engage staff in problem solving.

Source: Brody, 2005, pp.183–4

Brody also identifies supervision mistakes.

BOX 5.4

Supervision mistakes

- Micro-management, conveying a sense of mistrust and stifling opportunities for staff growth and development.
- Assigning projects that are beyond staff capacity—unless these are recognised as 'stretch goals' that are about learning through experience (rather than successful task completion).
- A lack of honesty in dealings with staff.
- Playing favourites.
- Encouraging cliques among staff.
- Creating an environment where there is only one way to do things.

Source: Brody, 2005, pp.185–6

We would add two things to this list. First, supervision is not performance appraisal. The supervisory encounter is about trust and honesty in describing one's work and shared problem-solving to address concerns and support staff development. Second, it is not a disciplinary process. While there will be some discussion on progress made and challenges encountered, if disciplinary procedures are required a separate process will be involved. Coulshed et al. (2006) provide an insightful description of supervision that highlights the various aspects involved: this is included in the readings list for this chapter.

Linkage
We explore performance appraisal and disciplinary procedures later in this chapter.

REFLECTION EXERCISE

Take a moment to think about your experience as a supervisee or supervisor. What worked well? What would you like to improve? Do you have any strategies to add to Box 5.3 or Box 5.4?

Staff well-being and supervision

We need to explore one final area related to supervision. Donovan and Jackson (1991) suggest that some employees in human service organisations feel that the welfare orientation of services should extend to staff. This would include accommodating staff who are not performing, and subjugating the needs of the organisation. While this may seem like a compassionate and caring approach, there may be negative consequences for all. The staff member will not be supported to recognise and respond to issues affecting their performance, other team members will bear practical consequences (such as an increased workload) and clients may experience inadequate and inappropriate care.

Managers may be able to make compromises in the short term, such as a leave of absence, training to address a skills deficit, or flexible work hours. Occasionally, staff groups may decide to provide additional supports—for example by opting to do more while a colleague receives a short-term dose of treatment or recovers from an accident. Both of these examples require a planned, deliberate approach where the rights and responsibilities of all parties and the conditions of the arrangement are clearly acknowledged.

Linkage
The practitioner profiled earlier in this chapter, Daryl Fitzgibbon, provides an insightful perspective on strategies to support staff well-being and development.

While staff welfare is a crucial concern for managers, the management perspective is fundamentally about the effect of staff needs on their work performance. For some issues, you may encourage staff to seek professional/practical supports outside the workplace, who are ultimately better placed to provide certain types of support. It is important to maintain a constructive and compassionate approach throughout. However, your management decisions must be based on the understanding that client welfare is the primary focus of the organisation (Donovan & Jackson, 1991).

Mentoring and coaching

Many senior people in health and human services organisations recognise the significance of mentors. Irrespective of where you sit in an organisation's hierarchy, you may find it beneficial to engage with a mentor or coach. This relationship is all about you—problems at work, underlying issues such as anger or lack of assertiveness that impact how you operate in the workplace and (importantly) how to get where you are going, activities to prioritise, networks to engage in, and areas taking too much of your time and providing limited return.

Mentors provide a wise and objective perspective on how to improve your situation, whether that's by promotion or by increasing your sense of satisfaction with the workplace. They are useful sources of support regarding specific concerns and in maintaining a perspective on 'what matters', in terms of your current role and your career path.

Specific issues may also be addressed through coaching. This will involve working with someone who has capacity in the area you wish to address, so you can develop skills through practical experience. Examples include becoming familiar with new software and observing group facilitation. These situations provide a useful way for staff to take on unaccustomed roles as teachers and learners; attending to an identified need with immediate benefits for individuals and the organisation.

Performance appraisal
Formal, systematic review of staff performance by employee and their manager; has bearings on decisions about staff development and career direction.

Staff appraisal and review

Performance appraisal is a systematic approach by which a manager reviews staff performance and provides feedback, leading to decisions about further development and career direction. Although supervision and feedback occur continually, having a formal process is important as it allows both manager and employee to reflect on the employee's performance, training needs and areas for development. Randhwa (2007, p.130) describes performance appraisal as involving:

- The periodic, formal evaluation of employee performance to inform career decisions.
- A formal, structured system to discover how and why the employee is currently performing and how performance can be improved to benefit the organisation and individual.
- Identifying, measuring and managing human performance in the organisation.

Performance appraisal works better if the job is well defined and understood by both employee and manager. This includes a detailed job description that addresses tasks, outputs and organisational context (how the position relates to others in the organisation). Regular supervision involves informal discussion on tasks and productivity related to the job description, and formal performance appraisal should be a natural development from this series of discussions. Having a written record is essential, and many organisations have standard templates. The record is a valuable summary of performance plans, achievements and directions—and it provides a useful point of reference when reflecting on progress and barriers encountered.

Weinbach and Taylor (2011, pp.228–32) describe elements of a 'fair' performance appraisal, which illustrate how the manager needs to operate for the benefit of the staff member and the organisation:

- Use previously understood criteria.
- Avoid comparisons with other staff.
- Provide an honest assessment of staff performance.
- Apply realistic expectations that are based on the staff member's experience and position.
- Account for problems in the work environment that have impacted on the staff member's ability to do their job effectively.
- Use appropriate criteria, including set items (such as quotas on service delivery or products delivered) in combination with subjective assessments of quality and attributes of the staff member's conduct (for example, collegiality, professionalism).

There is some variation in the extent to which performance appraisal is connected with processes about salary increases and staff promotion. There is some association between the two, but if performance appraisal is dominated by decisions about salary rates this may constrain the honesty and thoroughness of the approach. Some organisations separate incremental salary increases from performance appraisal and there may be a separate approach to promotions that is linked to a review of organisational structures. You may be able to appreciate the need to separate these processes in terms of the different objectives involved.

Discipline, incompetence and dismissal

As a manager, you may encounter employment challenges that range from underperformance to unprofessional behaviour. Extreme behaviours, such as breaching codes of conduct and ethics and criminal activities, require drastic action, and in these cases you are likely to work with other senior staff in the organisation to reach a quick and appropriate resolution. Our focus here is on more moderate situations; instances where staff are not fulfilling requirements of their position and management needs to take action.

Brody (2005) describes a number of situations where staff exhibit attitudes that are not helpful for them or the workplace. This may involve:

- Someone with no opportunities for promotion, who feels 'stuck' in their position, prompting dissatisfaction and a lack of motivation to perform.
- An employee who misses out on an internal promotion and experiences a sense of frustration and of being under-valued by colleagues and seniors.
- Someone who is risk averse, and new challenges cause high levels of anxiety and procrastination.
- A situation where there is a poor fit between an employee and requirements of the role. This can arise when the recruitment process sets up a particular expectation of staff capacity or when the role changes and a current employee does not 'keep up' with what is required.
- Someone who manipulates others to obtain standing in the workplace, for example by establishing cliques and pitting employees against one another or by being difficult to engage with—meaning little work comes their way.
- A new staff member, who is not familiar with expectations of the organisation and is generally unresponsive to work requests.
- Staff without a full understanding of their responsibilities and what is required to complete their work at a satisfactory level.

These challenges need careful attention, to achieve resolution by prompting positive changes in staff conduct or, where this does not occur, steps leading to staff dismissal. First, it is important to understand what is happening. This involves one or more conversations with the employee—perhaps as part of, or in addition to, regular supervision—where they are made aware of the concerns and expectations. Talking about actions the staff member can take to remedy the situation will provide a platform for change and the scope to monitor improvement. If the situation continues, the staff member may be issued with a number of written warnings that provide a factual description of the concerns, suggested actions and lack of progress. It is important to establish a record of these concerns early in the process, as a point of reflection and to enable disciplinary action, including termination, if this is required.

Management need to work with the employee to identify strategies that will bring their performance up to standard. This may include training, reclassification to a role with lower expectations, or the better articulation of what is required—including measures for performance monitoring. During this process of change, it is important to recognise the efforts and improvements made by the employee, operating in a professional and respectful manner throughout. However, if positive change does not result, management are duty bound to resolve the situation by taking stronger action. It is not feasible to retain a staff member who is not doing their job.

By way of summary, the following steps may be required:

1   Explain your concerns and your expectations. Identify and account for any mitigating factors. Establish a structure by which you can provide clear feedback on the staff member's performance, and gain agreement on the process.

2   If the situation does not improve, provide a verbal warning to the employee that your expectations are not being met and specify what is required.

3   One or more written warnings may subsequently be issued (possibly involving HR), which detail expectations of the role and how the employee is operating. It is important to focus on factual examples and to be accurate and neutral in your account of what has occurred.

4   The final step involves termination, where the staff member is asked to leave the organisation.

Throughout this process, it is important that you receive advice and support. Your organisation should have appropriate policies and procedures. You may need to debrief, in a confidential and non-judgmental environment. If the situation escalates you will probably experience considerable stress—both from actions of the staff member and the time needed to implement disciplinary actions such as those outlined above. This means you need to utilise resources of the organisation, including advice from senior management and from HR, and support from trusted peers. You should not feel alone, or operate in isolation. Following an agreed, professionally oriented process that encourages staff improvement, but includes an appropriate response to staff that do not fulfil their role, will lead to effective resolution of the situation.

The practitioner profile below is a valuable illustration of the many roles involved in being a senior manager at a busy health service. As you read the profile, try to identify points that are consistent with our consideration of workforce support and development.

Linkage

Having up-to-date and practice relevant policies will be invaluable if you need to deal with staff incompetence. You may wish to re-read the section in Chapter 3, on organisational policies.

PRACTITIONER PROFILE 5.2

CHERYL SOBCZYK

GENERAL MANAGER, PRIMARY HEALTH AND INTEGRATED CARE, BENDIGO COMMUNITY HEALTH

Position

The community health service includes community medical practices, nursing services, allied health and chronic disease management as well as a broad range of alcohol and drug services. Within my branch there are more than twenty funding streams and a workforce in excess of sixty staff, across five sites. My key portfolio areas as part of the executive team include service coordination and clinical governance. I am currently also managing the local super clinic as part of a management contract reporting to a board of directors.

Typical day

I commence the day checking my calendar of meetings and appointments combined with travel time between sites if required. I have access to a personal assistant three days per week and rely on her to manage my diary and prepare necessary papers and information. We check in as early as practical on her first day to prioritise invitations and organise rescheduling

(continued)

of appointments as required. At the end of the day, typically around 6pm I always review the next day to ensure I am prepared for the morning's appointments.

I typically attend meetings in Melbourne and routinely take the train. That enables me to spend two to three hours responding to emails and delegating work to my managers and assistants as needed.

Challenges

The primary challenge is finding the balance of commitment to meetings and appointments with adequate time to do the work! The ability to structure the day to reduce the need for appointments at different sites saves time, although travel periods are often useful to undertake voice-activated phone calls from the car.

One of the biggest issues when covering a broad range of services and organisational responsibilities is the large volume of communications that flood my email inbox. It requires discipline not to get bogged down responding to email at the expense of fulfilling other critical work.

Skills and qualities

- Advanced knowledge of policy and practice as it relates to key areas of responsibility. Capacity to critically analyse, think conceptually and provide leadership to inform planning, innovation and enterprise.
- Strong interpersonal and communication skills (written and verbal) that build and maintain relationships. Substantive human resource management as it relates to recruitment and performance management.
- Application of finance and business planning skills, including the ability to delegate responsibility appropriately.
- A passion for promoting community and organisational health and well-being, displaying values and promotion of a culture inclusive of integrity, respect, learning and innovation, environment and accountability.

Lessons learnt

The most challenging area has been learning the skills to manage poor performance and/or having to implement disciplinary action. Although I had learnt the basic theory and practice approaches to manage these issues it was not until I have had to put actions in place that I have learnt from and improved in my approach.

Staff conditions

Staff conditions
Normally founded on basic conditions set by government, and augmented with conditions put forward by professional associations. Conditions are set through negotiations between employers and staff representatives.

Staff conditions include salary rates, leave entitlements and so on. They are normally set through detailed negotiations between staff groups and employers, with input from government on basic conditions, as well as standards established by professional associations. The industrial landscape in Australia has changed considerably in recent decades and this is evident in the level of complexity and uncertainty surrounding workplace conditions.

Government as employer

Across many Western countries, major change in industrial legislation has occurred in recent decades, as governments strive to contain workforce costs and boost flexibility. In Australia, governments fund public services to such an extent that they are effectively a major employer, with a level of authority to shape workplaces according to their own agenda. They control the policy framework and can 'steer' organisations as they wish. With a political imperative to reduce taxation and demonstrate service efficiencies, workplace reform is considered important.

The introduction of enterprise bargaining in the 1980s and workplace bargaining in the following decade are both attempts to decentralise processes by which conditions are defined. This effectively means that employers have greater capacity to negotiate salary and leave conditions (for example), while employees will naturally strive to maintain (and possibly improve) their conditions.

Industrial organisations

As we explored earlier in this chapter, health and human service organisations involve a wide range of professions, from social workers to psychologists, and including medical doctors and administrative staff. These people have access to **industrial organisations**, which can be a group of employees/employers, a trade union, or any other group established for people based on a particular industry, trade, profession or employment (Office of the Anti-Discrimination Commissioner Tasmania, undated). Industrial organisations play a significant role for managers and workers; they provide a benchmark for workplace conditions and play a substantial role in negotiations.

Unions comprise workers who choose to be part of an industrial group that works to promote and preserve their workplace conditions. These unions generally have paid staff that provide advice and support for their members, and representatives that play an intermediary role during workplace negotiations. Some unions have large memberships, substantial resources and 'an established and influential role in organisational decision-making' (Jones & May, 1992, p.291). At best, workplaces and unions negotiate to reach a balance between the industrial rights of workers and organisational needs.

Negotiating conditions

We would expect that cost containment and service improvement are common goals of funders and providers; but there have been substantial concerns about the mechanisms used by funders to achieve change in this area. Outsourcing is one way to curtail labour costs—changing the composition of the workforce so lower wages and conditions are possible. The possibility of outsourcing may increase job insecurity, driving employees to comply with sub-standard conditions. The compromise position is one where conditions are acceptable to employees while also supporting the financial viability of the organisation. As you can imagine, this can be difficult to achieve and, when there is a decentralised approach to workplace negotiations, it falls to employers to value staff skills

Industrial organisation
A group of employees and employers, a trade union, or any other group established for people who work in a particular industry, trade or profession.

Unions
Organisations that represent their worker-members, and aim to preserve or improve workplace conditions. Union staff play an intermediary role during workplace negotiations and provide general advice and support for their members.

when considering industrial conditions. Therefore, industrial organisations have a key role in the negotiation of workplace agreements.

Donovan and Jackson (1991) explain that discriminatory practices in areas including recruitment, opposition to unionisation, attempts to destabilise the workforce, and classification of positions in a highly restricted and authoritarian/bureaucratic way, are examples of concerns about efficiency rather than effectiveness. Managers must find a balance between these joint challenges, so the organisation is viable and has the necessary staff to provide a service that is useful to the community. This will be advanced by workplace conditions that value and recognise the quality and extent of staff contribution within a rational approach to financial management.

Linkage
We explore financial management further in Chapter 8.

In 2010, the Council of Australian Governments established a Commonwealth statutory authority to deliver a national, coordinated approach to health workforce reform. This authority, Health Workforce Australia (HWA), aims to 'address the challenges of providing a skilled, flexible and innovative health workforce that meets the needs of the Australian community'. You may choose to learn more about the objectives, work plan and achievements of the authority by accessing the HWA website, which is included in the readings for this chapter.

SUMMARY OF KEY ISSUES

The workforce in health and human services is expanding. Much of the workforce is female and a substantial proportion is aged fifty-five years or older. Workers earn less, on average, than people in other industries. Addressing the workforce shortfall involves training, bringing in qualified workers from other countries, and strategies for staff retention and re-entry.

Sound processes for staff recruitment, selection, induction and performance review are useful for both managers and workers. Supervision, mentoring and coaching can assist with career development and staff retention while disciplinary procedures require an objective approach to resolve concerns while maintaining a respectful orientation toward both worker and organisation. Staff conditions are detailed in workplace agreements and impacted by conditions attached to membership of professional associations. These mechanisms are an important foundation in the determination of workplace conditions.

PRACTICE ACTIVITIES

1 The workforce

The information in this chapter shows there is considerable variation in the professions that make up the workforce. You are encouraged to read further, on particular professions or areas of work that may be of interest to you. Please refer to Healy and Lonne (2010, in the list of readings) who describe qualifications and characteristics of the workforce. Take a moment to reflect on what is happening in your industry.

2 Volunteers

Explore volunteer activity in your workplace or in an organisation with which you have some connection. First, seek out the volunteer coordinator (if there is one) and learn about policies and practices in the area. Then, talk to one or more volunteers about their motivation for being involved and their experience as a volunteer.

3   Interviews

Talk to five of your colleagues about their most recent recruitment interview. What worked and how could the experience be improved?

4   Industrial organisations

Read about the vision and principles of an industrial organisation that is relevant to your current or planned occupation. What are your conclusions about the organisation?

FURTHER READING

Volunteers in the workplace

This site has resources for volunteer programs and information on training and development:
www.volunteeringaustralia.org

Supervision

Coulshed, V., Mullender, A., Jones, D. N. & Thompson, N. (2006). Chapter 6, 'The Human Resource: Meeting the Needs of Staff', in *Management in Social Work*, (3rd edn), New York: Palgrave Macmillan, pp.161–91.

The social work and human services workforce

Healy, K. & Lonne, B. (2010). Chapter 5, 'Qualifications and Characteristics of the Workforce', in *The Social Work and Human Services Workforce: Report from a National Study of Education, Training and Workforce Needs,* Strawberry Hills, NSW: Australian Learning and Teaching Council.

Health Workforce Australia

Australian Government (2012). 'Information on a National, Co-ordinated Approach to Healthcare Reform', www.hwa.gov.au

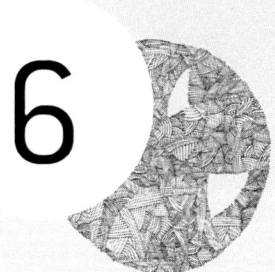

6

Strategic Planning for Practice

OVERVIEW

This chapter will:

- explore planning frameworks and processes appropriate for health and human services
- detail a strategic planning process
- describe a variety of planning tools
- discuss planning models, including emergent and participatory approaches.

In this chapter we look at the planning frameworks that shape and determine organisational direction, growth and success. Practical directions are offered for undertaking a comprehensive strategic planning process.

KEY TERMS

action plan

business plan

business profile

emergent planning

operational plan

participatory planning

program plan

project plan

strategic plan

Planning

Planning in health and human service organisations occurs at various levels, in numerous forms and is conducted by a range of people. Plans are incorporated at the client level, in action and individual program plans and case reviews; at the staffing level, in career development plans and performance appraisals; at the community level, in engagement strategies, collaborative planning and public forums; and at the organisational level in strategic, program and project plans, agency reviews and evaluations. Planning and evaluation are endemic to all forms of work in the health and human services sectors, and aspects of planning are encountered in each working day.

REFLECTION EXERCISE

Take a moment to reflect on your last encounter with a 'plan' at work. Who or what did the plan relate to? What kind of plan was it? Were you involved in developing the plan? If not, who was? What was your relationship to the plan? What was the purpose of the plan? Was the plan written or was it verbally expounded by an inspired colleague, or perhaps yourself?

Although we are engaged in planning and assessment processes in some form or another on a daily basis, many of us undertake limited training on how to develop, implement, monitor and evaluate plans for health and human services. It is often something consultants, CEOs, boards of governance, reluctant program managers and 'other people' do. And yet, one of the most powerful avenues for ensuring positive client outcomes, organisational success, and effecting change in an organisation, is through planning and review processes. Documented plans form an essential base for evaluation, accountability and quality control. Policies, both external and internal, are informed, developed, implemented and assessed through the various organisational planning processes. Importantly, when challenges and unexpected threats arise, plans provide a point of reference for checking whether or not actions have strayed from the intended path. At the same time, a plan can gauge how direction might be changed. Planning processes are fundamentally future focused and, as such, are effective mechanisms for bringing about organisational change.

Linkage
We further discuss the relationship between change and strategic planning in Chapter 9.

Responding effectively to a complex and challenging practice environment is not achieved with simplistic approaches. And yet, in order for organisations to function and operate successfully in a demanding and constantly changing climate, coherent, purposeful and manageable plans are required (Bryson, 2004). In this chapter we aim to articulate a participatory, user friendly *and* robust process that will be of practical use for developing organisational plans and translating them into action.

We begin our exploration of planning with the profile of Leanne Coupland who, as a director and member of the executive team in her organisation, shares responsibility for strategic and program planning and monitoring. Leanne refers to a consultative and participative approach, which involves developing plans 'backwards'. When you read Leanne's profile, reflect on what she means by this. How does this compare with the planning processes within your own organisation, or with which you are familiar?

PRACTITIONER PROFILE 6.1

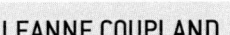

LEANNE COUPLAND

DIRECTOR—WORKFORCE AND PARTNERSHIPS, UNITING CARE GIPPSLAND

Background

Leanne is a qualified social worker who trained in the UK. Leanne spent several years working in generic children and family services teams, before moving to Victoria, Australia, in 2005. Leanne was recruited by the Department of Human Services and worked in Victoria's child protection system during a period of significant legislative change—Leanne worked closely with community service organisations to implement the required changes. Leanne now works for a community service organisation involved in the delivery of child, youth and family services. In addition, Leanne teaches undergraduates at a local university.

Current role

As a director with Uniting Care Gippsland, I am a member of the executive management team responsible for strategic direction and planning and operational oversight of agency programs and services, including supervision of field staff. The programs I am responsible for are primarily community development, and focus on vulnerable children and families. As an agency, we work across programs to harmonise services, therefore I am frequently involved in other areas of the agency, in particular our ChildFIRST and integrated family services teams. In addition to this I am also responsible for workforce issues, including staff health and well-being, work health, training and development, and student placements.

A typical day

Is made up of numerous things. Often there are meetings, both external and internal, team meetings, professionals meetings, case planning meetings, partnership meetings, internal planning meetings and the list goes on and on. Staff support is a huge component of my role and can involve supervision, support with a case, observed practice, consultation and discussion, or debriefing.

In addition to the above there are a range of administrative tasks that are required, such as reports to funders, legislative obligations, budget and finance reports, internal administration requirements.

Challenges

There are the obvious challenges in terms of funding and a lack of resources with which to support clients. The nature of short-term funding and therefore short-term contracts result in high staff turnover and the loss of good staff prior to the end of their contract and their program funding, as they attempt to find job security. The consequences are a disrupted service to clients and loss of program knowledge and continuity.

Partnerships and relationships with external agencies and/or service providers can at times be difficult to manage and time consuming.

Lessons learnt

I recall how as a beginning practitioner every decision I was required to make seemed to be urgent, or rather that was my perception. In hindsight, and with the benefit of practice wisdom, there are very few decisions that are truly urgent and which require an immediate response. The decision-making process is complex and often the extra time taken to consider the available options, debate a decision with a colleague and potentially identify suitable alternatives, is beneficial for all concerned. The decisions we make as practitioners, team leaders, managers and directors are significant and require our full time and attention in order to fully meet the needs of our clients.

A significant learning has been that I do not need to have the answer to everything, it is professionally acceptable to say, 'I don't know' or "I will need to consult with a colleague' or 'I will come back to you on that, I need to consider that further.'

Self-care is extremely important, if you want to provide the best possible outcomes for your clients, you need to provide the best possible care for yourself first.

Skills and qualities

The skills and qualities required are many and varied, the most obvious being organisational and communication skills. The diverse nature of both the role and the human services industry as a whole means you often need to switch between different tasks, jobs and roles. This requires sound organisational skills and the ability to communicate on numerous levels.

With regard to qualities, a high level of emotional intelligence is essential, again both in dealing with clients and services users, but also in interactions with other professionals, service providers, funders, external partners and staff. The ability to look back and reflect on practice is also essential; this enables us to become better practitioners and recognise changes and developments in our own practice as well as how best to support other less-experienced practitioners.

The ability to see alternatives and be open to other ways of doing things is critical, as is knowing when to ask for help and support, without perceiving it as a weakness or a failure on your part.

Planning approach at Uniting Care Gippsland

As an agency our planning processes are potentially a little different to the norm—two of our seven principles are consultation and participation. Therefore, in developing agency plans, including our strategic plan, we consult broadly with agency members (staff, volunteers and students) clients, service users and communities. We work from an outcomes-based planning platform: having done initial consultation regarding what is required, we work backwards from what the result should be.

Organisational plans

There are so many different plans in an organisation, it can be confusing to know which type of plan you are dealing with at a given time. Also, once immersed in a planning exercise you very quickly realise that there are plans within plans within plans!

REFLECTION EXERCISE

Think about Leanne's profile. How many situations in a typical day can you identify where Leanne might be required to work with a plan of some kind? Is it likely that these plans would interconnect in some way? How?

Leanne's reflection on her daily workload makes it evident that she does not have a lot of time to sit around drawing up complex and complicated plans, and yet she works for an organisation that places high importance on planning, and values consultation and participation in its planning processes. According to Mike Hudson, planning documents at every organisational level should contain objectives, performance measures, priorities and implementation time frames that are 'set out on as few sheets of paper as possible' (Hudson, 2009, p.148).

As we identified in Chapter 4, a key function of management is planning, and competency in the various dimensions of planning is essential for success at organisational, group and individual levels. As Hudson cautions, being able to keep plans manageable is also an important skill to develop. For managers and workers who are not located at the executive level, it can feel like an organisation is populated by an endlessly expanding web of plans that do not seem to have a lot to do with day-to-day practice. This sense is likely to be an outcome of cloudy definitions, confusion about purpose, lack of ownership caused by low participation in development, poor communication and, most significantly, neglect of plans once they are developed. Understanding the different types of plans, and what they are used for, can be a helpful place to begin.

Types of plans: Strategic, business, operational and program

Strategic, operational, program, project, business and action plans are terms that you have no doubt encountered. But how do they sit in relation to one another? Figure 6.1, opposite, offers a simplified illustration of the relationship between various organisational plans.

Strategic plan

Strategic plan
An organisation's blueprint for future operations over a defined period of time.

In general there is one overall **strategic plan**, which informs all other planning processes throughout the organisation. The strategic plan establishes the 'base' position of the organisation; it is the blueprint for operations for a defined period of time in the future. Even though the strategic plan defines the client group, the services that are offered and the distribution of resources, strategy is still required at divisional and program levels (Hudson, 2009).

The strategic plan is an overarching, 'high end' map, which:
- usually spans three to five years
- defines the organisation and articulates values and purpose, mission and vision
- identifies the current organisational position in relation to external *and* internal environments
- determines direction and duration—what the organisation aims to achieve in a defined future period
- identifies strategies for achieving goals and objectives
- prescribes how it will know when and whether it has achieved its aims
- identifies who will be responsible for actions arising from the plan.

FIGURE 6.1 Hierarchy of organisational plans and functions

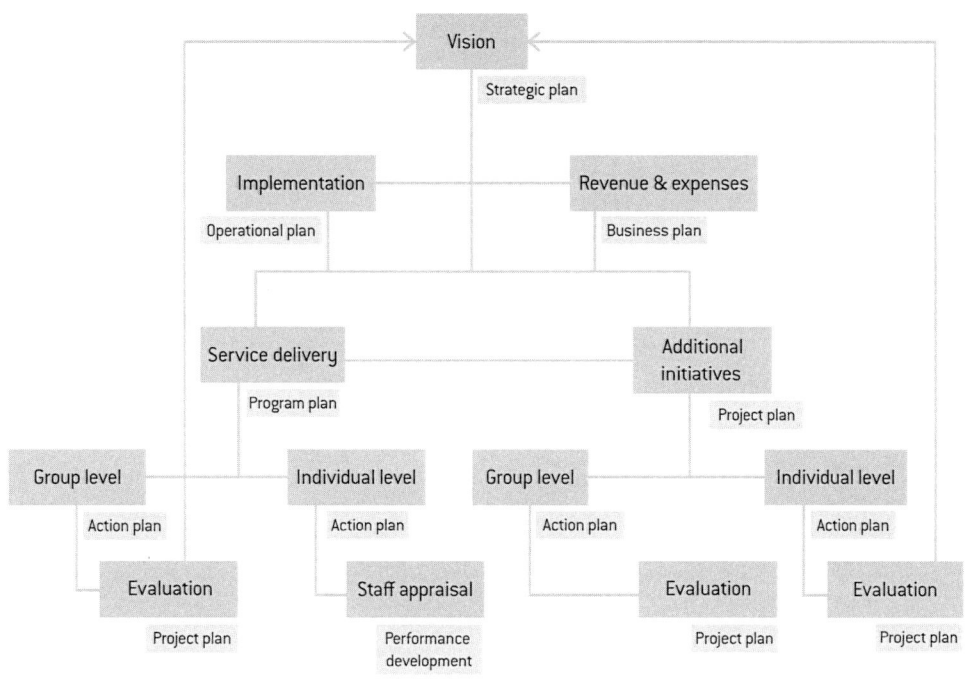

While senior executives and the board often develop strategic plans at the governance level, in order for the plan to be relevant and effective, all key stakeholders must be engaged and have the opportunity to participate and contribute. It is essential that they are clear about their position in the plan, and that they are able to taking some level of responsibility for implementation (Anheier, 2005). A useful method for engaging stakeholders and formalising their involvement is to use action plans.

Operational plan

Each phase of a strategic plan requires an **operational plan** that provides the details for enabling implementation. It outlines objectives and strategies for achieving milestones, identifies key indicators, justifies the budget on an annual basis and draws links between the strategic plan and organisational activities. In other words, it articulates how the strategic plan will become operational (Hudson, 2009).

The operational plan:
- flows from the strategic plan
- spans one year
- specifies day-to-day activities
- sets out what will be done
- identifies who will do what
- articulates benefits to the client group
- defines quality standards and key measures
- includes the implementation timetable
- details the budget.

Linkage
Action plans are discussed in more detail later in this chapter, together with the other types of plans arising from the strategic planning process.

Operational plan
A sub-set of the strategic plan that is focused at the individual program or project level.

Operational plans are usually prepared by service-level managers, in consultation with key stakeholders, and should be short, easy-to-read documents. They are often presented in a one-page table format (Hudson, 2009).

Program plan

A program is 'a set of planned activities directed toward bringing about specified change(s) in an identified and identifiable audience' (Smith, 1989, cited in Owen, 2006, p.26). A program is, in itself, a type of plan and a planning tool, and can be described as 'a complex system … a more or less self-contained package with its own goals, objectives, policies, procedures, and rules, and usually its own budget' (Weinbach & Taylor, 2011, p.307).

Program plans result from, and form part of, wider organisational planning processes, such as strategic and operational plans. A program can be identified by the inclusion of at least two key components: 'planning' and 'action' (Owen, 2006). A program plan is a design for the provision of a service that will meet client needs, in accordance with the strategic directions of the organisation. It is a unique future-focused assemblage of procedures and strategies which, in combination, have the purpose of achieving particular goals and objectives (Weinbach & Taylor, 2011).

A **program plan** is usually prepared by the program manager in consultation with management at the next level up, the work group and other key stakeholders.

A program plan:

- is informed by strategic and operational plans
- outlines the goals, strategies, implementation process, resourcing and evaluation methods for a particular service
- usually covers the duration of a particular program according to the funding cycle
- identifies the group of people for whom the program is to be delivered
- specifies the rationale for the provision of a particular service delivery approach
- details the process for delivering the program
- articulates how the program will be resourced
- describes how the program will be evaluated
- forms the basis for formative and summative evaluation.

Project plan

A **project plan** includes the same key features as a program plan, but for an event or activity that is not part of the organisation's ongoing service delivery program (Lewis et al., 2012). A project plan may be developed for a pilot or trial to test a new approach, or it may be related to an evaluation or other piece of research.

Project plans:

- aim to value-add to existing operations
- are not necessarily directly linked with programs arising from the strategic plan
- can arise from events that were unanticipated when the strategic plan was being developed
- are usually developed for one-off events

Program plan
A sequence of strategies, tasks and resources organised into a coherent framework designed to attain a shared goal; the key elements in this process are 'planning' and 'action'.

Project plan
Similar to a program plan, except it's for a specific project. The plan provides a detailed account of the project's aims, objectives, background, activities, stakeholders, resource implications and timeline.

Linkage
Project planning is discussed in detail when we look at project management and evaluation in Chapter 7.

- are time limited
- are often connected with evaluation or some form of trial.

Business plan

A **business plan** anticipates and details the financial resources and expenses required for implementing programs and projects. It examines the current financial situation of the organisation and uses this information to forecast performance over a defined period of time. Hudson (2009) observes that business planning involves a detailed analysis of the organisation's financial position in relation to the resources required to meet strategic objectives, fund programs and deliver services. The process of business planning often combines strategic and operational planning. A participatory process is not usually considered appropriate for the development of business plans, which are formed by upper-level executives in consultation with the organisation's financial managers.

A business plan:

- details the financial resources required for the organisational activities generated by the strategic plan
- combines elements of strategic and operational planning
- is developed at executive and governance levels
- is less dependent on consultative and participatory processes
- forecasts financial performance over a defined period of time.

Business plan
Examines the financial situation of the organisation, anticipating the financial resources required to implement the strategic plan and using this to forecast performance over a defined period.

Action plan

An **action plan** is generated and utilised at the group or individual level. But this does not mean that the action plan is insignificant. Action plans specify those responsible for achieving the actions relating to tasks within a program, project or operational plan. It is at this level that the strategic plan becomes concrete and is translated into practice.

The failure of strategic plans to achieve stated goals often stems from the lack of translating plans into actions. This can be attributed to oversight of the need to identify actions, assign responsibility and monitor progress. It is becoming common practice in many organisations for progress against actions or tasks to be regularly reported on at monitoring meetings. Action planning and monitoring is essential to linking strategy with practice. An action plan needs to be specific, and brief. As we mentioned earlier, a one-page table format provides a workable document (Hudson, 2009).

An action plan:

- is generated at the work group and individual levels
- identifies essential tasks, or actions for achieving goals and objectives
- details who is responsible for specific tasks
- provides a framework for monitoring progress in implementation of the plan
- links strategy to practice.

Action plan
Details of the specific tasks required to translate objectives into actions, generated and acted upon by teams and/or individuals at practice level.

As you can see, there are many types of plans. Plans are nested within other plans; they constitute large, complex, detailed documents (developed over long periods of time, by whole teams), and brief, simple, single goal documents (developed on the run by individuals and work teams). The multitude of plan types is matched by an equal number of planning approaches. Even though planning is a core management function, it has no good purpose in a health or human service organisation unless it ultimately results in positive outcomes for the client group.

Embarking on a planning process

Because plans constitute the methods, systems and processes that drive an organisation forward, it is advisable to ask before engaging in any planning exercise: *why* the organisation is undertaking the particular planning exercise, *what* and *who* the plan is for, and *how* key players will be involved.

Identifying and involving key stakeholders

Identifying key stakeholders and inviting their participation from the early stages of planning ensures plans are relevant and well informed (Bryson, 2004). Stakeholders are individuals and groups, internal and external to the organisation, with an identified interest in the outcomes of the particular plan. This might include, but is not limited to, funders, clients, workers and partner organisations.

No matter what type of plan, or its purpose, in organisational settings planning is not an isolated, individual exercise. The purpose of an action plan might be to guide a worker's career progression, but even though the negotiators are limited to the worker and their supervisor, the organisation itself is also a stakeholder. As such, the plan is prepared and monitored with reference to other tiers of organisational planning, through a consultative process.

Linkage
We further explore the importance of stakeholder engagement in Chapter 7, when discussing project management, and again in Chapter 9, when looking at managing change.

REFLECTION EXERCISE

Refer back to Leanne's description of the planning process in her organisation. How many and who are the stakeholders that she identifies?

Now think about a recent planning process in an organisation that you are involved with. Who were the key stakeholders, and how were they involved in the planning process?

Thinking beyond supervisors and managers is one way of ensuring participation across various levels and sites. A framework using micro, mezzo and macro levels can be helpful for making this assessment; these are outlined in Table 6.1.

TABLE 6.1 Levels in the organisational environment

MICRO	MEZZO	MACRO
Internal to organisation—'coalface'	Interface between internal and external environment	External to organisation
• clients	• the organisation	• governments
• workers	• managers	• funders
• programs within the organisation	• boards of management	• policy makers
	• partnership organisations	• communities
		• the public

The number of key stakeholders can become unworkable, so it is helpful to contain the list to those directly affected by the plan, and who may be able to represent a number of interested parties. Once the various stakeholders are identified, a decision needs to be made about degree of involvement: do they need to be included on the planning working party, or might it be more appropriate to inform and/or separately consult with them? This decision may be based on a number of factors:

- Specialist knowledge—whether they can offer insight into issues and problems that may not be immediately evident to others.
- Their experience and skills.
- Whether they will be directly impacted by the outcomes.
- Their willingness to participate.
- Their ability to contribute.
- Their capacity to participate.

The choice should not in any way be approached as an opportunity to exclude key stakeholders, but it is wise to select representatives for a working party who are able to contribute meaningfully to the planning process. There is no point in having token members on a planning group; everyone needs to have a role and areas of responsibility. If a stakeholder group is not included, other opportunities for participation should be identified.

As we have established, the strategic plan provides the framework and reference point for all other planning activities in an organisation, cascading to programs and service delivery areas (see Figure 6.1). We are now going to work through stages in a strategic planning process that aims to be inclusive, participatory and practical.

Linkage
The selection of stakeholders is discussed further in Chapter 7 when exploring project management.

The strategic planning process

Strategic planning arrived as an organisational management tool in health and human services with the introduction of managerialism. Although it's now widely accepted as a planning and change management practice, its corporate heritage still causes wariness amongst some about its real purpose and value. Even so, various frameworks based on the vast literature developed in the business sector have been adapted for application in human service organisations (Weinbach & Taylor, 2011); a list of examples can be found in the reading list at the end of this chapter. These models invariably establish a linear process with a number of common stages that utilise specific analysis tools:

1 Establish a planning process.
2 Identify key stakeholders and engage key personnel.
3 Define the organisation: clarify values, mission and core work.
4 Assess the external environment.
5 Analyse organisation in context and identify strategic issues.
6 Formulate desired future directions and strategies for their achievement.
7 Develop implementation, monitoring and evaluation processes.

Table 6.2, overleaf, elaborates on these stages by including actions and potential information-gathering methods. The addition, inclusion and/or exclusion of stages is often

Linkage
We address stages 1–5, as well as actions plans, in this chapter. The key elements of stages 6–8, including logic models and Gantt charts, are addressed in Chapter 7.

TABLE 6.2 Stages of strategic planning

STAGE		ACTIONS	POTENTIAL METHODS AND TOOLS
1	Establish planning process	Identify and engage key stakeholders	Stakeholder analysis
2	Define the organisation	Clarify values, purpose and vision	Communicate and consult across all organisational levels
3	Assess external environment	Map external environment	SPELT analysis
4	Analyse organisation in context	Assess organisation in its context Identify strategic issues	Business profile SWOC analysis
5	Formulate goals and directions	Identify objectives and strategies	Logic model
6	Develop implementation: operational/business/action plans	Engage staff across all organisational levels	Gantt chart Planning tools
7	Implement plan	Communicate and consult with stakeholders and key actors	Communication strategies: launches, bulletins, promotional materials, etc
8	Monitor and evaluate	Develop evaluation, monitoring and accountability frameworks	Monitoring and evaluation tools Stakeholder analysis Logic model Gantt chart

dependent on the size and complexity of the organisation and the context in which it is operating, as too is the choice of method for informing the planning process. Whatever process is selected, it needs to define the organisation, shape its identity and establish a pathway forward.

Before describing these key stages in the process, and tools that are commonly utilised in strategic planning, we present the following description, drawn from our case study research. It offers insight into a community health organisation's planning approach.

PRACTICE EXAMPLE 6.1

Planning process

Our 'quality and risk management' manager is responsible for coordinating planning. Basically, planning is connected to our quality-improvement working committee. The job of the working committee is to evaluate the planning processes that have occurred in the organisation for the previous twelve months and to make any changes. In actual fact, there are some changes that came out in the last two weeks. A new pro-forma has been developed that's just been released to simplify the planning process and to ensure that we have a higher level of compliance, because I have to acknowledge that despite being one and the same organisation, we don't have quite the compliance that we would like. We always want 100%, but it's not always there.

Developing the next strategic plan usually involves a retreat for the board of governance. They decide our priorities for the next three years. The plan then comes back and it's communicated down to the exec level and then it just goes down and down from there. So that's the organisational priorities taken care of.

In terms of the individual program priorities, we have a meeting to discuss those and include them as part of our overall document, but we also decide some of the key issues for us as a local provider, and we incorporate them in our planning process. That involves team meetings, and half- or full-day planning, sometimes both. We then have a full day of planning and decide what our key issues are, and then we come back three months later for an in-house planning day to see how that's going.

REFLECTION EXERCISE

Consider how the above description compares with the planning process described by Leanne Coupland.

What are some of the challenges for organisational planning that are revealed in this description?

How does this compare with the organisation where you are employed, or one with which you are familiar?

Establishing the planning process

Preparation at the front end can allay problems that might otherwise arise further down the track, when there is the risk of much hard work being undone as a result of oversight of a key factor. For the planning process to successfully proceed, a number of conditions must be met.

1   A sound rationale for undertaking the process.
2   Representation by a range of key stakeholders from governance board to clients.
3   Competent leadership and management within the organisation.
4   Commitment and sponsorship from all key decision-makers to develop, implement and monitor the plan.
5   Preparedness to engage with change.
6   Allowance for an adequate time frame.
7   Absence of organisational crisis and relative stability in senior management.
8   An effective communication strategy to ensure all stakeholders are kept informed throughout the process.

Source: Brody, 2005; Bryson, 2004; Hudson, 2009

As articulated in Practice example 6.1, many organisations approach strategic planning as the domain of senior management at the executive level. Whilst strategic planning is a governance function and responsibility, let us impress again that this should not override participation of representatives from all levels, including clients (Brody, 2005).

It is important to remain mindful, however, that 'whilst much work is done jointly, management is usually responsible for proposing the strategy and the board is always responsible for approving it' (Hudson, 2009, p.161).

Having identified key stakeholders and formed the planning team, the next step is to nominate a facilitator to lead the process. To enable an objective process and full participation by all stakeholders, this is often a role performed by an external consultant—this decision being determined by the size of the organisation and available resources. The team then needs to take care of 'housekeeping', such as:

- deciding roles and responsibilities
- establishing a time frame with milestones
- setting session dates
- identifying required resources
- specifying the planning approach and related tasks.

Defining the organisation

With all players in place, the first task of developing the strategic plan is to review and re-evaluate the organisation's purpose, values, goals and overall vision. This stage, often conducted away from the worksite as a retreat, performs a number of important functions. It brings the group together around the task at hand, and establishes a shared purpose. It is also an opportunity to 'take stock' of the current state of the organisation, and to assess the degree to which the goals of the previous strategic plan were achieved (assuming there was one). Collaborating on a shared vision for the future direction of the organisation is inspiring and motivating. This is particularly so for health and human service professionals, who have chosen their career because they want to improve people's lives, and contribute to a more just society (Lewis et al., 2012).

Vision

A vision statement is aspirational; it expresses an ideal future state of the organisation in terms of how its workers and other stakeholders want it to be identified. As an inspirational message, it is intended to motivate staff to strive towards its achievement.

Participatory planning
A process that involves various stakeholders in decision-making and the design and implementation of a plan.

A **participatory planning** process increases the likelihood of alignment with individual visions (Senge, cited in Lewis et al., 2012). In formulating the vision statement a key question is 'What is our ideal achievement?'

For example, the vision of Yoowinna Wurnalung Healing Service ('Our Safe Place'— Gunai/Kurnai language) is:

> To be a viable and accountable service that is responsive to our community's needs and works in partnership to create healthy, safe, prosperous and cultural communities.

Mission

A mission is a succinct statement of statement of role and purpose; it describes the work performed by the organisation, and as such focuses on the 'present and immediate future' (Austin & Solomon, 2009, p.326). In identifying the organisational mission, a key question is, 'Why does our organisation exist?'

For example, the mission of Yoowinna Wurnalung Healing Service is:

To provide a safe, cultural and spiritual environment, underpinned by the integration of Aboriginal teachings, to support and protect victims of family violence, and deliver specialised services for Indigenous men, women, youth and children that support the recovery and healing of Indigenous individuals, families and communities.

Source: Yoowinna Wurnalung Healing Service Strategic Business Plan

Values and guiding principles

Organisational values are concepts that express the principles and qualities of service delivery, which are upheld as standards for practice within the organisation.

These serve as guidelines for conduct, decision-making and program design. Values may be expressed as simply worded statements (as in the example provided in Chapter 3, from Parenting WA) or they may be articulated at some length. Some organisations list values only, some include guiding principles and values, while others only have guiding principles. A key question in identifying organisational values is, 'What are the qualities and attributes that guide our services and behaviours?'

For example, Yoowinna Wurnalung Healing Service has seventeen guiding principles, which include the following:

- All forms of family and community violence are unacceptable.
- We have a responsibility to show leadership in preventing violence.
- We are holistic, comprehensive, solution focused and client centred.
- We use a team-based and collaborative approach that respects the individual, their capacities and privacy.
- We act with integrity in our dealings with clients, government, our partners and with each other.
- We work well together and with our stakeholders in the common interests of justice.
- We are committed to ongoing professional development, evaluation and research, and strive to be a learning organisation that continues to improve all aspects of its business.

Source: Yoowinna Wurnalung Healing Service Strategic Business Plan, p.5

Vision, mission and value statements are often found on promotional materials, an organisation's website, and in annual reports and other official documents. Many organisations have them framed and displayed in the reception area. A criticism of these documents is that they can fade out of fashion, losing their currency in the fast pace of organisational life. A tired-looking vision, mission and values statement can communicate the antithesis of its intended meaning, as can an out-of-date website. If the organisation has a regular planning cycle, it is advisable to revisit these statements as concepts and guiding principles, as well as reviewing how and where they are communicated and displayed.

Analysing the external environment

For strategic planning to be of any value to an organisation and the clients and communities that it serves, it must be attentive to political trends and forces. These are identified by analysing the external environment. An environment analysis is informed

Linkage
We explored values at some length in Chapter 3, when we looked at organisational culture and ethics.

by the organisation's vision, mission and values, and asks what is necessary to know about the external context that will enable identification of issues and formulation of strategies towards achieving the organisation's goals (Eadie, 2006). A defining feature of an environmental analysis is that it examines issues that are beyond the control of the organisation. This process is also referred to as environmental scanning (Austin & Solomon, 2009; Gray et al., 2010).

A common approach to an external environment scan is to examine the 'political', 'economic', 'social/cultural' and 'technological' influences that affect the organisation, its client group and its services—commonly referred to as a PEST analysis (Lewis et al., 2012). Other frameworks include 'legal, or legislative' influences, resulting in the acronym SPELT (Field, 2010). Some add 'environmental', which produces the acronym PESTLE. We have adapted an approach based on the SPELT model proposed by Richard Field (2010). The analysis involves a number of steps:

1 Identify external environment influences on the organisation.
2 Map according to a 'current', 'medium term', 'long-term' time frame.
3 Identify the possible implications of each influence.
4 Assess the likelihood of occurrence according to a measure of low, medium or high.
5 Use analysis arising from the above steps to decide actions in relation to the influence: for example, consider further planning as a strategic priority, monitor or ignore.

Source: adapted from Field, 2010, p.128

Structuring the analysis of the identified SPELT factors according to a time frame can be useful for long-range strategic planning (three to five years). Classifying issues according to a time frame can also be very helpful for keeping the planning process focused on priorities and for scheduling strategic actions.

Table 6.3 maps influences on a (fictional) family support agency in a growth corridor on the western fringe of a capital city, according to a time frame (see steps 1 and 2 in the above list). Note that this table only maps one thread of external influence across the three time dimensions (current, medium and long term). In other words, in the first row demographic trends only are mapped. It is also important to note that an influential factor may impact in more than one area. For example, the introduction of DisabilityCare—National Disability Insurance Scheme will have, at the least, both economic and legislative consequences.

It is highly likely that a single brainstorm session on SPELT influences will produce dozens of influential factors. For example, in the above schema, for each of the five SPELT dimensions, three areas of influence have been identified. Even if each of these only produces one specific influential issue, there will be potentially fifteen requiring consideration. Therefore, it is necessary to identify the possible implications of each influence (step 3), assess the likelihood of their occurrence (step 4) and prioritise them for action in the strategic planning process (step 5).

The next step involves developing a business profile.

TABLE 6.3 SPELT analysis grid: Issues and time frame for a family support agency in a growth corridor area

AREAS OF INFLUENCE	CURRENT	MEDIUM TERM	LONG TERM
Socio-cultural: • Demographic trends • Attitudes to social justice and equity • Media	Influx of young families	Refugee youth settlement house establishment	Increased multicultural diversity
Political—government policies and priorities: • Local • State • Federal	Change in state government	Council elections	Federal election
Economic—resources: • Funding availability and processes • Accountability requirements • Global and local economy	DisabilityCare (NDIS) funds	Network agency partnerships	Funding consequences arising from change in state government and federal election
Legislative: • Federal and State Acts • Human rights charters • Legal compliance requirements	*Disability Act* *Children and Young Persons Act* *Equal Opportunity Act* *Family Law Act* Victorian Charter of Human Rights & Responsibilities NDIS		
Technological: • Information and communication systems • Reporting procedures • Data storage	Electronic data systems	National Broadband Scheme (NBS)	

Business profile

A **business profile** helps clarify the work that the organisation does and how it relates to its environment. It involves identifying:

- Clients: Who are you funded to provide services to? Who do you provide services to? Who accesses your services?
- Services: What work is actually done? What formal services (funded activities: roles and programs) do you provide? What informal services (unfunded activities: community engagement, guest speaking, media interviews) do you provide?
- Suppliers: Who are the businesses and organisations that supply goods and services, such as training, IT, accounting and other administrative support, catering, cleaning and printing services, that keep the organisation running?

Business profile
Develops a picture of the work of the organisation in relation to its environment by looking at clients, services, suppliers, partners and assets.

- Partners: Who are the organisations and services in your network that you depend on to deliver programs? Who do you have partnership agreements with? Who do you refer clients to?
- Assets: What tangible and intangible assets does the organisation have? Tangible assets include things that are owned, such as buildings, equipment, office furniture, information technology and library resources. Intangible assets can include the location of the organisation, goodwill and fundraising capabilities, staff morale, experience, expertise, and relationship with communities. It is important to understand your assets and to use these to overcome deficits.

If you have worked through these questions, and stages 1–3 (see Table 6.2) you will have developed a detailed picture of your organisation, and will be well prepared to complete the next step—the SWOC analysis.

SWOC analysis

SWOC is the acronym for strengths, weaknesses, opportunities and challenges. You may be more familiar with the term SWOT—in which 'threats' is substituted for 'challenges' (Lewis et al., 2012). Either way, this form of analysis is widely used for assessing how an organisation is positioned, and what might be needed for responding to factors in the external environment. It involves examining the things that an organisation does have some control over (internal weakness and strengths) in relation to those that it does not (external threats and opportunities).

Bryson (2004) observes that organisations often see challenges as threats rather than opportunities. Citing Weick and Sutcliffe he suggests that 'attending to challenges and weakness should be seen as an opportunity to build strengths and improve performance' (Weick & Sutcliffe, 2001, cited in Bryson, 2004, p.39). The table below illustrates the questions to be considered in each dimension of the SWOC analysis.

In some strategic planning approaches the external analysis component of the SWOC exercise—opportunities and challenges—is incorporated into the SPELT analysis and business profile described above (Allison & Kaye, 2005). Alternatively, in smaller scale strategic planning processes, for example in small agencies or where a strategic plan is being carried out by a program area or department within a larger organisation, the SWOC analysis alone can be sufficient. While a SWOC analysis can provide a useful

TABLE 6.4 Diagram for a SWOC analysis

	STRENGTHS	WEAKNESSES
Internal	What are the organisation's strengths?	What are the organisations weaknesses?
	What do we do well?	What are our areas for improvement?
	What resources and skills do we have?	What skills and resources are we lacking?
	OPPORTUNITIES	CHALLENGES
External	What are the opportunities that align with our vision, mission and values?	What might challenge or obstruct our aspirations?
	What challenges might we engage with?	What potential changes and/or risks do we need to be alert to?

focus in planning a brainstorming session, it is important to ensure that perceptions are measured against actuality, and that key stakeholders are consulted (Allison & Kaye, 2005).

Once the strategic issues are identified, it is time to determine future directions.

Formulating future goals and directions

To this point the analysis has developed a clear picture of the organisation and determined issues that *might* be addressed. Deciding what the organisation needs and wants to address or, perhaps more astutely, what it will not undertake, presents a major challenge in and of itself. According to Allison and Kaye (2005), this is when exploration turns to reality. It is also the point where a decision might be made about whether the planning strategy continues on a rational, linear, goal-driven path that assumes capacity to have some control and determination over future direction, or whether it diverges towards an emergent process. Ideally, elements of both will be incorporated. We take a brief detour here to consider what this alternative pathway might involve.

Emergent planning

Emergent planning involves working with opportunities and issues that emerge as a result of the complexity of the practice climate. The planning process is responsive, reflective, iterative and evaluative, incorporating factors that arise along the way. An emergent planning process does not seek to identify and fix goals and future directions, rather it relies on attentiveness to trends and arising issues in the organisation's environment, and responds to them innovatively and creatively.

With a well-developed appreciation of strengths and capacity, the emergent planning organisation fosters innovation and creativity, and encourages and rewards risk taking (even when an initiative 'fails'). Emergent approaches tend to be decentred, in that they recognise that collective efforts achieve greater results than those of individuals, and that all levels of an organisation have the capacity to lead the organisation in productive directions. Importantly, emergent planning attends to, and incorporates, relevant influences that arise in the course of the process. The concept of the learning organisation, introduced by Peter Senge in *The Fifth Discipline* (1992), exemplifies the organisational culture that fosters emergent processes.

Emergent planning is not simply making incremental changes in an ad hoc way; it aspires to innovation, and to being well prepared for responding to contingencies and risk taking. Emergent processes also involve drawing connections between aspects of the environment that may have previously been considered beyond the organisation's purview. For example, in Chapter 4 we read about a community health centre investing in a local nursery business as a training program for clients. While this may not be innovative for an organisation like the Salvation Army, which has a long history of establishing enterprises, these kinds of programs represent new fields for community health services.

Emergent planning models follow a similar process to the action planning cycle, which involves the 'plan, act, observe and reflect' spiral (Figure 6.2, overleaf). They also incorporate additional dynamism and openness to external factors, as illustrated in Figure 6.3.

Emergent planning
A 'ground-up' approach to planning that involves embracing opportunities and incorporating them into a planning cycle. The process is responsive, reflective, iterative, evaluative and inclusive.

FIGURE 6.2 Action planning spiral

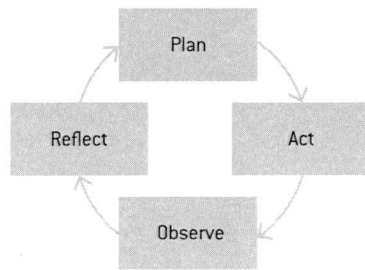

Source: Kemmis & McTaggart, 1988, p.11

Emergent planning promotes reflection and responsiveness rather than reaction. It is systematic and accountable, and requires acknowledgment of responsibilities and boundaries, and the need for monitoring and reporting—albeit in flexible ways. If an emergent planning direction is chosen, the 'strategic' planning process opens up at this point. Information is provided to resource work teams, opportunities for creative reflection are provided, and feedback processes are established.

If, on the other hand, the decision is to proceed with a goal-led approach, then strategic issues are identified, and these inform the desired future goals and directions of the organisation or program area.

FIGURE 6.3 Emergent planning spiral

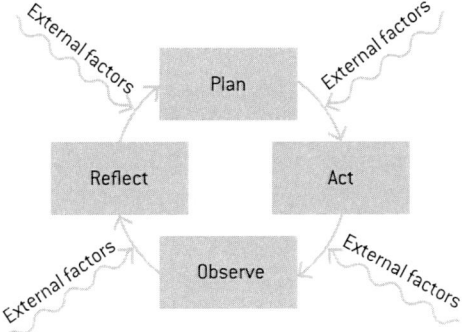

Developing organisational goals

At this point it is time for the planning team to sit back and review the information gathered about the organisation and its environment, and to make decisions about the strategic direction that it proposes to take in the next three to five years. All organisations have implicit strategies: get more funding, survive, deliver current services well, and so forth (Lewis et al., 2012). Lewis et al. observe that *strategic* planning is about carefully considering the actions that will move the organisation towards identified future directions, making them explicit and, therefore, more effective.

For each strategic issue that is selected, strategic goals are required. Goals are broad aims and strategies are the actions that will be taken to achieve the identified goals. Strategic goals are credible visions developed on the basis of identified strategic issues; they represent the main purpose of the organisation's mission. They are usually not measurable (Lewis et al., 2012) and are formed with reference to the vision, mission and values identified in Stage 2: *Defining the organisation* (see Table 6.2).

At the risk of labouring the point, we would like to reiterate that goals are only effective when they are shared and owned across the entire organisation. Strategic issues will ideally be discussed widely and openly, and input for the development of strategic goals will be sought from all work levels. Some examples of strategic goals for a (fictional) regional family support agency called Central Highlands Region Family Support Services (CHRFSS) might be:

1 To grow and expand its services in response to the population growth in the Central Highlands area.
2 To form a strategic partnership with the Central Highlands Community Health Service, with a view to jointly tendering for programs that reflect their shared interests and strengths.
3 To maintain a financially viable service over the next five years, with growth in program funding per annum.
4 To build and promote a learning organisation culture.
5 To be the organisation that most people in the Central Highlands first think of when asked to identify a key family support agency.

Once there is agreement about the organisation's strategic goals they must be translated into practice. This can be done in a variety of ways, depending on the organisational context. For large organisations, objectives may be developed at the executive level (always with consultation and input from stakeholders), or they might be devolved to programs.

Developing strategic objectives

Objectives are the measurable outcomes of the goals. So that they can be evaluated, they must be specific, measurable, achievable, realistic and time-framed (SMART). Objectives for achieving goal 1 above might be:

1 To establish a family violence prevention program by submitting a proposal to the next call for tender by the Department of Families and Communities to introduce early intervention programs in community organisations.
2 To jointly tender with the Community Health Service for at least one program suitable for co-delivery in the next twelve months.
3 To further explore the proposal to merge with the women's health service in this region over the next three months by conducting a feasibility study.
4 To initiate and conduct a community audit within the next twelve months to measure the changing demographic profile and emerging needs in the area.

These objectives are specific and measurable. Outputs are identified that can be realistically achieved, and they include time frames. Each one can be regularly monitored for progress, and evaluated at the end of the strategic planning cycle.

Linkage
We further discuss goals and objectives in relation to project management in Chapter 7.

The objectives, however, are not specific enough to ensure that action will take place. As discussed above, goals and objectives are only meaningful if they are translated into practice. Therefore, they must be converted into strategies, or actions, which detail how the objectives are going to be achieved and who will take responsibility for this.

Action plans

Action plans, which we discussed earlier in this chapter, outline specific and measurable strategies, and task responsibilities for achieving objectives. They are developed at the program, work group and individual levels. It is here that ownership is strengthened through participation in their formation, and where planning becomes practice. To briefly recap, action plans:

* are generated at the work group and individual levels
* identify essential actions for achieving strategic goals
* specify who is responsible for tasks
* provide a framework for monitoring implementation
* link strategy to practice.

TABLE 6.5 Sample action plan

ACTION	PERSON/S RESPONSIBLE	TIME FRAME
Exploratory discussions with potential stakeholders	CEO	One month: by next board meeting
Nominate person who will be responsible for preparing tender	Executive committee	Next exec meeting
Form steering committee to develop project plan in preparation for tender release	Nominated tender writer/s	One month after the board meeting
Steering committee meetings	Nominated tender writer/s	Weekly for half an hour throughout tender preparation period
Survey community and networks to determine need and appropriate programmatic response	Research and policy officer	Within two months
Liaise with Department of Families and Communities regarding the tender process	Nominated tender writer/s or steering committee representative	Throughout the first two months
Draft program proposal in preparation for tender	Nominated tender writer/s	Third exec meeting of the year (within three months)
Prepare tender documents	Nominated tender writer/s	Within two weeks of call for tender
Draft tender to exec for comment	Nominated tender writer/s	Three weeks after the call for tender
Submit tender	CEO	By tender due date

The *actions* in action plans are often expressed as strategies. These are the activities that must be undertaken in order to achieve the objectives. It is essential to identify who will perform the actions, the time frame and the desired outcome. For example, let's consider strategic objective 1 of CHRFSS—to establish a family violence prevention program by submitting a proposal to the next call for tender by the Department of Families and Communities to introduce early intervention programs in community organisations—and let's assume the call for tender is scheduled for release in three months' time. Table 6.5 outlines the actions that must occur.

Monitoring and evaluation

As we have already mentioned, it is important to ensure that the strategic plan is not thrown into the back of a drawer and forgotten until the next Annual General Meeting report is due, or when the board of governance commences a new planning cycle. It should not be a confidential document; everyone in the organisation needs to be aware of it, to understand how it relates to their own area of practice and, importantly, to feel that they can and are making a contribution to its achievement. One way to keep 'the plan' alive is ensuring action plans are included on meeting agendas, with a requirement for reports from those responsible for the identified tasks. Treat the strategic plan as a living document, make it look attractive and inviting to read, and make it visible. The strategic goals of the organisation also need to have a presence and to be referred to in performance appraisals and supervision sessions. It is surprising how difficult it can be to locate and identify the strategic plans in some organisations.

REFLECTION EXERCISE

Where is your organisation's strategic plan? What are the strategic goals and actions in your work area?

SUMMARY OF KEY ISSUES

This has been a lengthy and demanding chapter, because we believe that planning is a crucial function of management and leadership practice, and therefore deserves detailed attention. Unfortunately, it is often glossed over or overlooked as a key area of knowledge and skill development. This oversight contributes to poor implementation, and a negative spiral of unrealised strategic plans that attract complaints of having soaked up scarce resources in development, and end up with very little to show in practice (Lewis et al., 2012). The increasingly complex and changeable climate of the present and the foreseeable future (such that it is foreseeable) requires more flexible planning approaches. In this chapter we have presented a range of concepts, tools and strategies for working with the planning challenges and opportunities that surround your organisation and emerge from within it. In the next chapter we continue the discussion on planning, this time in relation to project management.

PRACTICE ACTIVITIES

1   Locate your organisation's strategic plan.
    a   How does it link with the work that you are doing?
    b   What role did you play in its development?
2   Design a strategic planning process appropriate for your organisation.
    a   Which stages will you include?
    b   How will you identify and engage key stakeholders?
    c   How will you select the planning team?
3   Visit these organisations' websites to view the vision, mission and values statement. Having accessed these, follow the links to their strategic plans.
    •   Ermha, a community-based organisation that supports people recovering from mental illness: www.ermha.org/about-us/vision-and-mission
    •   EACH, a multi-site organisation that provides health, disability, counselling, mental health and social services: www.each.com.au/about-us
        Explore the websites of other organisations relevant to your service area and view their strategic plans.
    a   How do the strategic plans compare?
    b   How many years do the plans cover?
    c   How long are they?
    d   How much detail is included?
    e   Do you find one format more accessible than another?

FURTHER READING

Examples of strategic planning models developed for health and human service organisations

Anheier, H. (2005). *Nonprofit Organizations. Theory, Management, Policy*. United Kingdom: Routledge, p.262

Austin, M. J. & Solomon, J. R. (2009). 'Managing the Planning Process', in Patti, R. J. (ed.), *The Handbook of Human Services Management* (2nd edn), Thousand Oaks, California: Sage, pp.321–37.

Brody, R. (2005). *Effectively Managing Human Service Organizations* (3rd edn), Thousand Oaks, California: Sage, p.59.

Hudson, M. (2009). *Managing without Profit* (3rd edn), Sydney, Australia: UNSW Press, p.164.

Lewis, J. A., Packard, T. R. & Lewis, M. D. (2012). *Management of Human Service Programs* (5th edn). USA: Brooks/Cole Cengage Learning, p.49.

Ozanne, E. & Rose, D. (2013). *The Organisational Context of Human Service Practice*. Australia: Palgrave Macmillan, p.218.

Developing strategy and strategic plans in the NFP sector

Bryson, J. M. (2004). *Strategic Planning for Public and Nonprofit Organizations* (3rd edn), San Francisco: John Wiley & Sons.

Hudson, M. (2009). *Managing without Profit* (3rd edn), Sydney, Australia: UNSW Press. 'Chapter 7: Devising Strategies to Maximise Impact', pp.145–73 & 'Chapter 8: Creating Competitive Services Strategies', pp.174–92.

Planning processes

Field, R. (2010). 'Planning and Budgeting', in Gray, I., Field, R. & Brown, K. (eds), *Effective Leadership, Management and Supervision in Health and Social Care*, Exeter, UK: Learning Matters Ltd. pp.120–41.

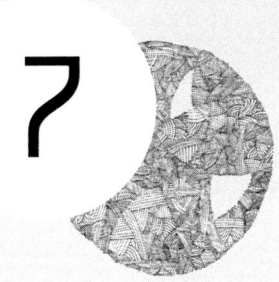

7

Project Management and Evaluation

OVERVIEW

This chapter will:

- clarify the difference between programs and projects
- describe methods and tools that enable project planning, implementation and the achievement of set tasks or goals
- explore evaluation as a form of systematic enquiry about the nature, delivery and effectiveness of a project, program or policy intervention
- explain two approaches to evaluation that are particularly useful for current and future practice, while also adding to the evidence base.

This chapter is about steps in project design and implementation, and the nature and usefulness of project evaluation.

KEY TERMS

communication strategy	need
empowerment evaluation	outcome evaluation
evaluation	output evaluation
evidence-based practice	program
implementation planning	project
logic modelling	project timeline

Project management

Distinguishing between programs and projects

You will recall from the previous chapter that Weinbach and Taylor define a **program** as a 'complex, integrated system that has been created to address some problem' that is 'more or less self-contained', with discrete goals and objectives and its own budget. Additionally, they state that the program manager's role is 'to advocate for the program; publicize it; monitor it; and, when an outside evaluator is not used, help to judge its overall value, worth, or merit' (Weinbach & Taylor, 2011, p.307).

An organisation usually has multiple programs, and there is a degree of competition for resources. Some overlap between programs is inevitable and this may result in territorial issues that management must try to resolve. It may be helpful to think of a program as a social system, which has a relationship with other social systems that make up the organisation. From this perspective it is easy to appreciate that the nature of one program will impact other programs (or systems) that make up the organisation (Weinbach & Taylor, 2011).

A program may comprise a number of projects, which have specific funding for set deliverables and operate over a limited time frame. Projects may not continue beyond contractual arrangements, although the program may survive—with a constantly evolving combination of projects that vary in intensity and priority as their contractual obligations are addressed by the program. In this respect, an area of work (the program) may be able to endure despite the vagaries of short-term or uncertain funding. This means there is increased potential for staff development and continuity, and for maintaining the organisation's expertise and profile, with scope to bid for funding opportunities as they arise. It does, however, create substantial challenges for managers as they seek to address requirements of existing projects, the cost of staff resources, and efforts to bring in money so the program can be maintained. Many of these issues have been canvassed elsewhere in this text; here our focus shifts to the processes involved in planning, implementation, and delivery at project level.

Projects

A **project** is:

> A unique, one-time work effort with a defined start and a defined end, the objectives of which are defined in advance by those who are paying the bill (and those who have vested interests) and are to be achieved by the use of finite and limited resources. Projects are temporary work, bounded by time, resources, and requirements

Source: McGhee & McAliney, 2007, pp.3–4

This definition needs modification to account for the funding and practice environments of health and human services. For example:

- The funder may set broad objectives (for example, for a national grants scheme), while organisations provide detailed objectives that align with needs of their client group and account for associated project activities.
- Project resources may be augmented by funding from other sources (for example, philanthropies, core funding).

Program
A complex, integrated system with discrete goals and its own budget.

Linkage
We encountered the definitions of 'program' and 'project' in the previous chapter, when we looked at types of plans; we expand the discussion of projects in this chapter.

Project
A unique, one-off effort, with a defined budget, time frame and set of requirements.

- The temporary nature of a project, as represented in contractual documents, may be part of the time frame for a much longer iteration of the project (for example, when an organisation is able to access multiple or subsequent funding streams that support project continuity).

Project types

Projects in health and human service organisations range from service provision to organisational development. They may be about:

- Developing new services, programs or technologies.
- Improving existing services, process and practices.
- Implementing new organisational structures and systems.
- The construction, installation and/or commissioning of new equipment and facilities.

Source: Dwyer et al., 2004, p.9

Each project requires its own management plan, although many of the processes and tools are generic and provide a structure that may be adapted to the specifics of project activities and context.

The project manager's role

Project management involves five processes: definition, planning, leading, monitoring and completing (Rosenau, 1998, in Dwyer et al., 2004, p.8). The project manager is responsible for:

1   Managing resources to deliver the project, the budget and time line, and implementation process.

2   Fulfilling traditional roles of management: delegating, negotiating, persuading, organising, co-ordinating, facilitating, and team building.

3   Detailing and executing the communications plan, with discretion regarding 'what to tell and to whom'.

4   Making decisions that enable the successful delivery of the project, within funding conditions and accounting for organisational constraints.

Source: McGhee & McAliney, 2007, p.7

One of the practitioners we first met in Chapter 5, Daryl Fitzgibbon, has provided some interesting comments on project management and evaluation. His thoughts are shown below, as context for our consideration of project planning, implementation and evaluation.

PRACTITIONER PROFILE 7.1

DARYL FITZGIBBON

CLINICAL MANAGER, WESTERN REGION ALCOHOL AND DRUG CENTRE (WRAD)

Preferred approach to project management and evaluation

- Projects inject some variety into workers' roles and often leave a legacy of enhanced understanding and capacity behind.
- Projects allow the creative to show their skill. The evaluation teaches the workers analytical standards and reporting requirements.

- All too often projects are evaluated as worthwhile but don't receive funding. Bookshelves are full of projects that at least provided research data.
- Research influences policy to determine practice modalities to feed into research to lobby government that more research is needed.

As you may appreciate from these illustrations of project management and evaluation, there are many uncertainties involved. What has seemed feasible on paper may not be realistic in practice. Broader issues such as staff turnover and competing demands on organisational resources may pose additional challenges. The project manager needs to combine flexibility with good planning and maintain communication channels with internal and external stakeholders so the project can successfully deliver a useful product that is valued by all.

Project planning

Throughout this text, we have emphasised the importance of a thorough and considered approach to management. Nowhere is this more essential (and perhaps underdone) than in the establishment phase of a new project. Table 7.1, below, outlines key stages in project planning and the associated benefits, along with some potential risks of poor planning.

TABLE 7.1 Core steps leading to a new project

NATURE OF EACH STEP	POTENTIAL BENEFITS FROM THOROUGH PLANNING	POTENTIAL RISKS IF NOT UNDERTAKEN THOROUGHLY
Assessing need for the project, in terms of the problem and associated service gaps	A detailed definition of need	An inadequate understanding of need and failure to account for services already provided/ remediation strategies that are already underway
Setting goals and objectives that are based on need in combination with evidence on effective responses	Clarity in what the project hopes to achieve that accounts for 'what works' and for obstacles that need to be recognised	Unrealistic goals and objectives that set the project up to fail
Developing an action strategy to deliver the project, including the consideration of alternative approaches	Activities are described, along with the sequence and timing for delivery	Lack of clarity regarding project activities
Developing a communication strategy to engage stakeholders	Stakeholders are identified Communication mechanisms are part of planning	The project is not supported by those important to its success and sustainability
Articulating resources for project implementation	A sound understanding of project requirements (staff and direct costs)	Insufficient or poorly matched resources
Finalising the project plan using clear and straightforward language	A concise document that outlines the intention and scope of the project	No record of the foundation for and design of the project

Let us consider the first of these steps, the assessment of need, in further detail.

Needs analysis

Need
A subjective assessment of a problem that is influenced by community standards.

As shown in Table 7.1, the foundation for a project is **need**—where there is a problem and no strategy in place for its remediation. While this may seem straightforward, our understanding of need is subjective and shaped by social, political and economic factors. In broad terms:

> It is important to evaluate existing conditions against some societally established standards. If the community is at or above those standards, there is no need; if it is below those standards, there is need. The difficulty comes in defining the standards. They are often vague, elusive, and changing.
>
> Source: Kettner et al., 2013, p.52

Bradshaw (1972, cited in Kettner et al., 2013, p.59) defines need from four perspectives:

- *Normative need*: as defined by experts in the field. Assessment involves the use of existing data and standards from comparable communities/expert opinion to establish a target that is judged to be appropriate to the community. Examples include the number of hospital beds per 1000 people or the caseload for a child protection worker.
- *Perceived need*: as seen by those experiencing the need. The main problem with this definition is that each consumer is operating from his/her own standard, which may fluctuate, and the needs they report may be symptomatic of underlying problems that should be further defined.
- *Expressed need*: assessed by the number of people who seek out services (sometimes called demand). For example, the waiting period to enter a residential withdrawal program. A major problem with this assessment is the substantial gap between those in need and those who seek assistance; the failure to account for overall need in the community.
- *Relative need*: based on needs and resources in one geographic area or community compared with those in another. This perspective is not based on community standards but draws from the concept of equity, the prioritisation of resource allocation based on who is in greater need.

As you may appreciate, each perspective on need has its own shortcomings. In deciding on your approach to defining need, you may combine aspects of these perspectives. Ultimately, the time and resources available for the needs analysis will determine the approach that is used for project development.

REFLECTION EXERCISE

As we have explored, need may be defined from different perspectives, which determine views on the importance for a particular project. Take a moment to consider how you would determine the need for a project and whether your approach could be improved by combining different definitions of need.

Goals and objectives

Having undertaken your analysis and arrived at a best estimate of need, you are well placed to identify the goals of your project and to translate these goals into activities. **Logic modelling** is a very useful way to translate the theory behind your project into a planning framework. It is a tool to organise your ideas in terms of planned objectives, activities and impacts/outcomes.

Logic models come in different shapes and sizes, depending on the nature of the project, characteristics of those involved in its design, the stage reached in terms of conceptual formation of activities, and completeness of the information available for the planning process. For example, logic modelling may involve an unformed 'mind map' that seeks to capture stakeholders' thoughts about appropriate objectives and activities to respond to the problem. It may result in a conceptual framework, where details are added by an external consultant and then checked by project stakeholders. The important elements of logic modelling are:

- identifying project objectives
- matching these to activities
- considering the evidence on what works, to modify activities as needed
- outlining outputs (what will be delivered)
- identifying outcomes (what will be achieved in the short and longer-term)
- defining markers of success.

Depending who is involved in project design and how advanced their thinking is, a number of sessions may be required to arrive at a well-developed logic model. Even then, the model will be revisited and refined during implementation.

The final point above, on defining markers of success, is the first step toward demonstrating that what you are doing matters in relation to the need you have identified. This means you need to arrive at identifiable measures of project success. We will return to this later in the chapter, when we explore the integration of evaluation with project management.

Figure 7.1 provides an outline of the categories to include in a straightforward logic model. As noted above, it is important to remember that the exact format of the model will vary according to the project. In addition, feedback loops may be included to reflect the intention to modify the model with the benefit of experience once the project has commenced. There are many examples of logic models on the web and one of this chapter's suggested readings (W. K. Kellogg Foundation, 1997) includes an array of diverse models. Taking a look at these models will help your understanding of the modelling process and the different styles of models that may be developed.

Logic modelling
A diagrammatic representation of the framework for a project, which is developed by those involved in project development and typically includes aims, activities, outputs and impacts/outcomes.

Linkage
At this point you might like to review the discussion on the formulation of goals and objectives in Chapter 6.

FIGURE 7.1 A simple outline for a logic model

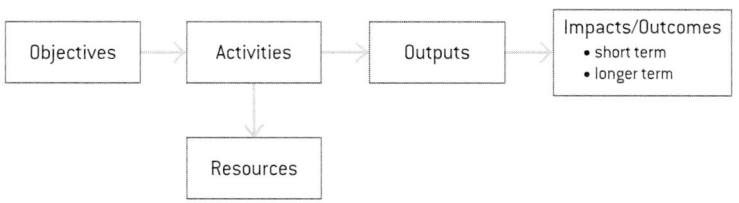

The logic model is a concise summary of the project that is useful for communication with internal and external stakeholders. The process of developing the model assists in building the rationale for the project and identifying the expectations—and this may extend to consensus building when multiple and diverse stakeholder groups are involved. Modelling will help to identify gaps in the logic of the project and underlying assumptions that may need clarification to avoid unrealistic expectations. Finally, it is useful for describing areas of enquiry for evaluation and review.

Using the evidence

Evidence-based practice
The integration of research evidence with practice expertise.

The approach of **evidence-based practice** is to use what we know about project effectiveness, and consider this in the design of future work. The value placed on existing knowledge reflects a commitment to an ongoing cycle of improvement, to avoid 'reinventing the wheel' by building on existing literature and practice wisdom (Wandersman et al., 2005).

There is some concern in the research literature about restrictions on what is understood to be valid evidence, involving a focus on research studies that meet restrictive methodological criteria. This focus overlooks practice-based expertise and knowledge obtained from theoretical and qualitative work. For project managers in health and human services, evidence from research *and* practice needs to be considered.

The context for project implementation is also important. There will be practical ramifications regarding resources (for example, if distance is a factor) and perhaps including the extent to which the service network is developed (for example, impacting ease of referral pathways). The project manager will account for these factors in fine-tuning the project model and deciding on resource implications, making decisions based on need, evidence, and their understanding of local conditions. Sackett (1996) provides a useful definition of evidence-based practice that is inclusive of different sources of information, involving 'the integration of best research evidence with clinical expertise and patient values'. Potential benefits of considering evidence-based practice in project planning include:

- Learning about the latest developments in the area of interest.
- Reflecting on current and past practice and what has been learnt.
- Having a foundation to justify the approach put forward for the project.
- Avoiding ineffective or outdated techniques that are based on tradition.
  You may have identified other benefits from this approach.

Practicalities

Project activities identified during planning give an indication of the resources needed for implementation. The anticipated time frame is another major impact on resources. Your conclusions about the practical requirements of the project will be tentative at this stage, as funding may be uncertain and other factors (that range from competing project demands on staff resources to how much funding will be received) need to be addressed during project establishment.

The project plan

After completing the needs analysis and logic modelling, along with the budget, you are ready for project initiation. It is important that you record the results and conclusions from these planning steps in a project plan. Common elements of this plan include the following:

- Broad aim of the project.
- Detailed objectives that are action oriented, identify the target group and include tangible outcomes.
- Background information on the identified need and potential benefits of the project.
- A description of what the project will involve: activities, outputs and outcomes. A version of the logic model may be included in this section.
- An outline of internal and external stakeholders that need to be considered in developing a communication strategy to support project implementation.
- Resource implications, including staff salaries and overheads, and direct costs.
- A timeline that allows sufficient time for establishment and maturation of the project so that outcomes may be achieved.

The final plan is one that is agreed to by stakeholders in the organisation. It may be used as the basis for one or more funding applications and is also a useful tool to inform communication activities targeting the community and key groups, such as advisory committees and senior management. In addition, the plan is a valuable record of the project origins and it provides a useful reference point as the project is implemented, as sustainability is considered, and during internal and external reviews.

Project implementation

Having developed the conceptual and resource-based framework ('the plan') and obtained approval for the project (for example, funding and organisational support), your focus turns to implementation. This stage is about revisiting the project plan to account for any changes in the context for project implementation or modifications deemed necessary, and gathering resources needed for the project to become operational.

Planning for implementation

Questions to consider during **implementation planning** include the following:

- What staff are suited to the project and are they available for the project? Which staff will be central to project operations (for example, coordinating, delivering service, gathering data on project activities and impacts)? Do you need to recruit for any project positions?
- How will the project interact with other activities in the organisation, for example, in terms of shared information, referral linkages, and common client groups?
- How robust is the budget? Are there costs you haven't considered? Have salary rates changed since the budget was constructed?
- Is your timeline realistic? How long will it take for the project to be underway?

Implementation planning
A process that addresses contextual factors, gathers resources, and clarifies the time frame for a project to be operational.

- What are the major risks to the project and what steps can you put in place for their remediation?
- How can you and the organisation support the potential success of the project (for example, internal management meetings, media, dissemination activities)?
- Where does the project sit in relation to other activities: does it belong with an existing set of projects (a program of activities that operates as a discrete system in the organisation) or does it represent something new—and what are the implications for establishing the project as a core activity in the organisation?
- What communication strategy is required to promote the project and encourage support from internal and external stakeholders?

During this establishment phase of the project, you will essentially build on the plan that has been developed to clarify uncertainties and address practicalities, thereby making the project a reality. The project team and their respective roles need to be developed. Mapping tasks against the project time frame will provide a structure for implementation and monitoring progress. Mechanisms for project oversight and review processes also need to be agreed upon and put in place.

The project team

Ultimately, the nature of the project team will be guided by the budget and the availability of current staff. You may need to recruit to specific roles as well. This means careful consideration of the skill set required for the project, different levels of seniority required for project implementation, and particular interventions—such as professional development and supervisory arrangements relevant to the work that is planned.

Other important aspects of the team are the extent to which staff work in harmony and their level of engagement with the project. As with any social group, team members will establish a natural hierarchy—operating in an environment of mutual trust and respect is important for team functionality and well-being. The level of project ownership that staff have will affect their motivation to take on challenging tasks and strive for high quality work.

The team structures in your workplace will influence the extent to which your role as project manager is defined or subject to change. In hierarchically oriented teams, staff are organised according to their function, and roles are very clear. Task allocation follows naturally and lines of communication and accountability are obvious. But this type of structure may impede innovation, and fail to provide opportunity for staff to demonstrate their full capacity.

Linkage
Some of the considerations raised here are also relevant to the section on staff recruitment and development in Chapter 5.

Another approach, using a matrix structure, draws from a broader program or departmental arrangement, where staff have designated roles in the organisation and they contribute to multiple projects simultaneously—sometimes in different capacities (for example, as coordinator, or focusing on a particular area of skill). This can pose challenges for all, with competing demands and role confusion at times. However, the matrix structure means increased flexibility in the wealth of skill and knowledge that is available across the staff group (McGhee & McAliney, 2007).

Communication strategy

Health and human service organisations are about people and the range of stakeholders involved—from those funding, providing and working with the project, to those targeted by the project. The various interests and perspectives of these stakeholders need attention throughout the project—without their engagement and support the project may fail.

A simple yet useful exercise is to identify stakeholders in the project in terms of their significance for project success and the likelihood that they will hinder or support the project (Dwyer et al., 2004). Examples include staff in the organisation, who may have capacity to block initiatives or enable their success in practical and political ways, and external stakeholders, who may have strong views about the area involved and what is needed. For example, support from nurse unit managers is important for a project targeting workforce development in hospital settings. In another example, community leaders may need to be actively engaged, in an ongoing way, in a project targeting a cultural minority. The advice and support these stakeholders provide will benefit the project design and facilitate community access.

The **communication strategy** will include mechanisms to engage those important to the project and hopefully subvert any negativity that may get in the way of project implementation. Table 7.2 provides an example.

Linkage
In Chapter 2 we explored external forces that shape health and human service organisations, underlining the importance of constructive and ongoing communication with project stakeholders.

Communication strategy
A process involving identifying and mapping project stakeholders and mechanisms in order to engage support, thereby enabling project success.

TABLE 7.2 An outline of a project communication strategy

STAKEHOLDER	INFORMATION REQUIRED	FREQUENCY OF COMMUNICATION	MEANS OF COMMUNICATION
INTERNAL			
Senior management	• Purpose • Importance	Intermittent; early on and prior to completion are important periods	• Briefing • Information in program reports • Information distributed (e.g., website, listservs, newsletters)
Program staff	• Purpose • Progress • Learnings	Intermittent; schedule into regular program meetings	• Presentations at meetings • Information distributed • Advisory group member?
EXTERNAL			
Funder	• Progress updates	As per contract requirements	As per contract requirements
Consumers	• Project orientation • Reinforce worth of project	Intermittent; early on and prior to completion are important periods	• Consultation with representatives • Information distributed (e.g., flyers, displays) • Advisory group member?
Organisations with links to the project	• Project orientation • Project links • Project progress	Intermittent; early on, scheduled intervals, prior to project completion	• Consultation • Information distributed (e.g., flyers, displays) • Advisory group member?

Linkage
We revisit stakeholder analysis in Chapter 9 when exploring change management strategy.

Mapping project activities

Project timeline
A diagram that maps project activities by time.

Developing a diagram or **project timeline**, which maps activities against the planned duration of the project, is useful to articulate what needs to happen and when. The timeline may also include governance and communication activities, such as project meetings and information sharing. A sample timeline is shown in Table 7.3 opposite. It is essentially a modified form of the Gantt chart, which is a project schedule that shows activities by time period and may map progress as the project advances. In each project timeline there will be some elements that are fixed and inflexible—such as contracted deliverables—while the exact timing for some activities may change following encounters with unforeseen events (for example staff shortages).

Progress and review

Typically, projects have set targets that outline the activities to be delivered. This may involve goals linked to project establishment (for example, recruiting staff, establishing memoranda of understanding with collaborating organisations) and include outputs such as the number of sessions provided. It may specify desired outcomes of these activities (for example, ranging from referral uptake to positive changes in client behaviour).

It is essential to have tools to record the work undertaken in setting up the project, and to measure activities and outcomes, so that you can demonstrate and reflect on progress, barriers and achievements. This is useful for monitoring progress, updating plans and deciding on future directions. This information is also invaluable for external reporting requirements and internal review processes. This brings us to the final section in this chapter, evaluation.

Project evaluation

The area of evaluation is substantial: many references have been developed on the philosophies, designs and techniques for data collection and analysis. You are encouraged to read further about these aspects of evaluation. Our focus is on fundamental aspects of evaluation planning, as well as empowerment and collaborative evaluation techniques, which are particularly useful for health and human services.

First, we present a practitioner profile of an evaluation consultant with many years of experience working with funders and providers. Next, we consider categories of evaluation. Then, we explore how the orientation of an evaluation is determined; what is the purpose of the evaluation and what questions need to be addressed? The section closes with a description of collaborative evaluation, a model that involves both staff and external consultants and has considerable potential for all project stakeholders. Throughout this section you are encouraged to think about project evaluation as a tool for management.

TABLE 7.3 Sample project timeline

MONTHS / FOCUS	1–3	4–6	7–9	10–12	13–15	16–18	19–21	22–24
Establishment, governance	Staff identified Resources in place Advisory group/s formed	Project meeting Advisory group meeting	Project meeting Advisory group meeting	Project meeting	Project meeting Advisory group meeting	Project meeting	Project meeting Advisory group meeting Sustainability planning	Project meeting
Communication	Information distributed		Information updated			Information updated		
Project activities	Tools Training Commence project	Number of sessions/ visits/other as per plan	Number of sessions/ visits/other as per plan	Number of sessions/ visits/other as per plan	Number of sessions/ visits/other as per plan	Number of sessions/ visits/other as per plan	Number of sessions/ visits/other as per plan	Number of sessions/ visits/other as per plan
Ongoing cycle of review and improvement	Reflection and suggestions for improvement		Reflection and suggestions for improvement		Reflection and suggestions for improvement		Reflection and suggestions for future work	
Monitoring and formal review	Systems for data recording Initial report			Annual report				Final report
Sustainability planning	Initial thoughts about project duration					Develop and implement sustainability plan	Implement sustainability strategies	Steps toward project continuation/ termination

PRACTITIONER PROFILE 7.2

DR SUE CARSWELL

INDEPENDENT RESEARCH AND EVALUATION CONSULTANT

Role

I am an independent research and evaluation consultant based in Christchurch, New Zealand. I have worked on a range of projects with a focus on evaluating social programs in the justice and health sectors. Clients include governments, community organisations and universities. The role includes tendering for contracts, design and project management of research and evaluation projects, data collection and analysis (qualitative and quantitative), report writing, publication and presentation of findings. I often work in collaboration with other researchers and evaluators and either subcontract colleagues to work on a particular project, or I am subcontracted as part of a project team.

Typical day

I am usually involved in a number of projects concurrently so a typical day involves a wide variety of tasks that cover project management, communication with project teams, stakeholders and participants, designing methodology and data collection tools, conducting fieldwork, data analysis and report writing. The evaluation of national services often means a considerable amount of travel to conduct fieldwork.

Challenges

A major challenge can be time management when juggling different projects and the demands of meeting tight contract deadlines. The nature of this type of contract work is that you can seldom afford to only do one or two contracts at a time. Complex projects with multiple stakeholders require time to consult and engage with the appropriate people in order to establish a robust project design, tools and a team that is ready to go. It is important to establish what can and cannot be achieved within specified time frames and what can be delivered to meet funders' own deadlines, for example, reporting to government, decisions on rollout of initiatives, making funding applications.

Lessons learnt

Working from home requires a considerable amount of dedication and the ability to self-manage. A constant challenge is maintaining a balance between work and personal life so it is essential to plan your time, stick to routines and book holidays that are work free! If you are managing your own research and evaluation business, ensure you develop efficient financial and administrative systems as these tasks can be time consuming.

Skills and qualities

The Aotearoa/New Zealand Evaluation Association is currently working on identifying evaluator competencies and I recently attended one of their workshops, which highlighted the following four competency domains:

- Contextual analysis and engagement
- Systematic evaluative practice
- Evaluation project management and professional practice
- Reflective practice and professional development

A number of skills and qualities fall under each domain, and key for me is an understanding of the context and clarity about objectives in order to respond with the right mix of team and project design. The ability to engage and manage relationships is also key to this role.

Preferred approach to project management and evaluation

My approach to evaluation and project management is consultative, ethical and culturally responsive, with the aim of designing and implementing an evaluation that will address the evaluation objectives within the restrictions of the available resources and time.

Sue Carswell has undertaken projects involving vulnerable groups and worked with Māori organisations and communities, maintaining a culturally appropriate method that accounts for shared ownership of the project process and findings. Sue has a keen understanding of protocols regarding working with first peoples and a strong appreciation of the importance of communication and relationship building as tools for collaborative evaluation. Later in the chapter we explore an evaluation that uses culturally responsive methods to examine an initiative involving Aboriginal Australians (see Table 7.5). First, let us consider what is meant by the term **evaluation**.

Evaluation is a systematic way of examining the usefulness of an activity. It is often prompted by funding bodies and involves external evaluators, while evaluation is also an important tool for organisations. It may be undertaken by project staff and include a collaboration with external consultants.

Ideally, evaluation is part of planning and implementation; to determine the need for an intervention and monitor its progress and for ongoing improvement as well as reporting. While evaluation may be challenging and confronting for already-busy staff who are trying to establish and run a project, it is best viewed as a way to inform the nature of the project, provide direction for its improvement, and demonstrate the success of what has been delivered. This is easiest if evaluation is built into planning, data systems and reporting mechanisms. It is most useful if seen as a tool within an ongoing cycle of reflection, action and change that is designed to inform and improve organisational practice.

> **Evaluation**
> A process of systematic enquiry to assess the value and merit of an activity.

REFLECTION EXERCISE

What do you think of evaluation? Write down the first thoughts that come to mind when the word is mentioned. Now reflect on those thoughts to explore what has shaped your views (experience, hearsay, other).

Types of evaluation

Project evaluation operates at different levels. Apart from assessing need, as we have already explored, it may focus on how the project has been implemented, on outputs (what has been delivered), and on outcomes (whether desired objectives were achieved). We explore these types of project evaluation briefly below.

Implementation

An **implementation evaluation** involves examining how the project looks in practice, steps taken to establish the project, and contextual factors that impact the extent to which planned implementation can be realised. This type of evaluation may also focus on sustainability planning, whether and to what extent management has been able to address project survival beyond the initial funding period.

MacLean and colleagues (2012) explored implementation effectiveness among 127 community-based projects addressing alcohol and drug problems. First, they reviewed the research literature and identified areas where barriers and enablers of implementation may occur, for example funding and staffing. Then project documents were examined to identify whether these factors had been experienced and if implementation had been effective. Table 7.4 shows factors that were often involved, with examples of enablers and barriers for each of the factors.

The factors in Table 7.4 are listed in order of frequency, with factors experienced by most projects appearing first. In other words, the most common factors that enabled project implementation were about:

- strong external communication and agency relationships
- having suitable staff and appropriate leadership
- thorough project planning and design
- strong organisational governance and capacity
- project sensitivity to service users and settings.

It is worth considering the correlation between these areas and the approaches we have explored elsewhere in this text, for example, communication, workforce development, leadership and planning. While good management will not resolve all concerns in project implementation, a systematic approach will enhance the potential for implementation success. In turn, this will support project delivery and effectiveness.

> **Linkage**
> The study by MacLean et al. reinforces the importance of elements of project planning that we explored earlier in this chapter.

Outputs and outcomes

> **Output evaluation**
> An assessment of whether intended project activities have been delivered.

An **output evaluation** assesses whether intended deliverables have been realised. It addresses questions about the activities that have been provided; examples include the number of episodes of care provided or clients engaged within the target demographic, as well as the type and extent of agency linkages that have been established or strengthened. Output evaluation tells us about *what* has been provided, but not about the effect of these activities.

> **Outcome evaluation**
> The review of short- and longer-term impacts and outcomes of a project to measure the extent to which intended results have been attained.

An **outcome evaluation** reviews short- and longer-term results of a project—to measure the extent to which intended results have been attained. For example, a project may aim to improve staff skills in data entry through training and recognition. Measuring skills before and after training, and differences according to recognition of positive change, will indicate the relationship between the project and skill development. In another example, a project targeting obesity among older people may involve activities to boost their self-esteem and improve their dietary habits. Evaluation measures are concerned with improvements in these areas. We should also document unintended impacts, such as increased social activities or exercise, which are also desired mechanisms for weight reduction.

TABLE 7.4 Enablers and barriers encountered during the implementation of community projects targeting alcohol and drug problems

FACTORS	ENABLERS	BARRIERS
External communication and relationships	Support from partner agencies or from participating communities; used existing networks	Lack of partner agency or community interest in or commitment to project; partner agency withdrawal
Staffing and leadership	Employed suitable staff or contractors; staff or management provided leadership; staff training activities undertaken	Delay in staff recruitment; staff or management turnover; staff lacked relevant skills
Project planning and design	Evidence-based model; good fit to needs; flexible design; appropriate scoping; holistic approach	Poor fit; inadequate scoping; poor timing
Governance	Organisation already experienced in project work; good policies and procedures; effective internal reference group	Lack of management involvement; reference group unrepresentative or ineffectual
Sensitivity to service users and settings	Model culturally appropriate; employed culturally/gender appropriate staff	Resources or approach not culturally appropriate; failed to engage specific demographic groups
Staff roles and communication	Staff engaged and enthusiastic about project; staff consultation mechanisms	Staff roles unclear; staff conflict; staff didn't prioritise project involvement; placed additional stress on staff
Participatory approach to service delivery/complexity of service users	Target group involved in development; used role models or peer approaches; activity-based approaches	Little participation; chaotic lives; challenging behaviours
Funding and resourcing	Well funded; using existing resources; gained additional funding; partner agency contributed resources	Submissions for ongoing funding unsuccessful; other funding problems
Research, evaluation, data collection	Well documented; effective data collection; ongoing research	Poor data collection systems; poor response to evaluation; data missing
Wider service system challenges	Not identified	Lack of other services; inter-professional problems; philosophical differences in addressing alcohol and other drug problems

Source: adapted from MacLean et al., 2012, p.62.

Linkage
This information may be useful in management reviews on whether projects should be continued, which we explore in Chapter 8 when looking at financial management.

Moving beyond outcomes, this information can be used to measure project efficiency—it can be combined with cost data to address questions about the merit of project expenditure relative to the benefits attained.

Determining the evaluation focus

Our perspective in this section is on project management that includes evaluation as a core activity. The first step involves determining the question/s you seek to address, which will identify whether the focus is on implementation, outputs or outcomes. Let us start by considering some fundamental questions for the project. Evaluation must also consider practical issues and the multiple perspectives involved. This involves an understanding of 'what works, for whom and in what circumstances, in what respects and how' (Pawson et al., 2005, p.21). The list of questions below illustrates both the grounded nature of evaluation and the range of queries that may be involved:

- How does this project work?
- Why has it worked or not worked? For whom and in what circumstances?
- What was the process of development and implementation?
- What were the stumbling blocks faced along the way?
- What do the experiences mean to the people involved?
- How do these meanings relate to intended outcomes?
- What lessons have we learnt about developing and implementing this project?
- How have contextual factors impacted the development, implementation, success, and stumbling blocks of this project?
- What are the hard-to-measure impacts of this project (ones that cannot be easily quantified)? How can we begin to effectively document these impacts?

Source: W.K. Kellogg Foundation, 1997, p.12

Once you have decided on the critical question/s the evaluation needs to address, planning tools can be used to identify what is being measured and how. The logic model is a good place to start as it captures the intended aims, activities and outcomes. This information can form the basis for identifying project targets and sources of information. You may wish to replicate the logic model to develop an evaluation framework by:

- Revisiting the project logic model and making adjustments based on the context for the project.
- Reviewing the planned achievements of the project (for example, in terms of inputs, outputs and outcomes) and whether these are realistic.
- Considering information-gathering mechanisms that are already in place (for example, service monitoring data systems and project reports) and adding particular tools to gather further information (for example, workforce surveys, diagnostic instruments).
- Deciding on the logic for the evaluation: the key focus, measures, data sources, processes and deliverables.

All the while, you will need to engage stakeholders (staff, leaders, project partners) in this process and be mindful of the resources you have for the evaluation.

A word of caution—evaluation is highly political. Each person will have their own view on the project and may be strongly vested in demonstrating its usefulness. Accounting for the different views involved and the politics of evaluation will require resources (time) beyond the actual tasks. Good communication throughout and encouraging shared ownership of the evaluation will assist in achieving a successful evaluation, which is ultimately about improving practice through a critical and constructive examination of what has occurred. We turn our attention now to two evaluation approaches that support shared ownership of the evaluation process and the application of evaluation findings.

Empowerment evaluation

Empowerment evaluation is an approach that strives to help stakeholders achieve positive results by increasing their capacity to plan, implement and evaluate their projects (Wandersman et al., 2005, p.27). As suggested by this explanation, empowerment evaluation is relevant to all project stages: planning, implementation, and the examination of effectiveness. The following principles are an important guide to the process and intent of empowerment evaluation:

1   Improvement

2   Community ownership

3   Inclusion

4   Democratic participation

5   Social justice

6   Community knowledge

7   Evidence-based strategies

8   Capacity building

9   Organisational learning

10 Accountability

Source: Wandersman et al., 2005, p.30

Empowerment evaluation
A capacity-building approach in which stakeholders are supported to develop skills and resources that enable effective project planning, implementation and review.

To read more about these principles and how they impact on project management and evaluation, please refer to the Wandersman et al. (2005) reference that is in the reading list at the end of this chapter.

Collaborative evaluation

Consistent with these principles of empowerment evaluation, a partnership may be developed between managers in an organisation and consultants with expertise in evaluation methodology. Table 7.5, overleaf, outlines two collaborative evaluations we have undertaken and the partnership roles involved. The first is a program targeting older Australians with alcohol problems, and the second is a community intervention against family violence that involves partnering with Aboriginal Australians. If you would like to explore this approach to evaluation further, see the paper by Berends and Roberts (2012) in this chapter's reading list, which is from an evaluation of a project that aimed to routinise screening and brief intervention for risky alcohol use in hospitals.

These evaluations demonstrate how the strengths and capacities of project staff and external consultants can be combined in an evaluation that is grounded in context, uses available material and resources, and focuses on what matters to project stakeholders. You will notice that project stakeholders were involved in all stages of the evaluation; it was their project as much as that of the consultants.

TABLE 7.5 Features of collaborative evaluation, two examples

OLDER WISER LIFESTYLES (OWL) PROJECT EVALUATION (MUGAVIN & BERENDS, JANUARY 2013)	THE GIPPSLAND COMMUNITY WALK AGAINST FAMILY VIOLENCE (LAMING ET AL., 2011)
PURPOSE AND OBJECTIVES OF THE EVALUATION	
Does OWL reduce risky alcohol use among people aged 60 years and older? • Reduction in risky alcohol use • Strategies supporting health and social well-being • Referral to health and welfare services as needed	• Successful and less successful action, features and products of the walk • Transferable approaches and actions • Contextual factors contributing to the success of the walk • Future strategies for best practice, knowledge sharing and partnership building between Aboriginal and non-Aboriginal communities and services
STRUCTURAL CONTEXT	
• Project started 18 months before evaluation • Interest in contributing to evidence base, for sustainability • External consultant recruited • Designated contact person at organisation	The original application to fund an evaluation involved members of the reference group that was subsequently developed, who were the 'key stakeholders, initiators and organisers of the CommUNITY Walk' (Laming et al., 2011, p.9). External consultants were involved from this point.
DIVISION OF ROLES AND RESPONSIBILITIES	
The evaluators: Developed and implemented a draft evaluation plan, for comment from project staff; met with project staff to discuss available data sources and suggest tools to use as part of daily practice; developed a database for staff; conducted interviews with project staff and external stakeholders; conducted follow-up interviews with project clients. *Project staff:* Provided input to the evaluation plan; included measurement tools in their entry interviews and added information to the database; asked clients about participating in evaluation; compiled project data and forwarded it to the evaluators; commented on progress reports and the final report.	*The approach:* A participatory approach was used, along with Aboriginal epistemology that advocated a holistic approach. *The team:* Partner investigators represented Aboriginal and non-Aboriginal services. The reference group met monthly, finalising evaluation questions and process, facilitating access for interviews and focus groups, hosting meetings and reviewing publications. Two consultants from the local university and a research assistant engaged in data collection and analysis.
EVALUATION PROCESSES	
Data collection processes: Specified and documented by evaluators; some data collected by evaluators and some by project staff. *Report processes:* evaluators prepared draft reports and project staff provided comment. *Report usage/dissemination:* Project staff and the evaluators delivered workshops and presentations at state and national conferences; the report has been distributed to interested groups and used to promote the project.	*Data collection processes:* The consultancy team gathered qualitative data from walk participants, organisers, reference group members, and representatives of key organisations and agencies. Evaluation sheets were collected from participants on the day they took part in the walk. *Report processes:* The reference group endorsed evaluation findings and associated publications. *Report usage/dissemination:* The report is available on the web; the consultants with reference group members have given a number of presentations at state, national and international conferences; the reference group has distributed copies to relevant stakeholders.

REFLECTION EXERCISE

You may wish to reflect on an evaluation that you are aware of, using the categories shown in Table 7.5. How did the process compare with that shown in the table? What would you do differently?

SUMMARY OF KEY POINTS

Project management involves activities at all stages of a project, from definition and detailed planning, to leading, monitoring and completion. Clarifying the level and nature of need is essential to inform the design and goals of a project. Logic modelling is a planning tool that assists in clarifying the project aims, activities, outcomes and measures.

Selecting a team according to project activities will maximise the potential for success, although this is not always possible. Including systematic communication strategies and establishing agreed timelines supports a shared understanding among stakeholders about what is involved. Collaborative evaluation is a useful tool to document project implementation and effects, contributing to knowledge about intervention planning and effectiveness, and providing direction for future work.

PRACTICE ACTIVITIES

1 Logic modelling

Think about a project that you have been involved in, or one that you would like to develop. Sketch a simple logic model for the project using the framework shown in Figure 7.1. Did you find this process helpful?

2 What matters in project implementation?

Take another look at Table 7.4, which shows barriers to and enablers of implementation among a sample of 127 projects. Focusing on factors where managers have limited control, think about strategies to minimise the risks to project implementation.

3 Evaluation

Find a logic model on the web and consider how you might go about evaluating whether the project has worked. You may use some of the tools and approaches we have explored in this chapter. Outline what you would do initially, to establish the evaluation.

FURTHER READING

Developing logic models

W. K. Kellogg Foundation (updated Jan. 2004). *Logic Model Development Guide*, Michigan USA: Kellogg Foundation.

Addressing implementation

Magnabosco, J. L. (2006). 'Innovations in Mental Health Services Implementation: A Report on State-Level Data from the U.S. Evidence-Based Practices Project', *Implementation Science*, 1, pp.27–41.

Implementation evaluation using a collaborative approach

Berends, L. & Roberts, B. (2012). 'Implementation Effectiveness of an Alcohol Screening Intervention Project at Two Hospitals in Regional Victoria, Australia', *Contemporary Drug Problems*, 39, pp.289–309.

Empowerment evaluation

Wandersman, A., Snell-Johns, J., Lentz, B. E., Fetterman, D. M., Keener, D. C., Livet, M., Imm, P. S. & Flaspohler, P. (2005). 'The Principles of Empowerment Evaluation', in Fetterman, D. M. & Wandersman, A. (eds.), *Empowerment Evaluation Principles in Practice*, New York: The Guildford Press, pp.27–41.

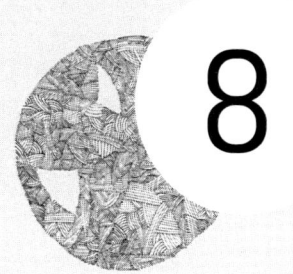

Financial Management and Quality Accreditation

OVERVIEW

This chapter will:
- consider strategies for financial management and approaches to budgeting
- describe processes for acquiring funds and steps involved in proposal writing
- explain accreditation and the implications for managers.

This chapter is about managing revenue and expenditure in health and human service organisations. We explore funding mechanisms and examine the nature and importance of quality accreditation.

KEY TERMS

accreditation

balance sheet

budget

financial management

forecasting

incremental budget

line-item budget

profit and loss statement

proposal writing

standard

total quality management

zero-based budget

Financial management

Streamlining financial arrangements is a shared goal of governments and agencies, to counter complexities arising from the existence of multiple and diverse projects, each with its own set of funding and reporting conditions. But health and human service organisations continue to be challenged by a lack of clarity in what is required to comply with contract conditions and in the consequences of failing to comply. Meanwhile, processes for determining salary and working conditions have undergone substantial change with the introduction of individual contracts and a shift toward contract-based and casual labour. All these factors come to bear on the role of service managers, as organisations devolve operational responsibilities. Carson and Kerr (2012, p.12) suggest that the decentralisation of managerial responsibilities has highlighted:

> An increased role for agency managers in managing contracts at the same time as the commissioning departments were being hollowed-out, leading to an increased need for workforce development, not less as has tended to be the case.

In this context, we have taken a highly practice-oriented approach to the tasks expected of managers in community sector organisations. Below, we outline some strategies that increase management effectiveness—to support financial viability and maximise the benefits from time devoted to **financial management**.

Financial management
Processes including the allocation and use of financial and material resources, activities leading to funds acquisition, and accounting for and reporting on resource utilisation.

Elements of financial management

As a manager you need to be aware of the income and expenditure in your workplace, ranging from the budget for specific projects and programs to financial circumstances across departments or perhaps the entire organisation. You may be involved in generating funds and be asked to explain and make decisions about resources and the future of specific projects and programs. In simple terms, financial management processes include:

- Planning the allocation and use of financial and material resources.
- Accounting for and reporting on resource utilisation.
- Activities leading to funds acquisition.

The exact nature of your engagement with these areas will depend on your position in the organisation and its size. As a CEO, or manager of a large department, financial management may involve having sufficient understanding to oversee financial staff and fiscal operations, and to inform planning and sustainability measures. As a manager of one or more programs, you are likely to be directly involved in budget development, management and reporting (Mayers, 2004). In either case it is important that you have a sound understanding of the fiscal status of your area and the costs of the services you oversee. Before exploring this area further, we return to one of the practitioners we met earlier, who provides a useful description of some ways that the funding environment affects her role.

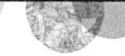

PRACTITIONER PROFILE 8.1

FIONA BOYLE

CHIEF EXECUTIVE OFFICER, GIPPSLAND CENTRE AGAINST SEXUAL ASSAULT (GCASA)

Financial management

Resources are always limited and this impacts on the ability to recruit and run programs that could enhance the organisation's operations. The impact of this is that time is taken looking for additional funding or ways that will support the organisation's core services. My organisation has been supported by government, in relation to a number of inquiries and commissions that have made recommendations on systemic changes for people who have experienced sexual assault and child abuse.

Strategies

Strategies to support your understanding and management of finances involve basic planning and attention to the way that information on finances is presented. In other words:

- Have you established a routine for reviewing finances on a regular basis?
- Do you understand the internal processes by which finances are organised and income and expenditure flows are governed?
- Does your organisation use plain language and transparent tools to share information about finances?

Wagner (2012) has documented five strategies to teach health physicians about financial management. These can be readily adapted for management in community services.

1 *Reviewing basic financial reports and key metrics regularly,* asking: what does cash flow look like; how is revenue trending; are there any outliers in expenses; and what is the forecast for cash flow in the next month (or more).

2 *Using benchmarks that you consider important.* This may include productivity measures on things like the number of clients seen and services provided, and extend to income targets based on predicted revenue and expenditure flows across the financial year.

3 *Exploring the consistency between planned and actual expenditure in the context of performance against benchmarks.* Are there particular factors that have an unanticipated drain on resources? Is it possible for you and your staff to 'work smarter' without sacrificing the quality of work and well-being of staff?

4 *Periodically reviewing your area and enacting decision-making processes to support effective function within budget constraints.* Examples include recruiting new staff and funding professional development programs—both of which will increase the capacity of your most important resource, staff.

5 *Using brief and transparent financial reports* that include only key information, while detail can be accessed through electronic records. Interpret these reports in the context of your expert knowledge about your area of work; for example, fluctuations in service activity or changes in personnel.

Obtain a recent financial report from your organisation or an organisation that you know. (The annual report usually has a financial summary of the year.) Is the report brief and easy to understand? Does it reflect your understanding of how the organisation is functioning?

Readiness

Beyond these specific strategies, there are some fundamental mechanisms that will support your readiness for financial management:

1   *Consider whether you need training*—perhaps related to the software that is in use or the database that has been established for the organisation. Do you need to upskill more broadly so you have increased confidence about your capacity for financial management?

> **Linkage**
> Training that is matched to position requirements is important for staff development, as we explored in Chapter 5.

2   *Explore if all hidden costs are factored into financial planning.* This may include program overheads which allow for things like staff training and networking and include a contingency weighting, for contracts that are delayed and projects that need to be refined as they progress from trial to establishment phase. Even if the exact contingency cannot be defined at the outset, it is useful to include this clause in determinations of required income.

3   *Be prepared to rethink how you 'do business'.* Are there better ways? How can the organisation be engaged in a process of reform and change? For example, a reflective approach may avoid reactive decision-making about freezing staff positions, or reducing resource allocation for team building or strategic planning activities.

Case example 8.1 outlines a case from the USA, where innovative management led to improved services and reduced costs, making health care more affordable, effective, and responsive to patient need. In reading through the case, you may wish to ponder the extent to which services were improved, and the real costs—both financial and in terms of staff well-being. If you would like to learn more about this case, see the list of readings for this chapter for the full reference.

CASE EXAMPLE 8.1

Improving financial performance in hospital settings

THE SITUATION

Shrinking payments for health services, and a management review of five hospitals and twenty-three clinics and related services that showed about $150 million in unexplained cost variations.

THE RESPONSE

Hospital chief operating officers were made responsible for the financial performance of all hospitals, supporting their drive to 'identify and implement evidence-based best practices and consolidate administrative services' (p.2). Examples include the consolidation of pharmacy management and purchasing structures, and revising emergency department protocols to cut waiting times and increase volume, along with avoiding unnecessary diagnostic tests and providing lower-cost preventative oriented services to minimise readmissions. Cutting costs is explained as 'part of a comprehensive effort to improve the patient experience' (p.3), through strategies such as reducing the number of steps in admission processes by coordinating patient flow out of and into the hospital. Another strategy is to use lowest-cost settings and providers for service delivery, without compromising the quality of care.

THE OUTCOME

Substantial savings, better care, and a budget situation that supports organisational viability.

THE CONSTRAINTS

Executive leadership is essential and some initiatives may require additional expenditure at first, with savings over time.

Source: Larkin, 2012

Having considered some general aspects of financial management we now turn to an essential planning tool, the budget.

Budgets

A **budget** is a quantified plan, expressed in financial terms, which addresses a defined period of time. It expresses the organisation's strategic plan in measurable terms. Always an estimate nearing reality, the budget describes the cost implications of activities by clarifying available income and required expenditure. Budgets assist with operational planning as managers must consider the balance between resources and expenditure and the need for action when a shortfall is projected. They may also prompt planning decisions about the feasibility of commencing new areas of work as well as maintaining current activities.

Skilled managers will try and maintain a balance between flexibility and accountability in the budget. Flexibility will allow a responsive approach to unforeseen events such as staff changes, project delays and new income. Accountability is necessary to ensure a sound understanding of whether activities are operating within or beyond their resources.

The budget plan is most useful when reviewed periodically (for example, each quarter), with major revisions each year/across multiple years. Individual project budgets are often combined into program- or organisation-based budgets. They are sometimes used to compare performance across different parts of an organisation and this may be reflected in perceptions about management effectiveness. Budgets may be structured in different ways; some pertinent examples are described below.

The line-item budget

The **line-item budget** involves detailing staff and material resources needed for activities. There are generally four categories of expenditure in health and human services: staffing; direct costs; program costs; and indirect costs, or organisational overheads. Staff salaries are for the people who are providing, managing and supporting

Budget
A quantified financial plan for a defined period of time; describes the cost implications of activities by clarifying the expenditure required and resources available.

Line-item budget
Commonly used for projects and programs, this details the staff and material resources (time and money) needed for activities. The four categories are generally staffing, direct costs, program costs and organisational overheads.

planned activities. Direct costs involve things like equipment, computer software and travel, and will vary with the nature of activities. Program costs refer to staff leave entitlements, work cover, and staff time for non-project activities. Organisational overheads include practical resources like rental and upkeep of the premises, car hire, telephones, computer equipment and printing. In larger organisations, these overheads may include expenditure to cover the cost of executive positions and associated expenses.

Linkage
The importance of detailing project activities and associated resources is emphasised in Chapter 7.

The tables below provide templates for a line-item budget. Table 8.1 is for revenue. This includes anticipated and received income, as well as in-kind contributions—possibly involving partner organisations and volunteers.

TABLE 8.1 Line-item budget template, income

INCOME—PROJECT X, MARCH 2014–MARCH 2015	
SOURCE OF ANTICIPATED INCOME	**AMOUNT ($)**
Submitted proposal	
Received income	
Seed funds (internal)	
Government contract	
Philanthropic grant	
In-kind contributions	
Partner organisation A	
Partner organisation B	
Community group (volunteers)	
SUB-TOTAL	$
GST	$
TOTAL	$

The second part of the budget, in Table 8.2, shows expenditure. This is expressed in terms of salary, direct costs, program and organisational overheads. Sometimes program and organisational overheads are combined.

TABLE 8.2 Line-item budget template, expenditure

EXPENDITURE—PROJECT X, MARCH 2014–MARCH 2015			
EXPENDITURE ITEMS	**COST PER DAY/ITEM**	**FTE/NO. ITEMS**	**AMOUNT ($)**
Salary costs			
Project manager			
Clinical workers			
Administrative support			
SUB-TOTAL SALARY COSTS			$

EXPENDITURE ITEMS	COST PER DAY/ITEM	FTE/NO. ITEMS	AMOUNT ($)
Direct costs			
Venue hire			
Travel			
Promotional material			
External consultant			
Other			
SUB-TOTAL DIRECT COSTS			$
Project overheads @ 20% of salary cost			
SUB-TOTAL PROJECT OVERHEADS			$
Organisational overheads @ 20% of salary cost and project overheads			
SUB-TOTAL GST ORGANISATIONAL OVERHEADS			$
Total GST exclusive			$
GST			
TOTAL GST INCLUSIVE			$

A number of other financial tools provide information for the project budget, such as award rates for staff salaries, set amounts for direct costs (for example, petrol allowances for vehicles or accommodation), and overheads set by the organisation.

The level of detail in a budget will depend on the complexity of the activity you are planning and the size of your organisation. In a small organisation, a single line-item budget may be sufficient for all projects. Larger organisations may separate the budget into program areas and have a master budget that includes totals from each program. As the manager responsible for a particular program, you will be expected to stay within your budget. The totals provide a clear indication of which areas of the organisation are doing well financially and areas that are under strain.

The incremental budget

A common approach to budgeting is to use an **incremental budget**. This is developed on the basis of the previous year's budget and assumes that income is stable and only a slight adjustment is required (to account for inflation). Shortcomings of this approach include the mismatch with contract-based income, which has a limited time frame, and the lack of opportunity to review and update activities in line with organisational goals (Mayers, 2004).

Incremental budget
A budget based on the previous year's budget, with the assumption that income is stable and only a slight adjustment is necessary, to account for inflation.

The zero-based budget

Zero-based budget
A budget that is determined prior to each fiscal year; expenditure must be justified regardless of current or past financial conditions. Planned expenditure generally needs to be completed within the funding period.

Zero-based budgeting has become more common in health and human services as organisations adjust to uncertainties in the funding environment. Budgets are returned to zero each year and planned expenditure must be justified in terms of anticipated and received income. This expenditure needs to be completed within the funding period—otherwise it is likely that funds will be absorbed at the organisational level. A result of this is often a rush of spending just before the end of a financial year, for example, in formal financial commitments to planned activities, purchasing equipment and other resources that have been budgeted for but not yet actioned (Weinbach & Taylor, 2011).

Some organisations operate on the basis of received (assured) income and unless funds are signed off before the start of the financial year then expenditure cannot be justified. This is problematic when programs operate within a soft funding environment, as contracts may be formalised at random points in the year. An organisation that lacks flexibility will curtail the entrepreneurial potential of a program because contracts are not in place before the beginning of the fiscal year. More innovative, and context relevant, budgeting practice involves having a budget plan that combines certainty with expectations about the future. This involves a combination of received and anticipated budget planning, involving revenue that is in place as well as additional estimated funds.

Forecasting
The use of past experience to estimate the future availability of funds, while accounting for contextual factors.

Forecasting is a common method, where staff predict future revenue based on past experience.

Finally, it is worth considering budget planning for development activities, such as piloting a new project or introducing a new position to strengthen organisational operations (for example, quality assurance, internal review). These strategies need to be valued by, and of potential benefit for, all parts of the organisation given the budget impacts involved. Ideally, managers will be involved in the decision-making process and kept informed about the financial progress that has been made.

Hidden costs

Budgets are an excellent way to clarify the cost of activities and inform grant proposals and implementation plans. However, some items are often overlooked, particularly in preparing budgets for specific projects. From our experience in preparing and managing budgets we suggest considering the following questions as you prepare and finalise your budget:

- Have you allowed for staff time in preparing the funding proposal, attending interviews about the planned project, and finalising contract negotiations?
- And what about management time? This may include time to develop and maintain relationships with external stakeholders and ensure there is support for project activities across different levels of the organisation.
- What about professional development for staff? Does your budget include funding for staff to attend seminars, training, or network meetings that will enhance their capacity to undertake the project successfully?
- Have you allowed for increased costs as new salary rates come into place and staff advances occur?

- Have you allowed for non-project staff time (for example, attending internal meetings, supervision, annual leave)?
- Have you included time for unforeseen contingencies such as delays in implementation and changes to the project?
- Have you allowed for all direct costs, for example, long-distance telephone calls, catering for stakeholder meetings, or advertising project activities?
- Have you included funds for evaluation?

A thoroughly considered budget is a useful resource to guide planning and expenditure. It is also useful if you need to justify expenditure on unusual items (for example, paying for external specialists or holding a meeting off-site) and to assist in deciding on future budget needs. Regular review is important to understand what is happening financially and decide on adjustments that may be needed.

A major challenge for middle managers is dealing with different project time frames and funding conditions. This translates to times of high and low demand for staff resources and limitations on the continuity of projects and, by default, positions. However, the skilled program manager who is supported by their organisation will be able to plan *across* projects to make the best use of staff resources and develop a program of work that consolidates project activities.

> **Linkage**
> Management includes an ethical obligation regarding financial viability while addressing staff conditions, as we discussed in Chapter 3.

The simplified budget

While detailed budgets are very useful for planning, the budgets used in internal meetings and those submitted as part of funding proposals are often summary versions. Some funders stipulate the format for the budget and this may include combining staff salaries and overhead costs. At organisational level, program budget totals may be a single item in the overall budget. As noted above, the critical factor is the bottom line.

Reporting against the budget

The final element of budget planning is the report of *actual* income and expenditure; the account of what has transpired and how this compares with original expectations.

The **profit and loss statement** is a summary of financial performance over time (usually monthly, quarterly or annually) and it is often used to monitor how the organisation is tracking against the budget plan. It provides a summary of income for a defined period and subtracts the expenses incurred in the same period to calculate the surplus or loss. Community sector organisations do not seek to make a profit, in contrast with private organisations, but there is still strong interest in knowing that expenditure has not exceeded income. A close match between the two, with some reserves, is the desired norm.

The organisation's **balance sheet** will provide a summary of the financial balances at a specific point in time, often the end of the financial year. It is used to guide decisions about whether activities operating at a loss should (and can) be supported by other areas. For example, an activity may require additional resources because it is in development or has suffered unexpected setbacks. Perhaps the activity can be modified to reduce costs. In addition, management may decide that operating at a loss in the short term is acceptable as longer-term benefits (for example, building expertise in the area) are likely. Conversely, a valued program that has operated at a loss for some years may have to be ended.

> **Profit and loss statement**
> A summary of income and expenses for a period (usually monthly, quarterly or annually) to monitor how a project, program or organisation is tracking against the budget plan.

> **Balance sheet**
> A summary of the financial balances at a specific time, often the end of the financial year; used to guide decisions about whether activities operating at a loss can be supported by other areas.

The practitioner profile below is an extension of Chapter 3's profile of Geoff Soma. Geoff provides a clear illustration of how central financial management is to his role as CEO. Financial management activities range from development and monitoring to reporting and integrating this understanding into the management of day-to-day activities.

PRACTITIONER PROFILE 8.2

GEOFF SOMA

CHIEF EXECUTIVE OFFICER, WESTERN REGION ALCOHOL AND DRUG CENTRE (WRAD)

I am active in the preparation, monitoring and interpretation of budgets. I also have regular input into profit and loss reports and balance sheet reporting.

I am responsible for the preparation of project budgets and monitoring and also grant application financial information. I work closely with the treasurer in relation to this area and monitor the general financials on a regular basis.

I believe that it is really important to have a working understanding of all finance-related matters as they are involved in fundraising, service contracts and day to day related matters.

Funds acquisition

Linkage
We explored different sources of funding in Chapter 2.

It is very likely that you will encounter situations where you have a role in funds acquisition, by preparing proposals, promoting the organisation, and perhaps developing relationships with influential people in the community.

Seeking donations and sponsorship

Initial deliberations about funds acquisition involve considering possible funders and their priorities, along with their history of funding in your area of work. Having some funding to cover part of the cost is a useful way to demonstrate that the project already has some viability.

Approaching foundations for funds is a process that involves a number of stages. For example:

- Many foundations require an introductory letter of interest, which may include a one- or two-page proposal outlining 'who you are, what your concern is, what you propose to do, and how much funding you seek' (Brody, 2005, p.316).
- Always follow up written communication with further contact, via telephone or email.
- You may offer to provide a presentation to the foundation staff or board, and suggesting a meeting is worthwhile.

Broader activities are critical to the success of these specific efforts. Ideally your organisation will have a board and executive staff who are opportunistic and strategic about promoting the good work being done and the potential to do more. This involves informal conversations around regular meetings and deliberate strategies such as media interviews and presentations. Having high-profile patrons, projects and staff members, along with a constant media presence, is useful. Holding special events, such as the launch of a new activity or celebration of project success, is another way to inform potential funders about the value of the work you do.

Formal resources, including a lively and informative website, newsletters, brochures and annual reports, along with use of listservs, twitter and similar strategies will help build the organisation's profile. Hopefully, your organisation will have dedicated staff to support these endeavours.

Supporting current and former donors

In addition to cultivating possible new funders, it is important to be responsive to those who already support your organisation. Make sure you convey your appreciation and engage them in what you are doing. Ask your funders to visit the organisation, perhaps during a special event or to see the impact of their financial support. You may develop a long-term relationship with one or more representatives, keeping them informed about project activities, progress and outcomes.

Finally, it is important to consider instances where funding may be available but it is not desirable. First, the amount may be insufficient to justify the administrative work involved, which means your organisation will essentially operate at a loss. Second, it may represent a threat to the image of your organisation. Examples include companies seeking to build the trustworthiness of their products or manufacturers that wish to position their brand as being safe or superior to alternatives. The standing of your organisation in the community and among major funders (including government) and, more fundamentally, the importance of being true to the values of your organisation, will guide what is appropriate in these circumstances.

Writing funding proposals

Preparing proposals for application to an external funding body involves many areas that have been outlined already, particularly budget preparation and project planning. As with these activities, a proposal should demonstrate the need for the project and identify the objectives, activities and desired outcomes. It should also describe resource considerations and steps toward implementation. In addition, you will need to be mindful of what the funder is seeking in how you structure the proposal and the level of detail you provide. In particular, you need to be aware of their priorities (for example, in terms of target groups, intervention types, and principles underpinning project models). Other factors to be addressed in **proposal writing** include the readiness of your organisation to take on this work, and the costs and benefits involved.

As a consequence, there are a number of areas to consider prior to completing and submitting the actual proposal. In deciding whether to prepare a proposal, you may wish to consider the following:

1   Are the principles and focus of the funding scheme consistent with your organisation's strategic plan? Do they match the mission, competencies, goals, and profile of your organisation?

Proposal writing
The steps involved in preparing a submission for an external funding round to match the requirements and expectations of funding guidelines and priorities.

2   Does your organisation need the work? Do you have capacity (staff, management, practical resources) to implement the project? Are you well placed to build this capacity in a short period if the proposal is successful?

3   Does this scheme provide an opportunity to obtain support for an activity/project you have already identified? This could be a partly developed project that has been identified during staff discussions and it may include an innovative service with demonstrated success that is in place elsewhere.

4   Is it strategically important to engage with the funding scheme? For example, when a scheme is likely to morph into recurrent funding or where it may expand into a large area of work.

5   Are the conditions for the scheme realistic? This may include the objectives put forward, the criteria for success, and the time frame for implementation and demonstrated outcomes.

6   Are you familiar with the funder? Does your organisation have a good relationship with the funder/a record of successful funding from them?

7   What is the logical place for the proposed work to sit in your organisation? Which staff will champion the project and should they be involved in writing or critiquing the proposal?

8   What is needed to strengthen the proposal? This may include developing a proposal with partner organisations, demonstrating your expertise in the area, or showing how this project will benefit from being housed by your organisation.

Once these preliminary considerations have been resolved, work on the proposal can begin.

Elements of a proposal

Linkage
Tools for project planning, including logic modelling, are explored in Chapter 7.

Since the advent of competitive tendering, many funding proposals have become minor tomes, as bidders seek to address all criteria put forward by funders and demonstrate the advantage they offer over other organisations. Some elements of a proposal are generic and they can be replicated/adapted for individual schemes. In addition, funders are likely to provide a template for proposals, stipulating the order of items, how the budget is presented, and information on staffing and possibly referees. In some cases, the word length for each section is spelt out. In others, a project logic framework may be involved—where you detail aims, activities, outputs and outcomes. A good initial step is to examine what the funder is seeking and what has already been prepared (for example, in other bids) that can be adapted for this proposal.

The heart of the proposal is the design and description of the project, including aims, objectives and indicators of progress and success. Supporting items include letters of endorsement from referees and collaborating organisations, along with information on your organisation's accreditation status and capacity to manage and respond to risks that may arise during project implementation. Table 8.3 outlines what is commonly needed in a proposal.

TABLE 8.3 Common elements of a funding proposal

ELEMENT	OUTLINE
Title	Relevant to the broad aim of the funding scheme. May include a short and catchy title.
Information on the organisation	Business and financial arrangements and who to contact regarding the proposal.
Summary	Brief, conversational and to the point. Will the funder know what you are planning and at what cost to them? Have you highlighted the unique strengths of your organisation and key staff who will be involved?
The organisation	A one- to two-page spiel on the purpose of your organisation and its strengths.
The team	An introduction to staff and their expertise, along with their roles in the project.
Background	A carefully written and evidence-based section demonstrating that you understand the issues and know about the challenges involved, along with potential strategies for their remediation.
	This is a good place to mention other projects that you are/have been involved in that demonstrate your specialist knowledge and track record.
Project description	Detail on what you intend to provide, linked to objectives and matched to deliverables and outcomes. This may include specific targets, resource requirements and staff contributions, along with equipment and other materials that are necessary for the project to occur. A timeline of activities and milestones for implementation is useful.
Budget	Detail on items of expenditure and costs, including FTE positions and salary rates as well as direct and indirect expenses.
Appendices	Information about your organisation that supports the proposal.
	Other elements that support your bid, such as letters of endorsement or evidence on the success of related projects.

In describing the project, you need a balance between demonstrating your expertise and providing sufficient information so the funder will appreciate what you are proposing and why. This can be challenging, and internal review of the proposal, in addition to working through a number of drafts to reach the final proposal, is helpful. In simple terms, you may consider whether you have clearly addressed the following points:

- *Problem:* Why is this project needed?
- *Goals:* What are you going to do, in broad terms?
- *Objectives:* What are you going to do, in concrete, measurable terms?
- *Approach:* How are you going to do it?

Source: Miner et al., 2011, p.31

While not essential to all proposals, the following may also be useful:
- *Evaluation:* How will you demonstrate progress against your objectives?
- *Value adding:* What do you bring to the proposal that adds to the resources provided by the funder?
- *Sustainability:* What steps do you propose (or have in place) that will support the continuation of project activities beyond the current funding round?

Effective proposals

Questions such as those shown below may be used to assess the effectiveness of proposals and they are worth reflecting on during proposal development:

- Does the project team have demonstrated competence in the area?
- Is your organisation aware of and supportive of the planned work?
- Have you presented a strong argument about the need for this project and what it will deliver?
- Is the proposal feasible?
- Are there other funds/in-kind support that will supplement what is being proposed?
- What is the scope for sustainability of the project beyond this funding round?
- Is the proposal attractive to look at and easy to read? Have you avoided jargon, while addressing the funder's requirements?
- Is the budget realistic, transparent, and does it address budget requirements specified by the funder?
- Have you explained how you will record the results of the project and communicated this to the funder?

Supporting activities

Developing a relationship with your potential funder is essential. This involves making contact prior to submitting the proposal, so you are clear on what is sought and have provided an indication of your interest and capacity. Contact following submission is a mix of dealing with practical issues (did the proposal reach its destination? when might you expect to hear something?) and making the most of formal opportunities (interviews and presentations) to show that:

Linkage
In the last chapter we considered the importance of communication for successful project management. In Chapter 10 we further explore the essential role of communication within and beyond the organisation.

- you know what you are doing
- what you are offering is what is needed
- you are well placed to deliver what you have offered
- you are professional, flexible and reliable.

Managers in funding organisations, like the rest of us, seek a positive engagement with their counterpart during the selection process and project implementation, and in the realisation of their objectives. In our experience, the most important aspect of the funding process, from development to implementation and resolution, is communication.

Your organisation's profile

As touched on earlier, a broad set of activities will assist in building the funder's awareness of your organisation. This includes having high-profile staff on board and patrons who praise your work, along with the informal networking that occurs in practice, policy, and academically oriented meetings and engagements. A common concern for health and human service organisations is the failure to celebrate the good work that is being done. Does your website promote your work? Do you disseminate markers of success such as positive outcomes for clients or the successful delivery of new and innovative programs? Are you actively engaged in spruiking the projects in your workplace and why they matter? These efforts will provide a platform that supports specific proposals during the review process.

Proposal review

The first step in proposal review is to determine whether administrative requirements of the funding round have been met. For example, was the proposal submitted on time, in the right format, using the designated template? Further to this, does your organisation meet eligibility criteria, such as not-for-profit or accreditation status, and does it have the necessary insurance? Once these items are addressed, a committee will start the review process. The committee will generally include senior staff in the relevant policy area, those in associated areas who can provide an independent yet informed assessment, and staff that look after conditions of procurement and contract administration. One or more external parties may also be involved. They generally start by scoring the proposals against stipulated criteria and this information forms the basis for short-listing and final selection.

Funding information generally includes a set of objectives that proposals must address, or there may be a set of evaluation criteria and associated weightings. A hypothetical set of items is shown in Table 8.4.

TABLE 8.4 Possible criteria for the evaluation of a funding proposal

CRITERIA	WEIGHTING
1 Proposed project is evidence-based and addresses objectives of the initiative	50%
2 Personnel have a track record of excellence in this or a related area of work	20%
3 Demonstrated understanding of challenges in this area of service delivery along with strategies supporting success	10%
4 Evidence of innovation	5%
5 Demonstrated organisational capacity to deliver quality products on time and within budget	10%
6 Value for money	5%
Total	100%

As you may appreciate, judgments against these criteria are quite subjective and there is a strong reliance on the perspective of committee members. In turn, their views may be affected by broader factors such as the organisation's profile. Sometimes short-listed applicants are invited to an interview where they have an opportunity to expand on their proposal. This may involve a formal presentation and it is often about clarifying elements of the proposal. Knowing your work and being ready to articulate why it is so important and how it fits within a broader program of activity is important at this stage.

Linkage
Chapter 7 has some
useful planning tools
for this stage of the
process.

Each application for funding is an opportunity to learn about the process and build relationships that may prove beneficial for later submissions. Maintaining a positive and constructive perspective will assist in getting the most from your efforts. If successful, your work has really just begun: resourcing the project and planning for implementation will now be the focus.

Before turning to accreditation, we meet a community health practitioner, who provides an insightful perspective on the many tasks involved in managing projects and staff in this busy environment.

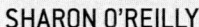

PRACTITIONER PROFILE 8.3

SHARON O'REILLY

CLINICAL SERVICES MANAGER, BAYSIDE MEDICARE LOCAL

Position

My background is as a clinician—nurse and psychotherapist working in the alcohol and drug sector in direct clinical service delivery. I am currently employed as the Clinical Services Manager for the Bayside Medicare Local. The Medicare Local Model is a new initiative of health sector reform impacting primary health in Australia. The aim of the Medicare Local Model is to integrate primary health services in the community to effect better access and outcomes for clients. My role involves the management of a community based specialist drug treatment service specifically focusing on people with complex needs and marginalised populations. Additionally the role involves the management of a mental-health nurse program, with a pool of mental-health nurses working in the community—in GP clinics with clients with severe and persistent mental-health issues. The role includes the management of a range of projects that do not involve direct clinical service delivery, so the role is diverse.

Typical day

A typical day involves checking in with the clinical services initially. It may be that trouble shooting both client and staffing issues needs to be sorted out to progress with the day. I am generally involved in at least two meetings a day on site or with other stakeholders or government departments. In my peak body role I am a representative voice for the alcohol and drug treatment sector; in my Bayside Medicare Local role I am the representative of the clinical services—alcohol and drug and mental health for the catchment, which services a population of 65,000. Provision of supervision over clinical services, project management and clinical practice review are also important aspects of my role.

I am involved in the executive of the Bayside Medicare Local so I participate in the strategic development of the organisation. So, my day is generally prioritising a range of scheduled and unscheduled commitments in an effort to meet the objectives of all programs, while maintaining a cohesive and harmonious staff group. From time to time there may be a critical incident that has to be managed and reported, with the process of staff debriefing and support foremost in this instance. Occasionally there may be an issue related to drug use or mental health in the local community that requires a media response—I am one of the 'go to' people for these responses. From time to time I am involved in writing articles, conference abstracts and presentations and funding submission or tenders. So, depending on the external environment and the time of year, these areas of work may take priority over day-to-day management.

Challenges

One of the greatest challenges is how to rapidly prioritise demands on my time, meeting staff needs so that client care is attended to. I often receive random requests for reports on a range of issues from population health, emerging issues and trends etc., for higher level strategic responses, or media requests for comment on a particular emerging issue. I have to juggle priorities constantly, so remaining focused and alert is the key.

Skills and qualities

Basic management skills are fundamental to the job. Empathy for the community that you work with is essential, as is a high level of emotional intelligence so I am able to respond as best I can in any given situation. Recognition of how to use opportunities that are highlighted through failure or lack of anticipated successes is essential. A strong sense of perseverance in the face of adversity and the ability to model this to the staff group is important. Finally, and most importantly, a sense of humour and a capacity to laugh at yourself is essential.

Lessons learnt

When I started out as a manager I wish I had a greater understanding of the structural organisational requirements related to staff and program management. When I transitioned from a clinical to a management role, resources were not available to provide me with those management frameworks. It is a common assumption that if you are a good clinician you are automatically competent at higher level work. Over time I have studied further in this area and been trained in specialist areas of management. My day-to-day experiences in a clinical management role have also developed and informed my practice.

I have also learnt that thinking you are in control of a situation is not a reality; you do the best you can and make the most of the opportunities that present. Also, lack of success in a range of circumstances can be helpful in informing how to best go about challenges in the future—learn from failures to build success.

Accreditation

Formal accreditation is a process involving self-assessment and independent review, to assess whether an organisation meets approved standards of care. These **standards** define the quality of care that services are expected to provide: some apply to organisational functions and generic aspects of service delivery, while others are specific to particular types of service (for example, aged care or disability).

Accreditation focuses on compliance with the standards and mechanisms for continuous quality improvement. There are generic standards, those specific to particular services, and others that carry an expectation of innovation and excellence. Organisations are expected to engage in a cycle of reflection, action and review that contributes to an environment of learning and improvement.

The accreditation process is ideally embedded in operational management and part of regular discussions on how the organisation is performing. A formal accreditation review occurs every few years and it combines an internal process of self-assessment with an external process that is managed by an independent body and often includes one or more peer reviewers. You may recall the discussion on accreditation in Chapter 5, when

Standard
An explicit statement of the level of care consumers should be able to expect from services.

Accreditation
A process used to assess whether the quality of services provided meets approved standards of care.

the Productivity Commission recommended the establishment of a national evaluation and monitoring framework, as a vehicle for regulating how services operate and to what effect. The accreditation process may be seen as an evolution of this development. The standards framework stipulates expectations and the accreditation review process examines the extent to which organisations comply with these expectations.

Administering organisations

The Quality Improvement Council (QIC) is a major standards and accreditation body that involves more than 450 organisations from Australia and New Zealand in a three-year cycle of review and improvement. Organisations that are interested in being involved contact one of the licensed providers employed by QIC and enter into a contract with the council. The contract includes resources to support the organisation's readiness for formal review and there is an opportunity for staff to be trained as reviewers.

The council has developed a set of standards that are applicable to most community-based services. There are 18 standards, which address three areas: building quality organisations; providing quality services and programs; and managing the external environment. Box 8.1 includes a summary of these standards.

BOX 8.1

Health and Community Services Standards, 6th edition, Quality Improvement Council

QUALITY IMPROVEMENT AND COMMUNITY SERVICES ACCREDITATION (QICSA)

Section 1	Building quality organisations
Standard 1.1	Governance
Standard 1.2	Management systems
Standard 1.3	Human resources
Standard 1.4	Physical resources
Standard 1.5	Financial management
Standard 1.6	Knowledge management
Standard 1.7	Risk assessment and management
Standard 1.8	Legal and regulatory compliance
Standard 1.9	Safety and quality integration
Section 2	Providing quality services and programs
Standard 2.1	Assessing and planning
Standard 2.2	Focusing on positive outcomes
Standard 2.3	Ensuring cultural safety and appropriateness
Standard 2.4	Confirming consumer rights
Standard 2.5	Coordinating services and programs

Section 3	Sustaining quality external relationships
Standard 3.1	Service agreements and partnerships
Standard 3.2	Collaboration and strategic positioning
Standard 3.3	Incorporation and contribution to good practice
Standard 3.4	Community and professional capacity building

Source: www.qic.org.au (used with permission)

The council also endorses standards put forward by other organisations, which are specific to particular areas of work. Examples include standards from the Centres against Sexual Assault (Victorian Government), Te Wana Programme Mental Health Standards Module (Health Care Aotearoa NZ), and psychiatric support services (Government of South Australia).

Each standard is broken into specific items, which form the basis for internal audit and action to ensure compliance prior to external review. Examples of these items range from ensuring policies are up to date and accessible, to systems for storing medication.

The QIC has recently merged with its licensed providers (Quality Improvement Community Services Accreditation Incorporated, Quality Management Services) along with Quality in Practice (a subsidiary of Australian General Practice Limited) to form a new company, the 'Quality Innovation Performance' (QIP), which will become a subsidiary of Australian General Practice Limited. The new company will provide accreditation for all types of health and human services.

Accreditation in the community and broader health care sectors is an expanding area and the QIP aims to provide 'streamlined, value adding accreditation services across the entire health and human services continuum from community services and primary care to secondary and tertiary health organisations' (Quality Improvement Council, 2013). Streamlining accreditation and review processes, to include different service types and settings for delivery, may provide for a more efficient system.

Implications for managers/readiness for accreditation

Unsurprisingly, activities supporting the accreditation process work best when the whole organisation is involved. One approach that supports this perspective is **total quality management (TQM)**. A basic premise of TQM is that service quality should be defined by the needs and wishes of clients.

TQM uses the principle of participative management and holds that staff will operate better if they have a role in decision-making in areas that affect them and their work. Decision-making groups are formed, with membership based on the 'knowledge, experience and/or expertise' that members can contribute to a decision (Weinbach & Taylor, 2011, p.68). Not everyone is involved in every decision, and group membership relies not only on individual capacity but also power structures that have been established in the organisation.

In this approach, leaders initiate improvements in the organisation and the responsibility for their implementation is shared among all levels of staff. In practical terms, managers will find themselves being held accountable for identifying areas

Total quality management
A process of improvement that stems from the premise that service quality should be defined by the needs and wishes of clients. Initiated by leaders in the organisation and involves all members, including clients.

needing attention and those with scope for innovation, as well as reporting on advances that have been made in the implementation of identified improvements.

The involvement of trained peer reviewers in the accreditation process is consistent with the principle of participatory management. A review process involving someone with practice experience in a similar service may be more accepted than using reviewers who are not familiar with the service content.

The perspective often missing in this process is that of the consumer. Accreditation requirements may include standards about consumer input to decision-making, and consumer feedback processes, but there are many areas of health and human services that need to do more work on adequately representing and considering consumer perspectives. Before continuing our exploration of accreditation, we shall look at what is involved in managing service quality in an alcohol and drug centre.

PRACTITIONER PROFILE 8.4

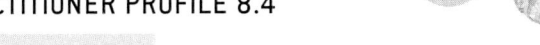

MELISSA ELLIOTT

ASSOCIATE DIRECTOR OF QUALITY, TURNING POINT ALCOHOL AND DRUG CENTRE, EASTERN HEALTH

Position

In the past three years my role has been as an Associate Director of Quality ('quality manager') within a large health service. The quality team consists of approximately twenty staff. The team is made up of people from different backgrounds and the quality directors have specialised in the areas of risk, safety, patient relations and reform. A significant amount of time is spent meeting with the broader quality team to discuss the development and implementation of new systems and processes. My role is to then review, adapt and implement the new systems into my program area.

My role entails working with a program to ensure it:

- establishes and sustains operating systems that are consistent with the organisational performance management framework and the clinical governance framework
- effectively participates in strategic, service and operations, and business planning processes, and complies with planning and reporting requirements
- effectively manages risks in accordance with the risk management system
- achieves its continuous improvement targets and priorities in accordance with the continuous improvement framework, methodology and reporting requirements.

I manage patient quality and safety in accordance with the patient quality and safety management system including:

- standards for patient quality and safety including policies, guidelines, standards of practice, performance indicators
- development and implementation of the patient experience of care program, and consumer, carer and community participation
- incident management (monitoring and management of variation and error in the quality and safety of clinical care)
- monitoring and evaluation of safety and quality of clinical care, including audit and legislative compliance.

Typical day

A typical day can entail long periods spent at the desk writing reports, reviewing incident documentation, undertaking audits, documenting, and developing practice guidelines to support staff in performing their role and attending meetings.

My program has increased in size over the past twelve months with the addition of two new services. This has resulted in my role being involved in increased service planning, accreditation responsibilities, incidents to review, development of practice guidelines, and gap analysis etc.

Throughout the day I work collaboratively with the management staff to ensure key systems and processes are clearly documented and continuously improved. This involves individual and team meetings with senior staff to ensure the development of policies is consistent with the needs of the program.

Challenges

As a quality manager it can feel like we are constantly introducing a new system or process and it can be difficult to keep abreast of the continuous change ourselves, let alone ensuring staff are aware of the change.

Sometimes my role can be perceived as the driver for developing systems and activities to get us through accreditation, when continuous improvement should be part of routine work and recognised as part of an organisation's strategic vision.

The role of a quality manager can be quite a solitary one; at times the activities are supported by upper management and other times they are seen as an unnecessary burden.

Linkage
Change management is explored in Chapter 9.

Skills and qualities

A quality manager needs to have a solid knowledge of health care standards to support the program/area in meeting the appropriate standards, guidelines and legislation.

The individual needs to embrace organisational change, as the health environment is constantly shifting to meet new strategies and priorities. This role is often involved in developing and implementing new system processes and at times is seen as responsible for changes in direction. The person plays the role of a foot soldier delivering the message, and it can seem like a battleground out there at times. This role requires the ability to persuade and sell the new package.

In this role it is crucial that individuals work collaboratively with the senior staff across the organisation so that service planning and the implementation, monitoring and evaluation of service objectives occur. It is therefore necessary to develop effective working relationships with managers and staff to implement a client-focused team approach to ensure continuous quality improvement is embedded in the organisation.

Lessons learnt

I have had over twenty years' experience in the field of health—seventeen years at a large teaching hospital, and the last five years in a smaller centre which is part of a large health service. Of my twenty-two years, sixteen have been spent in management roles and I have learnt to adapt to the ever-changing health system and expectations of the management role. Coping with change is routine in the health sector and I have learnt to view change as a positive aspect of the workplace.

Evidence on accreditation

While tremendous energy is being expended on accreditation, evidence on its effectiveness is limited and somewhat conflicted. An international review of the literature in this area suggested possible benefits from accreditation in terms of improved organisational processes (Hinchcliff et al., 2012). However, the key finding is that high quality research examining the benefits and limitations of accreditation is needed.

In our experience, the process has encouraged a more reflective approach to service quality. Conversely, risk management and quality assurance may overwhelm strategies directly related to client care. In addition, the limited nature of the review process precludes a truly rigorous evaluation of organisational function and effectiveness. While accreditation does not strive to achieve this latter objective, it may obscure problems in organisations that have been given a 'clean bill of health'. As with many processes that aim to improve services, the quality and commitment of managers and leaders in the organisation, along with the capacity for dedicated resources, are critical to make the most of accreditation.

REFLECTION EXERCISE

The above practitioner profile highlights what is involved in a quality management role along with particular challenges that may be encountered. Read through the profile again, noting factors that may help or hinder accreditation.

SUMMARY OF KEY ISSUES

Regular review, benchmarks, reporting, and ongoing planning and adjustment are important for financial management. Budgets are quantified financial plans and they require both a systematic approach (which accounts for all income and revenue) and flexibility to accommodate unforeseen developments.

Funding opportunities should be reviewed to determine the organisation's capacity to provide what is needed. Proposals are often structured according to the conditions put forward by funders, and having some generic material that can be adapted for specific proposals will reduce the work involved in developing individual proposals. Activities that promote the organisation are important to support the review process and each application for funding is an opportunity to document organisational potential and learn about the submission process.

Accreditation is a review process aimed at improving the quality of services, and includes regular external review. The benefits of accreditation may be maximised by embedding development and review processes into all aspects of service management and operation.

PRACTICE ACTIVITIES

1   Income and expenses

Many organisations include a summary of income and expenditure in their annual reports. You may wish to explore how this information is presented by accessing an annual report of an organisation via their website (see, for example, www.adf.org.au). It is worth noting the categories used and the main sources of funding, and considering the management implications for budgeting and funds acquisition.

2 Funding proposals

A useful way to become familiar with funding proposals is to examine one that has been completed by a colleague. If possible, read through the funder's documentation as well. How would you rate the proposal?

3 Getting to know accreditation

Is your organisation involved in accreditation? If so, it would be useful for you to speak to the individual or group that is championing the process and consider the relevance of this work to your role. You may also wish to explore the website of the Quality Improvement Council for further information: www.qic.org.au.

FURTHER READING

The basics of accounting

Mayers, R. S. (2004). *Financial Management for Non-Profit Human Service Organizations* (2nd edn), Springfield, Illinois: Charles C. Thomas.

Financial management challenges

Carson, E. & Kerr, L. (2012). *Marketisation of Human Service Delivery: Implications for the Future of the Third Sector in Australia,* Paper presented at the ISTR Conference, Siena, Italy.

Working with others to increase project potential

Larkin, H. (2012). 'Smart Money Management', *Trustee: The Journal for Hospital Governing Boards, 65,* 13–14, pp.19–20.

Miner, J. T., Miner, L. E. & Griffith, J. (2011). *Collaborative Grantseeking. A Guide to Designing Projects, Leading Partners, and Persuading Sponsors,* USA: Greenwood.

PART
3

CONNECTION AND ENGAGEMENT

The practice cases in this part are:

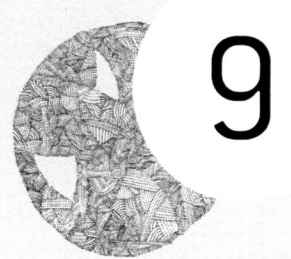

Change Management

OVERVIEW

This chapter will:

- describe different types of organisational change
- explore reasons for engaging with, and making, the choice to change
- discuss 'tried and true' approaches and new trends in managing change
- consider strategies for managing change in complex organisational environments
- encourage reflection on issues of power in the change process.

This chapter is concerned with managing change successfully and ethically in the current context of health and human services. On completion readers will be familiar with different types of change and factors to consider when making choices about introducing and responding to organisational change.

KEY TERMS

anticipated change	force field analysis
change drivers	market research approach
change management	planned change
community audit approach	stakeholder analysis
emergent change	unplanned change

Change in context

Constant, rapid and frequently unpredictable change characterises contemporary life. Change signals innovation, new ideas and better practices, and represents a fresh start; it is exciting and inspiring. Change can also be confusing, disempowering and exhausting. What feelings and reactions do you have when you think about going through significant change in your personal or professional life?

Throughout this text we have explored many topics, skills, issues and methods that are linked to managing change. For example, Chapter 1 discussed the development of ideas about management since industrialisation changed the way work is organised. In Chapter 2 we explored external contingencies that impel organisations to change, such as the introduction of new public management to the health and human services, and the effects of the resultant shifts in policy and funding processes. In Chapter 3 we considered the importance of creating a positive and flexible organisational culture that is responsive to innovation, change and growth. In Chapter 4 we reflected on issues relating to power and authority and the role of leadership in taking organisations towards new directions, and in Chapter 5 we discussed succession planning. Chapters 6 and 7 looked at planning, analysis and evaluation tools for setting strategic directions and translating goals and visions into practice, and Chapter 8 observed the changes to quality assurance mechanisms arising from the introduction of accreditation standards. Here, we look at responses towards change and different types of change, some 'tried and true' **change management** strategies, actions and effects of power, and recent approaches that take account of the complex and change-driven world in which we live and work.

Change management
A systematic and structured process of moving people and organisations from one state to a desired future state.

The relentless drive for change in organisational environments has translated into change management becoming a dominant function of managing organisations, and it is now widely recognised as a defining leadership capability. Almost everyone you encounter in the community services sector has a story to tell about a recent or current significant organisational change process. Unfortunately these stories are rarely positive, suggesting that knowledge, skills and practices in managing change—particularly in relation to the use of power and authority—requires attention (Hughes & Wearing, 2013; Ozanne & Rose, 2013). To begin, let us reflect on the way we think about change, and how this perception affects our response to it.

REFLECTION EXERCISE

Think about a significant change that you have been through in either your personal or professional life during the past two years.

1   What feelings and reactions do you have when you think about it?
2   How positive and/or negative and/or neutral are they?
3   How did the change come about; was it your own choice or was it imposed?
4   How did you perceive the use of power and authority in the change process? Was it a disempowering experience for you? If so, why do you think this was so?
5   Does it make a difference if it is yourself or someone else who makes the decision that change is needed?
6   Write down three words that you associate with change.

Attitudes and feelings towards change

Change sits at the heart of practice in health and human service organisations. Influencing positive change in the lives of clients defines the work of community sector professionals (Ozanne & Rose, 2013). As we observed in Chapter 2, a distinguishing feature of community service organisations is the value placed on improving individual, community and social well-being (Lewis et al., 2012). Practice theories and models are guided by goals to establish the most appropriate and effective ways to transition from a problematic or undesirable situation to a more desirable state of affairs; such as overcoming addiction or abuse, exiting homelessness by finding stable housing, or improving well-being by accessing health services.

Despite competency in dealing with varying degrees of change and crisis in the lives of other people, practitioners often have a less than positive response to, and experience of, organisational change in their own workplaces. Objections by workers frequently relate to being overwhelmed with the rate and demand of change, and concerns over negative impacts for the client group and themselves. Hughes and Wearing suggest that much of this resistance is linked to the disempowering effects of the recent rapid pace of change impelled by managerialism across the public service sector, and its implementation as a top-down process, with limited opportunity for participation. At the same time, they observe that managerialist changes reinforce the need for workers to remain committed to their professional values by participating in organisational change for the ongoing benefit of their clients (Hughes & Wearing, 2013).

Even though—or perhaps because—much recent change in health and human services has been led by a managerialist agenda, there has been a shift away from scientific management approaches, which treat change as a necessarily imposed technical process, and a shift towards attending to the way people respond emotionally to the idea of change, and how this affects their engagement with it. Of course, this is largely dependent on the type and dimension of change.

Types of change

There are myriad types of organisational change. Ozanne and Rose observe that change can be 'symbolic and real; planned and unplanned, incremental and sudden, major and minor, externally and internally driven' (2013, p.205). Other writers distinguish between change as a continuous process related to the growth or development of an organisation, and change that is discontinuous with the past and innovative, such as a new type of service, or a new organisation or service system (Osborne & Brown, 2005).

The type of change also varies according to purpose, organisational culture and climate, timing, staff morale, resources, policies and processes, levels of participation, management and leadership skills, and the internal and external environment. These factors influence whether or not the change is experienced as positive, and therefore they need to be considered when selecting an implementation process (Lawler & Bilson, 2010).

The following practice example describes a change scenario. As you read it think about the various types of change that might be involved.

PRACTICE EXAMPLE 9.1

Complexities of change in statewide reform

In 2011, amid a declining public sector budget and rising demand for services, the Department of Human Services in Victoria (DHS) determined that a new approach was needed in the way people with complex and ongoing needs were case managed. The challenge to reduce costs and increase services required not only changes to service delivery, but also to the structure of the department.

The document that communicates the rationale and outlines the proposed changes, 'Human Services: The Case for Change' (State Government of Victoria, 2011), identifies the need to make the transition from a welfare response to a 'more personalised and holistic response', and notes that this will require 'breaking down the silos that had grown up around specific areas of disadvantage'. The reforms were implemented in December 2012.

This statewide transformation involved major structural change, for example, service system regions were redefined and geographical boundaries were redrawn. This was accompanied by commensurate adjustments to the organisational structure. Middle management positions were reduced, and front-line workers were increased.

Changes were also made to service delivery. Previously, cases were allocated on the basis of client type being matched with a particular service area, such as children, youth and families; disability; or housing. In the new system, service is provided on the basis of individual need: clients can now access services, as appropriate, from across all DHS areas. For example, a client with an intellectual disability under the 'old' system would have been allocated to disability services, and would have been case managed by a disability services worker, with access to 'disability' services. Now, a client with an intellectual disability might receive services from the areas of housing and/or children, youth and families, as well as disability, together with the option to access a range of external service providers, according to the services that they choose themselves, and according to assessed need.

This multi-level, multi-dimensional change is contextualised within wider statewide reforms that encourage partnership arrangements and seek to build an integrated community service system. The guiding vision is for all public services to work together to provide a holistic response across the community and government sectors.

Linkage
As this chapter continues, we will return to this practice example to reflect on aspects of organisational change linked with it.

This complex scenario includes many elements of change, with implications across the entire organisation (which is obviously a large bureaucracy) and the wider service system, and at multiple levels, from clients to state government. You may have experienced government-driven, sector-wide restructuring in your own area of work.

REFLECTION EXERCISE

How many different types of change were you able to identify in the practice example? It may help to think about areas of change—where might changes have been necessary in the transition from a 'silo' to a holistic service delivery structure?

You may recall the discussion on different forms of power in Chapter 4. What forms of power do you see operating in this scenario: power *with*, power *over* and/or power *for*? Which aspects of the changes would you consider to be productive operations of power and which might be oppressive? Who will benefit from these changes?

Types of change are often described in competing terms. Above we listed 'symbolic and real, incremental and sudden, major and minor' change (Ozanne & Rose, 2013). Tolbert and Hall (2009) refer to 'technical and adaptive', and 'transformational and incremental' change, and Donovan and Jackson (1991) describe 'routine and crisis' change. This tendency to arrange types of change as oppositional pairs is perhaps reflective of the forces of resistance and compulsion that inevitably occur when any form of significant change is proposed. After all, at its broadest level, change is defined as a shift from one state to a different state. If we return to the concept of power discussed in Chapter 1, which understands power as a productive action—a force or energy that causes things to happen through a will to produce and enable—it is clear that the presence of change is evidence of power in operation. In other words, change occurs through the actions of power. This is why forces acting upon and resisting one another are heightened and highlighted in transitional states, particularly when the change is significant, and when change is seen and experienced as advantaging some and disadvantaging or marginalising others.

Capacity to predict change can have a profound effect on how it is received, whether or not it is positive, and the success of its implementation. The degree to which an organisation and the people within it are able to exercise control (power) over the rate, intensity and form of the change is linked with opportunity and ability to prepare for it.

Anticipated and emergent change

A popular way of describing the difference between types of change is to use the oppositional binary—planned and unplanned change, with planned change considered to be preferable to unplanned change. **Planned change** is deliberate, and results from systematic organisational processes, such as strategic planning and quality cycles. **Unplanned change** often, but not always, emerges from outside the organisation, with little warning; the organisation, program area or work group is required to respond to circumstances that were not anticipated, planned or desired.

Osborne and Brown (2005) describe unplanned change as **emergent change**. We also use this term because it challenges the negative connotations that 'unplanned' elicits. Additionally, even though the call to change may be unexpected, a planned approach can always be applied in response. Relatedly, our preferred term for change which is planned is **anticipated change** because, in our view, it is the predictability of the drivers for change, rather than the implementation process, that distinguishes these two types. In the health and human services, skills and knowledge for positively managing both anticipated and emergent change are essential for successful organisational development.

Anticipated change assumes a higher degree of control at the organisational level, involving a linear, rational process, such as:

1 Identifying and assessing the need for something to be done differently.
2 Determining how this might be best addressed.
3 Costing the change.
4 Designing a strategy for implementation.
5 Monitoring the effects of the change.
6 Making adjustments according to evaluation and feedback.

Planned change
Change that is implemented through a managed planning process.

Unplanned change
Change that results from unanticipated events, and for which no planning process is implemented.

Emergent change
Occurs as a result of external factors, or arises with little warning. There is usually no (or limited) opportunity for influencing the nature of the change, or planning for its implementation.

Anticipated change
Change which is planned for in advance.

Linkage
This sequence may seem familiar from Chapters 6 and 7, when we looked at strategic and project planning models.

It can be helpful to consider the above six-step process according to three decision-making phases:

1   Deciding that change is required and what change is needed.
2   Deciding how the change will be resourced, implemented and monitored.
3   Deciding the need for further change.

Table 9.1 aligns these six planning steps with the three-phase decision-making process. Although this is a simplified schema, focusing on decision-making in relation to the planning process highlights the choice that is involved. Importantly, wherever choice is exercised, there is opportunity to decide not to proceed.

TABLE 9.1 Planning and decision-making process for change

PLANNING STEPS		DECISION-MAKING PHASES	
1	Identify and assess the need for change.	1	Identify whether change is/is not required.
2	Determine how this might be best addressed.		If change is needed, determine nature of change.
3	Cost the change.	2	Identify resources.
4	Design implementation strategy.		Determine how change will be implemented and monitored.
5	Monitor and evaluate the change	3	Identify need for further changes.
6	Make further adjustments according to evaluation and feedback.		

To change or not to change?

In an environment characterised by constant change, and a culture that invests so much value in it, there is a high risk of organisations engaging in change for the sake of change, rather than because it is the best solution to the identified problem (Tolbert & Hall, 2009). It is also important to act cautiously and not leap to assumptions about the type of change required. Pressure to engage in change is exacerbated by the perception (and often the reality) that these decisions are out of the control of the manager and/or the organisation.

Adopting a planned approach for responding to emergent calls for change can assist to mitigate these traps. This can also contribute to shifting the power base, increase your sense of control and, importantly, help to avoid unnecessary change, which might be costly in terms of fiscal and human resources, organisational credibility, and in the consequences for client groups. Some believe this propensity to engage in change for the sake of change is evident in the way governments have implemented major structural reform in departments and services, when a focus on processes and attitudes may have been more appropriate (Checkland, 1999, cited in Lawler & Bilson, 2010).

For this reason it is important to be adequately informed, to exercise careful consideration, and to take a planned approach to change implementation wherever possible. Various approaches can be applied to decision-making about anticipated change; here we outline two popular options: strategic planning and survey approaches.

REFLECTION EXERCISE

Consider the above thoughts on 'change for the sake of change' in relation to the description of the restructure of the Department of Human Services in Practice example 9.1.

The strategic planning approach

Strategic planning has become a popular management process for identifying how, where and why an organisation needs to change.

Strategic planning, as we have identified, utilises a range of organisational environment analysis tools, which assist in orienting the status quo of the organisation and informing direction; these include SPELT and SWOC analysis. Before expanding, it is worth spending a few moments reviewing what these acronyms stand for, and how they are applied.

Linkage
Strategic planning is discussed in detail in Chapter 6.

REFLECTION EXERCISE

Complete the details for SPELT and SWOC in the table below. Reflect on the advantages and disadvantages for each. How might each of these analysis tools inform change?

TABLE 9.2 SPELT and SWOC analysis review

	SPELT	SWOC
Full term		
Application		
Advantages		
Disadvantages		

As we have acknowledged, strategic plans provide a practical, logical and clear map for a shared organisational direction. Ideally built on an informed and comprehensive analysis of the internal and external organisational environment, and developed through a participatory process, they establish and articulate organisational values and vision, outline areas for growth and development, and inform program and operational plans. Kettner et al. (2013, p.37) observe:

> To be effective organisations periodically need to step back, examine what they are doing, and determine whether changes should be considered if they are to be effective, especially in ever-changing environments.

In terms of capacity to effectively bring about organisational change, strategic planning has come under criticism because it is too often based on a hierarchical framework, and controlled from the governance and executive level—an exercise of power *over*, in other words. Another criticism, which we have also previously noted, is concern over the strategic plan becoming an end in itself, and thus failing to be implemented (Lewis et al., 2012). Furthermore, although driven toward a vision of the future, the environment analysis (SPELT and SWOC) on which the plan is founded is frequently contained in the present, and this hinders innovative change (Osborne & Brown, 2005). With the current health and human services environment changing so rapidly, a three-to-five-year plan cannot accurately reflect or anticipate unexpected, externally imposed requirements to change. One way that organisations are addressing the unpredictability of the environment, without abandoning a strategic approach, is to incorporate a capacity to respond to contingencies within the strategic plan.

To be effective, managerialist approaches to planning for change need to be well informed and relevant; this requires decisions based on thorough research into need within and beyond the organisation. Ideally, data relating to service-user needs and program performance will be incorporated into decision-making, and workers from across the organisation and community stakeholders will have an opportunity to contribute and participate in meaningful ways (Kettner et al., 2013).

Survey approaches

Using surveying in planning for change involves gathering data generated within the organisation. Osborne and Brown (2005) describe this as the market research approach. Another method involves surveying the needs of community beyond the organisation and current areas of service delivery. This is known as the community audit approach.

Market research approach
Gathering and analysing organisational data to determine whether client needs are being effectively met.

The **market research approach** was developed by Kotler and Andreason (Osborne & Brown, 2005) and involves gathering and analysing organisational data to determine the extent to which client needs are being effectively met. Findings are communicated in easy-to-read formats to key personnel, and then used to inform the development of a plan of action. The process is costed throughout in relation to available resources.

Researching the 'market' or 'target group' is integrated to some extent into all well-planned change processes; for example, in Chapter 7 we discussed this approach in relation to needs assessment. At the same time, it has been criticised for being demanding on financial, time and staffing resources, and because it is limited by a primary focus on current service users and immediate context, rather than potential and future projections. The survey method is predominantly about managing incremental change through monitoring service delivery, and measuring expressed and felt need. It does not aim to respond to wider community needs, nor to strategically position the organisation (Osborne & Brown, 2005). On the other hand, as we also discussed in Chapter 7, the rising emphasis on quality assurance, evidence-based practice and program evaluation promotes the importance of monitoring service effectiveness and measuring need, making this a pragmatic option for determining requirements for evolutionary change.

Community audit approach
A survey method that seeks information about community perceptions of need, demographic details and other services to assist in determining the most appropriate and beneficial programs and services for the community.

Community audit approaches are in many ways similar to market research or needs assessment in planning. They differ in that they extend surveying beyond the organisation to seek community perceptions of services and programs. Such models are informed by community development principles, and a high degree of emphasis is placed on stakeholder engagement and participation. In some versions, information is not only gathered about the services that a community would like to have provided, but demographic data is also used, along with service system mapping to assist in objectively determining the most appropriate and beneficial programs and services to introduce.

A community audit involves:

- the community as researchers
- studying the community holistically, using a variety of methods
- looking beyond problems and needs to identify strengths and assets
- seeking to bring about change, not just responding to issues.

In the current climate this form of surveying is often conducted by government to decide policy and funding directions, although the extent to which the community is able to actively participate beyond a consultative role is often a topic of criticism.

Community auditing can inform small-to-medium-scale organisational change, such as the decision to introduce a new type of program or service area outside the previous remit of the organisation. At the same time, community auditing, particularly when conducted by governments and external funders, can have the effect of bringing about large-scale, structural and unplanned change for organisations.

The introduction of the National Disability Insurance Scheme: DisabilityCare, for example, in changing the way support services in the Australian disability sector are engaged and funded, will consequently cause many services to change how programs are structured and services delivered. The trend to integration and collaboration, and person-centred service delivery, as outlined in the reform of the Department of Human Services, has also created profound change for organisations in this service system environment—it has affected how they provide services and how they work with other organisations.

These widespread system reforms encompass anticipated and emergent elements that arise during the change process. Although the above two changes began with a plan, as they unfold, new elements will arise and new plans will take form in the process of implementation. Before we move on to explore emergent change, please read the practitioner profile below. Sharon Fisher describes her approach to managing change in the restructure of the Victorian Department of Human Services outlined in Practice example 9.1. As you read Sharon's description, reflect on what we have been saying about different types of change. Observe also how Sharon is approaching the management of a complex change process involving elements of emergent and anticipated change.

Linkage
We take a detailed look at community engagement in Chapter 10.

PRACTITIONER PROFILE 9.1

SHARON FISHER

AREA DIRECTOR FOR OUTER GIPPSLAND, DEPARTMENT OF HUMAN SERVICES, VICTORIA

Position

I have recently commenced this role, which was newly created in line with the whole-of-department transformation to strengthen local community planning and achieve improved social and economic outcomes for vulnerable individuals, families and communities. To achieve

(continued)

this, DHS has recently undergone a whole-of-organisation restructure resulting in the creation of a head office focused on policy and program design, four divisions across Victoria focused on strategic direction and performance, and seventeen local service areas consisting of three multidisciplinary staffing teams focused on client-centred and place-based practice and local initiatives. The new area model consists of multidisciplinary teams, which combine housing and disability accommodation services, disability support, housing assistance and disability support services, and agency management and community capacity building. The child protection program currently sits beside this new area model, but will be integrated over the next eighteen months in keeping with the client- and family-centred approach.

My role is to lead and deliver this new structure and practice approach in Outer Gippsland, which incorporates the local government areas of Wellington and East Gippsland. I plan to achieve this by focusing on the following four key areas:

- strengthening client-centred practice
- building community capacity
- developing staff capacity and capability
- streamlining and strengthening systems and processes.

A typical day

Given this is a very new role, much of my time is focused on establishing relationships across the new local leadership team, their staff teams and the new divisional executive team. This is a critical time in the transformation, which requires regular communication and consultation at all levels of the organisation, feedback as to the opportunities and risks, active participation on numerous working parties to continue the design and implementation of the structure and model. This includes staff training and continually working up and down the organisation to start shaping the strategic direction, key areas of work and their associated performance and evaluation measures, and establishing various planning and implementation mechanisms to progress this work. I also have responsibility for providing briefings and responses to relevant government ministers, attending to DHS client complaints and procedural appeals or investigations, and occasional media engagements.

This internal work is balanced with a wide range of external meetings with executive managers from community and emergency service organisations, executives and senior managers across all levels of government and related sectors, and my active participation in a range of cross-sectorial planning meetings. In keeping with our commitment to client-centred practice and place-based work, my team and I have commenced meeting with local community members and resident groups to understand their experiences and commence co-designing responses that are accessible, achievable and enabling for individuals, their families and the community.

Challenges

Keeping a complex and highly visible human services organisation operating whilst implementing this scale of change is not easy. My challenge is to maintain a balance between governance and its associated administration and the people who plan and deliver the programs, and the lived experience of the individuals, families and communities we support. It requires a constant interface between the strategy and operations, and a need to balance leading vision, growth and development with quality accountability, assurance, practice improvement, performance and risk management. This requires a multi-level team approach and I am fortunate to have the support of a very talented and cohesive executive and local management team and an outstanding executive assistant.

One of the constant challenges in establishing a multidisciplinary approach, both within DHS and in collaboration with external agencies, is statutory programs, such as Child Protection and Youth Justice, and the interface with voluntary programs, such as disability housing services or community programs, such as Child FIRST. Notwithstanding the challenges posed by distinct legislative frameworks, differing program and practice parameters, and varied program cultures, there is a real opportunity to bring this together through the DHS transformation focus on client-centred practice, common client and multidisciplinary case planning and place-based initiatives.

Lessons learnt

A lesson I have learnt over time is to respect, listen, learn and build from the power and potential of local relationships, knowledge and experience.

Skills and qualities

Skills:

- Clear, considered and respectful communication.
- Ability to develop constructive, cohesive, collaborative relationships and networks at all levels of organisations and communities.
- Ability to analyse, plan, engage, enact and reflect.

Qualities:

- Respect
- Optimism
- Resilience
- Engagement
- Reflection

Strategies for managing significant change

In managing change I have adopted a multi-dimensional top-down/bottom-up approach, which aims to actively communicate and consult at all levels in relation to the vision, goals, rationale and operational impacts of the change. This involves providing open, clear and consistent communication and opportunities for feedback, sharing research, evidence and stories, maintaining a focus on staff performance and business continuity, engaging with our community and sector partners and demonstrating a willingness to consult and adapt as required. In my experience, this multi-dimensional approach ensures that people feel valued, informed, and supported to adjust their perspective and practice, whilst remaining effective in their role and actively engaged in the change process.

REFLECTION EXERCISE

1   What are some of Sharon's strategies for managing change?
2   Can you identify Sharon's change management process?
3   Would you do anything differently?
4   Have any strategies described so far in this chapter been utilised by Sharon?
5   What presence might emergent change have in this scenario?
6   How does Sharon make use of power?

Emergent change

Emergent change arises when an organisation is compelled to respond to a sudden, unanticipated change in the external or internal environment. The **change driver** might be a shift in government policy, defunding of a program, environmental disaster, a health epidemic, social pressure related to a moral issue, economic fluctuation, the loss of one or more key workers in a critical service delivery team, or pressure from a staff team for urgent action regarding client needs. Change drivers are often construed as having a negative impact, but organisations also often have to respond to unexpected opportunities, such as funding becoming available to deliver a new service, or to conduct a special project. In either case, there is no opportunity to anticipate or plan for the specific change event, and limited scope to influence the nature of the change. In short, it is: 'Change that is thrust upon the organisation by circumstances that it can neither control nor, sometimes, predict' (Osborne & Brown, 2005, p.6).

While this type of change is often referred to as unplanned change (Ozanne & Rose, 2013), as explained earlier, we prefer the term 'emergent'. This is because, although the impetus for the change might be unanticipated, and the circumstances chaotic and crisis driven, planning begins with an organisation deciding to respond to the request for change. This is a crucial point.

There is a prevailing discourse that portrays organisations as victims, caught in the flux of rapidly changing external forces, at the beck and call of governments, funders and powerful stakeholders. To be sure, there is much veracity in this image: increasing complexity and change are a reality of the health and human services environment, and to survive, organisations must develop ways of working with unpredictability, while complying with demands from major funding sources, such as government. On the other hand, it is important to recognise that there are always choices; an organisation can choose to do nothing, to resist, or to respond and change. Once a decision is made, the planning process for working with emergent change has commenced.

Strategies can be put in place in advance for managing emergent change when it does eventuate. These might include: risk management planning, succession planning, building flexibility into strategic planning, and fostering a learning organisation culture (Osborne & Brown, 2005). One of our case study interviewees describes below how, in their organisation, decision-making is delegated to program managers to enable responsiveness when unanticipated opportunities emerge.

Change drivers
Internal or external factors that cause an organisation to make changes to services, structure, policy or operations.

Linkage
We discussed emergent planning in Chapter 6; here we consider emergent change.

PRACTICE EXAMPLE 9.2

A strategy to manage growth

We plan for them [unexpected opportunities], and in actual fact it's part of our managing growth strategy, so managing growth and looking at opportunities as well as limitations on what we're currently doing … basically the organisation has said there are elements of planning that we don't always know beforehand are going to happen and therefore we leave it up to the judgment or view of the managers. There's also a lot of goodwill and trust placed in the managers to make decisions for themselves. At the exec. level there's a deliberate attempt not to interfere with that.

This example draws attention to the importance of an organisational structure that encourages initiative and innovation by supporting managers who are not at the executive level to make decisions, choices and take action. The above organisation has been particularly successful at expanding the number and range of programs over a ten-year period, growing from a local to statewide, and now interstate service. This was not achieved by controlling organisational change from the top down.

Osborne and Brown (2005, p.39) observe that emergent change recognises that 'top-down, planned change minimizes the learning that goes on across the organisation … which could enable it to change and innovate more effectively in the future.' This illustrates how emergent change engages with the productive qualities of power, by enabling the contribution and participation of workers at all organisational levels.

Managing change successfully

Despite perceptions to the contrary, organisational change does not 'just happen'. The events that give rise to the change may seem to emerge from nowhere, but the establishment of a different way of doing things is no accident; it requires intent and deliberate application. At the core of successful change sits a well-managed process, and this requires a convergence of a facilitative organisational culture, effective leadership and the cooperation of key stakeholders, preferably through maximising power *with* and power *for*, and minimising power *over*.

Successful change management is often seen as dependent on organisational culture, and leadership style and skill. Peter Senge's paradigm of the learning organisation (Senge, 1992), in which hierarchical and controlling organisational structures are dismantled and workers are engaged in a continuous learning cycle, is held aloft as an ideal model for fostering creativity and innovation; enabling organisations to be adaptive and proactive, rather than reactive, to change (Creed, 2011).

That said, the degree to which a health or human service organisation is able to operate as a learning organisation is limited in the real world. A prevalence of hierarchical structures, staff burnout from the intensity and demand of constant change, service delivery targets, accreditation standards, statutory requirements, and service provision—which ethically and legally, cannot afford to take risks with clients' health and lives—all inhibit the full realisation of Peter Senge's ideal learning organisation (Osborne & Brown, 2005). Alternatively, the principles behind the concepts of the learning organisation, in particular the ethical and equitable use of power and the reflective learning cycle, have much merit and value in the successful management of change (Hughes & Wearing, 2013). Despite delivering services and adhering to professional regulations, health and human services workers are required to have and develop skills in initiative, creativity and innovation in their practice; these skills can also be fostered and encouraged in organisational development.

REFLECTION EXERCISE

Spend a few moments thinking about the practice examples and practitioner profile above.

1 What capacity for innovation, initiative and creativity is there in Sharon Fisher's role?
2 How important do you think 'lack of interference from the exec.' is for initiative and innovation?
3 Are innovation, initiative and creativity essential ingredients for achieving positive change?
4 Does all change necessarily include privileging the needs and wants of some over others? If so, whose needs within the organisation should be privileged?

The ability to bring about large-scale, positive and innovative change is associated with the concept and skill of transformational leadership. Transformational leaders are considered to be capable of motivating and inspiring workers and work teams to reach for exceptional goals and targets, by overriding their own self-interests (Bartol et al., 2011). In a change-weary and -wary culture, people who exhibit skills in big-picture thinking, and are bounding with energy and inspiration can be assets—when they can be accessed. At the same time, it can be a challenge to find individuals with these qualities in a sector that is not replete with charismatic leaders. In large part, this is because the values and nature of the work in the health and human services sector do not tend to support overt individualism.

On the other hand, the hierarchical structure of many organisations and the arrangement of workers into practitioner-led teams offers opportunities for the application of transformational leadership principles at the work-group level. Here, more positive forms of power can be accessed and utilised by all team members, who are encouraged to take on leadership roles and participate in change agendas. As Mary Parker Follett recognised a century ago, participatory and inclusive approaches are far more likely to result in the successful implementation of change (Hughes & Wearing, 2013; Ozanne & Rose, 2013).

Addressing barriers to change

Addressing attitudes and emotional responses that cause resistance to change frames a number of change management approaches. Two enduring models, which have seen many variations, are Lewin's three-step process and Kotter's eight-step model.

Lewin's three-step process: Organisation as organism

Kurt Lewin conceptualised the organisation as an organism, with a natural tendency to maintain equilibrium, or homeostasis. When confronted with a disrupting force, like the requirement to change, the organisation—essentially those within it who are not party to the force for change—will resist, and try to maintain the status quo (Cameron & Green, 2012).

The three steps in Kurt Lewin's change management process are:

1 Unfreezing: this stage involves defining the present state, identifying the need for change and imagining the successful change outcome. This stage incorporates surveying and needs analysis. Forces for and against the change are analysed using force field analysis. Potential resistance to change is identified.

2   Changing: mobilising participation in the change process, and bringing about the change; acceptance by most that change is necessary.

3   Refreezing: stabilisation after the change has been achieved, celebrating and rewarding success, and establishing the new state as standard organisational practice.

Source: adapted from Cameron & Green, 2012; Ozanne & Rose, 2013

These three steps can also be conceived as: planning, implementing and consolidating (Heller, 1998)—see Table 9.3.

TABLE 9.3 Stages in managing organisational change

STAGE (HELLER)	STEP (LEWIN)	PROCESS
Planning	Unfreezing	Mapping the change. Identifying need, rationale, desired outcome, and obstacles.
Implementing	Changing	Mobilising participation, engaging in change process.
Consolidating	Refreezing	Stabilising post-change. Celebrating success.

Force field analysis

Lewin's three-step process incorporates **force field analysis**, which involves identifying the forces (actions of power) that drive and resist change (Bartol et al., 2011). Information is compiled into two lists: the first comprises data about the forces promoting the change (driving forces), and the second lists oppositional (resisting) forces, which are seeking to maintain the status quo. A comparison is then made, measuring which forces for and against are dominant. Table 9.4 illustrates a force field analysis for relocating an organisation to larger premises. Driving and resisting forces are listed in relation to one another, with the size of arrows representing the degree of strength of opposing forces (Cummins & Worley, 1997). Rather than increasing the forces that are driving the change in order to overcome resistance, Lewin proposed that the most effective strategy is to focus on reducing resistance. This analysis is usually conducted at the group level, in a meeting of stakeholders, such as a focus group.

Force field analysis
A method for identifying and analysing the degree of influence of the forces for and against a proposed change event, with the purpose of reducing resistant forces.

TABLE 9.4 Force field analysis diagram for relocation of organisation to larger premises

DRIVING FORCES	DESIRED CHANGE STATE	RESISTING FORCES
More space		Current premises adequate
More programs, more staff		Current workloads and skill levels adequate
Better access for client		Everyone knows where current premises are
Time: lease due to expire		Cost: new premises more expensive

In the above example, the main resisting forces are the desire to maintain current staff team and workloads, and the increased costs of relocating. Therefore, minimising these concerns by attending to the valid reasons behind them will result in the forces for change becoming predominant. This is widely regarded as an effective method for drawing attention to the dynamics of power relationships in change situations, for involving stakeholders in problem-solving resistance to change, and also for evaluating whether or not it is wise to proceed (Hughes & Wearing, 2013). The values underpinning health and human services practice, together with participatory management approaches, encourage the use of force field analysis for highlighting the concerns of individuals and groups who might be marginalised by the drive for change. This includes these stakeholders in the change process and, if exercised with genuineness, enables their needs to be acknowledged and addressed.

Stakeholder analysis

Stakeholder analysis
A process that identifies who, out of significant individuals and groups affected by a proposed change, is likely to support the change and who might resist.

Another approach to launching a change management process is **stakeholder analysis**. This involves identifying the significant individuals and groups that will be affected by the proposed change, and determining which of these are likely to support the change and those that may resist. The change implementation process then harnesses the support of those who are potential champions for the change.

Linkage
We looked at using stakeholder analysis in Chapter 7, as a communication strategy to gain support for a project.

Importantly, the process also involves identifying strategies for addressing the concerns of resistors, and adjusting the implementation process so that potential barriers are minimised. This may mean speeding up or slowing down the change process so that resistant stakeholders can be persuaded to take a more positive view (Gray et al., 2010; Osborne & Brown, 2005). Steps involved in stakeholder analysis include:

1   Identify all possible stakeholders in the change.
2   Estimate the degree of influence each stakeholder might have over the change process.
3   Identify the most influential.
4   Identify which of these are supporters and resistors.
5   Harness the support of change champions.
6   Address the concerns of resistors.
7   Adjust implementation strategies accordingly.

Source: adapted from Gray et al., 2010; Osborne & Brown, 2005; Ozanne & Rose, 2013.

Linkage
In Chapter 10 we explore approaches to stakeholder engagement.

This approach can be a useful and practical method for engaging with community, harnessing support and addressing resistance to change, especially when sensitive and complex issues are involved. Caution needs to be exercised, to avoid the manipulation of stakeholders and the consequent creation of mistrust (Osborne & Brown, 2005).

Kotter's eight principles of change management

Another strategy that has been highly influential in managing successful large-scale transformational change is John Kotter's eight principles of change management. In summary, these are:

1   Establish urgency.
2   Form an influential guiding team.

3 Create a vision.
4 Communicate the vision.
5 Empower others to act on the vision.
6 Plan for and create short-term wins.
7 Consolidate improvements and plan for further change.
8 Institutionalise new approaches.

Source: Kotter, 2011a

While the above strategies for successful change management contain many useful elements, they are largely based on change deriving from the insight and vision of a single leader, or a few members of an executive management group, who hold positional authority (and therefore it is assumed they know what is best for the organisation). These approaches are also dependent on a stable, predictable organisational environment that enables follow through on a linear-rational process—from the top down. Most significantly, they are founded on the assumption of resistance. This is hardly surprising when many workers, who are, after all, key stakeholders, experience organisational change as imposed from above—something they have little choice about and limited opportunity to actively participate in determining. This leaves them feeling marginalised and excluded from decision-making processes in situations that have potential to significantly impact on their own and their clients' well-being.

Bringing about change successfully and positively

For change to be successful in today's health and human service environment, attention needs to be given to participation across all levels, emotional and attitudinal responses, and multiple, rather than singular, trajectories and processes (Hughes & Wearing, 2013; Osborne & Brown, 2005; Rafferty et al., 2013). There is increasing attention on the affective elements of change, such as attitude and emotion. Although emotion is often seen by managers as a source of resistance and a barrier to change, emotions are now recognised as key aspects in promoting positive attitudes. Emotional responses can also be helpful in identifying valid concerns about the marginalising and disempowering effects of change and the misuse of power (Heath & Heath, 2011; Rafferty et al., 2013).

The majority of the workforce in a health or human service organisation is located at the direct practice level. Given that this workforce outnumbers those at the executive level, it stands to reason that their willing cooperation in the change process is essential. For workers to embrace change, however, some basic elements are required. Rafferty et al. (2013) observe that in order for change to be successfully implemented, and intended outcomes achieved, workers must be change-ready, and this requires holding a positive attitude. To this end, the proposed change needs to:

• Make sense: the change rationale must be clearly articulated and have a logical connection with the work of the organisation.

- Be achievable: workers need to feel like they have the required skills and workload capacity to carry out the change. Organisational capacity, support and adequate resources are required.
- Demonstrate positive outcomes: positive outcomes for individuals affected by the change (clients, staff and community) must be evident.

Source: Rafferty et al., 2013

It is important to reinforce this final point: that the values underpinning practice across the health and human services—to improve the well-being of clients and communities—must inform the bottom-line rationale for organisational and service system change.

We close this chapter with further insights from Simon Ruth, who we first met in Chapter 2. Simon shares his approach to managing change, which involves being attentive, prepared, perceptive, and knowing when the timing is right. He also draws on the wisdom of Peter Drucker to reinforce the observation that people, not plans, are the key to successful change.

PRACTITIONER PROFILE 9.2

SIMON RUTH

DIRECTOR—COMPLEX SERVICES, PENINSULA COMMUNITY HEALTH

Skills and qualities

- You need to have a good memory, particularly for figures, processes and history. Organisations, particularly large ones, shift and change. Funding agreements alter with no notice, key staff move on and things are often not written down. If you are able to recall why things are the way they are and what has been tried previously, you can impact on how things will be in the future.
- You need to be able to sit patiently and wait for things to happen. Although you may see a great need for change, others who get to make the decisions may not have the same priorities as you.
- You need to be able to cope with change. In an environment of constantly striving to do better, change is inevitable and you need to be able to flow with it. You need to be able to compromise and know when to let something go.
- You need to be able to read the politics of a situation. Whether looking at the government or your own organisation, you need to be able to understand more broadly why things are happening. If you can be aware of key people's positions on certain matters you can save yourself a lot of time and pain. You also need to be able to read the broader political environment. To recognise changes in language and policy shifts. If you can pick up on these early and include them in your own program you can be seen as a leader by funders.
- You need to be able to listen. Not only to government, but to staff and consumers. Often people just want to be heard and it is important when dealing with staff or consumers one on one that you are able to hear what they are saying so that you can be better informed when managing risk or developing new programs.

Lessons learnt

- I've learnt to be patient and I've learnt to not go into difficult meetings on an empty stomach. Being hungry can give you a short fuse, which is never helpful.
- I've learnt to keep all my emails, both sent and received. People shift jobs and people forget things and it helps if you can produce evidence of agreements or discussions.
- I've learnt to not be so serious. You get a lot further if people like and trust you so it's important to get along with people and be compassionate and understanding.
- Peter Drucker is reported to have said 'culture eats strategy for breakfast'. If you're attempting to change the organisation or the program you need to focus on shifting culture, not just creating a well-thought-out plan.

SUMMARY OF KEY ISSUES

Work in the health and human services is characterised by change; it lies at the heart of practice within an external environment undergoing constant change. Writers on this topic have observed a pervasive sense of change fatigue among workers, who feel overwhelmed by its relentless pace, which they feel they have little or no control over. Marginalisation from decision-making exacerbates feelings of disempowerment.

There are many types of change. Two predominant forms that we discussed are anticipated and emergent. Emergent change is increasing, thus organisations need to be positioned to respond to, and work with, unpredictable opportunities and challenges as they arise. Fostering a workplace culture that is able to embrace change requires awareness of the use of power and the dynamics of power relationships; workers must feel engaged, validated, capable and resourced to show leadership and participate when change presents.

PRACTICE ACTIVITIES

1 Types of change

Define what is meant by 'emergent' and 'anticipated' change.

2 Managing emergent change

Imagine that you are the CEO of a community service organisation that employs thirty staff across five program areas. You have just been advised that one of the programs will lose its funding in the next round. Six of the most skilled and valued workers are employed in that program. In the last strategic planning cycle, this program area was marked for expansion but now it looks like it will completely disappear, along with staff who had been given training in anticipation of receiving additional funding.

Outline a strategy for how you would respond to this unwelcome news. How would you go about managing this change?

3 Force field analysis

Draw up a force field analysis based on your imagining of the arguments for and against the following scenario.

You are the manager of a residential unit that is staffed twenty-four hours a day, seven days a week. You have been directed to introduce a significant roster change, which will require staff who have been working the same roster for the past ten years to change their work patterns. All staff will now have to share weekend and overnight shifts, whereas in the past these shifts were separately covered by 'day', 'night' and 'weekend' staff. You have three months to complete the change process.

FURTHER READING

Creative approaches to change management

Lawler, J. & Bilson, A. (2010). *Social Work Management and Leadership. Managing Complexity with Creativity,* London and New York: Routledge.

Osborne, S. P. & Brown, K. (2005). *Managing Change and Innovation in Public Service Organizations,* London and New York: Routledge.

Creating conditions for positive engagement in change

Heath, C. & Heath, D. (2011). *Switch. How to Change when Things Are Hard,* London: Random House.

Rafferty, A. E., Jimmieson, N. L. & Armenakis, A. A. (2013). 'Change Readiness: A Multilevel Review', *Journal of Management, 38*(1), pp.110–35.

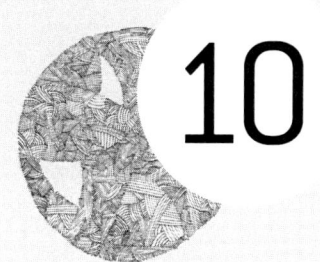

Communication, Community Engagement and Collaboration

OVERVIEW

This chapter will:

- define and explore communication, community engagement and collaboration as management processes in health and human service environments
- highlight the responsibilities of managers in leading genuine communication and engagement with stakeholders and communities
- consider the concept of organisations as 'networks of conversations'
- emphasise the importance of community engagement for embracing diversity.

This chapter explores communicating, collaborating and engaging with community as intertwined processes fundamental for building positive service system environments and responsive health and human service organisations. It considers processes and conditions for supporting effective communication, and inclusive, participatory practices, with emphasis on the importance of engaging with diverse stakeholders and communities.

KEY TERMS

collaboration

communication

community engagement

community of interest

community of place

community of practice

geographic community

interdisciplinary team

multidisciplinary team

service provision

transdisciplinary team

The importance of communicating for connection

Health and human services are reliant for success, survival and everyday functioning on collaborative practices within and beyond their organisation—in teams, across programs and agencies, and with communities (Taylor et al., 2013). Managers, as boundary spanners and leaders, are required to play an essential role in forging and maintaining meaningful connections with these various stakeholders. In many areas of the community services sector, organisations are now compelled, through policy and funding structures, to actively participate in integrated service system networks and to form service delivery partnerships. Globally, governments have begun regarding collaboration—between governments and with community—as strategically essential for achieving policy goals, enhancing service system responses and bringing about system-wide change. The extent to which this is rhetoric rather than reality remains a matter of some contention (Foster Alter, 2009). Attention to the development of knowledge and skills in communication and engagement is fundamental for organisational leaders if they are to achieve genuine collaboration.

At the service system level, differing degrees of collaboration are reflected in intra- and inter-organisational engagement practices, which in turn affect the extent to which stakeholders feel listened to and included as participants. Effective community engagement, as both concept and practice, is fundamental to building democratic partnerships that involve citizens, communities, organisations and governments (Dale, 2011). Without successful communication and considerable organisational commitment, genuine community engagement and collaboration remain elusive ideals (Foster Alter, 2009).

Although these three practices—communication, community engagement and collaboration—are distinct concepts, as processes towards achieving the goals of inclusion and participation for better client outcomes, they form an interdependent triad. To better appreciate their separate potential we begin this chapter by teasing them apart a little. We then consider the notion that organisations are 'networks of conversations' and, as such, are held together by communication. Finally, we explore strategies for community engagement, with emphasis on the importance of prioritising engagement with diverse communities. Throughout, we draw on a number of practitioner profiles, each of which illustrates the centrality of these processes in organisational leadership. It is made abundantly clear in these practitioners' descriptions of their core work, that community engagement and managing communication, in a variety of dimensions, comprise a significant portion of a leader's working day, not least because these activities are critical to forming collaborative partnerships for successful **service provision**.

The first practitioner profile is a contribution from the Disability Services Commissioner, Laurie Harkin, AM. The insight into his commitment to engaging widely with community and external stakeholders provides an apt foreground to this chapter.

Service provision
The practices, methods and modes by which an organisation offers services to clients.

Linkage
The Victorian Disability Services commission can be accessed at www.odsc.vic.gov.au

PRACTITIONER PROFILE 10.1

COMMISSIONER LAURIE HARKIN, AM

DISABILITY SERVICES COMMISSIONER

Position

Laurie Harkin is Victoria's inaugural Disability Services Commissioner (DSC). As an organisation, the office of the Disability Services Commissioner promotes and protects the rights of people receiving disability services in Victoria. It provides an independent and accessible means for people with a disability to make complaints about the services they receive, and works with disability service providers to improve the ways that complaints are responded to. The DSC researches ways to improve outcomes for people with a disability and to improve disability services' complaints systems. It also provides capacity development activities for people with a disability, their families and disability services through a variety of education and information modes to drive organisational and cultural change.

Typical day

With more than 300 registered disability service providers in Victoria, a key task of my role involves relationship management across the constituency and the broader disability sector. I make regular visits to disability service providers throughout Victoria. These visits provide me with an opportunity for direct discussions about key issues and challenges across the sector, and those specific to the particular organisation I am meeting with on any given day. I generally spend one to two days a week on my regional visit program. When I am not conducting regional visits, I spend a significant amount of time meeting with other stakeholders, including senior officials within relevant government departments.

I also meet on a regular basis with key senior staff of my office about issues of relevance that require consideration, and about ensuring that the work that we do is meeting the ever-changing needs of the people we serve and the sector in which we work.

Challenges

It can be disturbing to hear some of the lived experiences of people with a disability who have brought their issues to us to assist in their resolution. The challenge faced by all in the sector is to behave in ways that deliver rights-based person-centred support services to people, ensuring all are treated with dignity and respect. Great opportunities exist, and in many cases are being addressed through forward-thinking organisations and the people who comprise them in challenging paradigm stasis.

Lessons learnt

My assumption that I understood the disability services sector and the generally positive view I held about the character of the work could have been better placed. When confronted with the reality of the service system I recognised I had a more positive view than might reasonably have been held. On reflection, an even closer connection to the lived experiences of people with disabilities would have added value and provided greater insight into how our work was designed and implemented in the early days.

Skills and qualities

It is beneficial to have experience in a range of social and community services, including disability services, so as to contextualise the work that we do at DSC. An integral part of this

(continued)

job requires the ability to build and maintain effective working relationships both within and external to the organisation. In addition, a job such as this requires the ability to influence and lead change, to be a thought leader and always to be able to think strategically. As the head of a statutory body, it is imperative that one brings people management skills, empathy and the ability to communicate and work in a team environment.

Communication

Communication is a concept and practice with which we are all familiar. As discussed throughout previous chapters and demonstrated by the various practitioner profiles, managers and leaders (and indeed health and human service professionals at all levels) spend most of their time communicating, whether with stakeholders, peers, their own supervisors, clients, or the community (O'Flynn & Wanna, 2008; Taylor et al., 2013).

Communication is the means by which civilisations, societies, cultures and individual identities are formed; it is how organisations are led and managed and great endeavours are achieved. In short, communication is intrinsic to human survival. And, although communication is something that the overwhelming majority of us are constantly practising (we are engaged in a form of communication right now), those who work in community services fields know that poor communication lies at the centre of many personal and social dilemmas. Concomitantly, good communication is often the key to resolution. But despite its everydayness, communicating our intentions clearly and effectively is not something that we always do well, and therefore it cannot be taken for granted.

Communication happens in a variety of ways, through speech, script, image, sound, touch, emotion and even taste. Work in the health and human services involves all of these modes, each of which can adopt a plethora of forms. But no matter the context, a communication event necessarily involves a message being sent and received.

Communication
An exchange of information between parties using a shared language. Communication may be conveyed in a variety of forms: verbal, sensory, physical, emotional, technological, etc.

Linkage
In Chapter 7 we looked at how to develop a communication strategy for successful project management.

REFLECTION EXERCISE

1   Think for a moment about your day. When did your first communication take place? Did it involve you communicating a message to someone else, or were you receiving a message? Was it an exchange between two people, or did it involve technology of some kind, an alarm, or the ring of your mobile phone or perhaps your first email, or maybe it was your cat or dog looking to be let outside or fed?
2   How many other forms of communication have you engaged in today? You might like to make a list. Which involved exchanges with other people, and which involved an exchange of information with technology, or objects?
3   When you arrived at work or your place of study, what messages did you receive as you entered the building? (Can you recall looking in Chapter 1 at the way architecture sends messages and shapes the possibilities for the extent of human behaviour?)
4   How did you feel in response to the messages that you received? How accurate do you think your interpretations were?

In addition to the sending and receiving of a message, successful communication also involves accuracy of perception. Trevor Tyson observes that good communication involves more than exchanging information, it requires an accurate transfer of meaning, with the goal of achieving 'an understanding between the sender and the receiver whereby the meaning received is the same as the meaning intended' (Tyson, 1998, p.77). This can be particularly problematic in organisational contexts, when people must pass on messages they did not originally generate across a number of levels and in a variety of mediums. If you work in an organisation, it is quite likely that you are familiar with this phenomenon.

REFLECTION EXERCISE

1   Reflect on the last organisational communication that was sent to you. How did you receive it? In what form was it delivered? How many people had handled it before you received it? Did it require you to take any action? What did you do with the information when it was received?
2   How many communications do you receive and how many do you send in the course of a working day?
3   How many of these communications are exchanged: a) in person; b) by phone; c) by email; d) in hard copy; e) by mail; f) by fax; g) as a poster; h) by other means?
4   How many of these communication exchanges are related to managing and leading?

Cheryl Sobczyk, whom we first met in Chapter 5, reflects on some of the consequences of information technologies in management.

PRACTICE EXAMPLE   10.1

The increasing importance of IT for health and human service managers

The large volume of email traffic in my day requires learning skills to manage effectively. The ability to participate in blogs, Skype or teleconferencing facilities is important, as these are becoming significant time management and communication tools. Ready access to online information and use of electronic systems management (software) options are assisting not only clinicians and clients but also managers in streamlining reporting and management responsibilities.

Linkage
Further profiles in this chapter also discuss the impact of IT in managers' daily communications.

Communicating effectively in various modes using a range of personal skills and technologies is fundamental to health and human services work. Leadership positions in particular depend on well-developed capabilities in engaging at individual, group and community levels.

Community engagement

Community engagement can be described as the range of practices undertaken by an organisation to form meaningful connections with the communities within which it is located and for which it provides services. Community engagement activities may involve communication exchanges through networking, promotional activities, newsletters, e-bulletins, partnership agreements, stakeholder committees, boards of governance, and surveying at group or individual levels. The following vignette from our case study research illustrates an approach to community engagement adopted by

Community engagement
Practices undertaken by an organisation with the aim of forming meaningful connections with the communities and stakeholders it interacts with.

family violence support workers at the commencement of a new program offered by an Aboriginal healing service.

PRACTICE EXAMPLE 10.2

Engaging with community to build confidence in accessing family violence services

Before most of our team came on board I thought nobody wanted to deal with family violence in a really strategic or holistic way that supports the community. I thought: we can do that. We can run forums. We can run the camps. We can do the awareness-raising through safety forums, through school holiday activities, across the spectrum. The managers acknowledged that would be really good and so they released money to cover transport or groceries or whatever.

That sort of stuff was evolutionary for us, but I suppose the basic premise was to find out what the community want—you have to go and sit down with people. Initially when the Healing Service started, we were having cups of coffee and tea with people in their houses. Then their extended family would come when we were there. Then we started seeing other community people come in. They started bringing in biscuits and cups of tea, bringing bread and meat; we'd have little barbecues. What had happened along the way was that as we were working in partnership with other agencies, they started wanting to know more, saying 'so that's how you engage with people'.

Working closely with communities and other services in the external organisational environment is a distinguishing feature of the community services sector. But what does 'community' mean?

Defining community

Fiona Gardner (2006) identifies two types of community: a geographic community and a community of interest. Both have relevance to health and human services, and they share defining features, such as a commitment to the group, a sense of belonging, and a collective capacity for meeting the needs of individual members. Gardner also draws attention to community being defined through subjective experience. In other words, we know when we belong to a community because we feel part of it (Parish et al., 2006). This is reflected in the meaning of community for Aboriginal and Torres Strait Islanders peoples, for whom community is strongly linked to the subjective experience of family relationships and spiritual connections to country and place.

Geographic community
A community that comes together because of, or is defined by, physical location.

Community of place
A form of geographic community that is defined by ongoing interactions of the members due to their proximity.

Geographic communities are defined by physical location. This might be identified cartographically, for example: the planet, a region, a nation, a state, a local government area, a city, a township or a suburb. Population density, environmental features or socio-economic characteristics may further define these mapped communities, such as rural, coastal, urban, peri-urban and remote. Other forms of geographic community are shaped in relation to function, and defined more by architecture than natural environment. These include communities within housing estates, apartment buildings, prisons, care facilities, hospitals and boarding houses (Gardner, 2006). These are also referred to as **communities of place**, because the members are in proximity to one another.

In some organisational networks, clients in the same program areas form a community, especially through group work programs and in residential settings. You will already be recognising that there are multiple layers to community; they nest within, overlay and intersect with one another. Bryan Smith (1994) and Juanita Brown and David Isaacs (1994) offer another lens. They propose that, given the right conditions, organisations can become communities by facilitating the joining of individual workers in the pursuit of a common goal for the greater good. In fact, at the risk of becoming overly convoluted, communities are in themselves forms of organisations.

Adding yet another layer, **communities of interest** emerge from shared concerns, ideas or activities. These might develop and be sustained in physical locations, for example a community of artists, musicians or students. Or, they may arise among people who, sharing the same chronic health issue, form a support group which meets regularly. Communities of interest do not depend on members being in the same location. A burgeoning arena of community is groups that communicate and meet virtually via information technology, such as on Facebook, Twitter, blogs, discussion forums, etc.

A **community of practice** is a subset of a community of interest. This type of community can form naturally to address a particular interest, share knowledge and build skills, such as a young parents' group, or it might be facilitated through service organisations that are designed to improve practitioner skills, provide networking and mentoring opportunities, and enhance service delivery (Smith, 1994; Brown & Isaacs, 1994). Another example is house supervisors of government and community-based residential services located throughout a particular service system region, who meet on a monthly basis for peer support and to jointly explore issues and challenges encountered in their roles. They may also communicate through an online discussion forum and some members might attend meetings using remote communication technologies.

We now live and work in a world where communication technologies have expanded the means and opportunity for forming communities: communities are no longer as dependent on physical proximity and face-to-face communication. But these virtual communities pose challenges for the way we conceptualise the direct delivery of services (Hughes & Wearing, 2013). Organisations are faced with rethinking communication protocols, and the management of information flow and access in a digitised world. For managers seeking to facilitate effective engagement in the contemporary world, it is essential to have an appreciation of the diverse meanings of community, as well as an ability to utilise the ever-expanding options for communicating with communities via communication technologies.

Community of interest
A community that forms because of a shared interest, whether in a physical location (for example, a community of students) or not (for example, groups that 'meet' via social media).

Community of practice
A type of community of interest with a specific focus on learning through sharing skills, building knowledge and improving practice in an area of mutual interest.

REFLECTION EXERCISE

1   Consider the meaning of community. How many different communities do you belong to?
2   Draw a map of the various communities that are associated with your organisation, or an organisation with which you are familiar. Do these connect with one another? If so, how?
3   Are these geographic communities, communities of interest, or communities of practice? Or all three?

Engaging with communities

Just as there are many types of communities, with new forms continuously evolving, there are also varying approaches, degrees and levels of community engagement. In the profile below, Allyson Walker, whom you met in Chapter 2, offers her insights and strategies for engaging with the members of community who use the service that she manages. As you read Allyson's words, observe how and what forms of communication she employs. Think about which of her practices might be helpful for you to adopt when managing your own relationships with community stakeholders.

PRACTITIONER PROFILE 10.2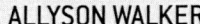

ALLYSON WALKER

MANAGER, SOCIAL AND COMMUNITY SERVICES, DANDENONG AND DISTRICT ABORIGINES CO-OPERATIVE

Engaging with community

- When working in the Aboriginal community it is extremely important to engage with the community. As manager I'm open to community coming into the office and having a yarn. We could yarn about work or it could be about family and our connections.

- Respect the silence. Sometimes when we chat we need that time to reflect on what's being said so just let that happen.

- Don't be in a hurry; make a cuppa tea and sit outside.

- Build relationships with the community members. As they get used to you they will open up about what is important.

- It's not always about work, sometimes they just want to ask how are the kids and how are your grandparents and tell you about their family too.

- Respect and acknowledge the elders: find out who they are and value them.

- Pop in and visit existing groups such as women's group, playgroup or youth. You will become known among the community attending the groups and it shows you care and support the group and its progress. It also means you are aware of what is happening at the groups.

- Attending activities gives you the opportunity to have that informal yarn with community members and also for them to raise any issues they may want you to be aware of.

- Put good news stories into the newsletter and contact the newspapers to promote good news stories.

- Knowing the local stories, history, people and groups is important, as ignorance is not a good reflection on you.

At the policy level, Australian state governments have defined community engagement as: 'A planned process with the specific purpose of working with identified groups of people, whether they are connected by geographic location, special interest or affiliation, to address issues affecting their well-being' (State Government of Victoria, 2013a). This is framed by the principle that community engagement is an inclusive process and, as such, is necessarily committed to embracing diversity. There are, at the same time, levels and degrees of engagement; these include but are not limited to informing, consulting, involving, liaising and collaborating (State Government of Victoria, 2005a, p.10). Box 10.1 articulates these concepts.

BOX 10.1

Levels of community engagement

Informing: one-way communication advising the community of organisational actions, available services, or other information deemed important.

Consulting: seeking the views of community about relevant issues as part of a process of program and service development, or to build community awareness and understanding.

Involving: inviting community participation in a range of ways to ensure understanding of issues and concerns, and inclusion in decision-making.

Liaising: mutual communication between the organisation and community, intended to maintain links, identify and address issues and ensure clarity in communication.

Collaborating: forming partnerships to develop shared goals, and working together on strategies for their achievement.

REFLECTION EXERCISE

How do Allyson's community engagement strategies align with these levels of community engagement? What might Allyson's approach have to offer these levels of engagement?

We end this section on engaging with communities with the profile of Rachel Mackay. Rachel's reflections on practice refer to a number of forms of community engagement and she identifies a range of communication modes, including social media. In fact, the Bsafe program that Rachel describes centres on the use of digital information technologies to deliver services. Note also that Rachel emphasises the critical role of good communication in successful community engagement.

PRACTITIONER PROFILE 10.3

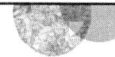

RACHEL MACKAY

PROJECT COORDINATOR, BSAFE PROJECT AND FAMILY VIOLENCE SUPPORT SERVICES TRAINING FACILITATOR

Position

Like many people, I have two facets to my role at Women's Health Goulburn North East. I am the project coordinator for the Bsafe Project, a personal alarm system for women and children escaping family violence, and I also facilitate training in family violence. My role with Bsafe

(*continued*)

has changed over the years, from coordinating and reporting on a pilot project, to overseeing the development of a sustainable model, and liaison with services, media and government departments.

The other facet provides an opportunity to facilitate training that increases awareness of the complex dynamics of family violence, how to respond, and the gendered nature of family violence. The training is provided to specific groups such as rural financial counsellors and emergency services staff (post natural disasters) and to those working in fields that have the capacity to identify and respond to family and domestic violence and abuse.

A typical day

I must juggle each of my roles within every day, so I have to remain organised, structured and plan ahead! In the morning I liaise with a colleague to modify the 'Family violence after natural disasters' training scheduled for the following week and plan for the resources and travel time needed. Then I telephone or email other Bsafe coordinators in the region and liaise with the product supplier, VitalCall, for the purchase of new Bsafe units. I meet and report to my manager, reply to email requests for training and check the Bsafe Facebook and Twitter accounts. I update the Bsafe database when new referrals are received and email monthly reports to police and family violence services.

Challenges

There are, of course, challenges. It has been frustrating lobbying for the Bsafe technology to be incorporated as part of a rural response to family violence. The political issues between Commonwealth and State responsibilities for ongoing funding have taken precedence over women's and children's ongoing need to remain safe in their homes, and their lived experiences of abuse.

Working in a rural setting, travel can be a challenge with many hours spent on the road. Add to this the eternal struggle and juggle of being a mother and managing childcare and work. There is also a sense of isolation, from training and other opportunities that only occur in metropolitan areas. Issues are often considered with a metro 'flavour', with minimal consideration for what it means for women in rural and regional settings. In the past few years we have had to live with droughts, floods and bushfires all impacting on our work and lives.

Lessons learnt

Trust yourself and your inner voice. It is always right. If you are coming from a place of compassion, which does not assume you know a person's story, then you will always work well with people.

Skills and qualities

- The ability to plan ahead, troubleshoot and think through your priorities on a daily basis are the key skills when working on a range of diverse projects.
- You need compassion and passion.
- A belief in what you are doing and the ability to return to the core of your vision.
- Listening and learning from colleagues.

Engaging with the community

Knowledge of local services, systems and demographics is crucial. Thinking outside the square is also important when engaging with communities. Some issues are complex and for others the way to engage is simple. Planning is also important for me but you cannot plan other people's responses, so I also like to remain flexible. You need the ability to think on your feet! Lastly, communication is key, so develop a communication strategy and stick to it to keep people informed.

Collaboration

At a broad level, **collaboration** involves two or more parties working together towards a shared goal. Success in attaining the goal depends on duration, context, purpose and process. Janine O'Flynn (2008) raises the concern that, although the term is now commonplace in public policy and practice discourse, it is more difficult than ever to locate a coherent definition. She argues that coordination and cooperation do not sufficiently constitute collaboration; that it is more than simply 'working together'. According to O'Flynn, collaboration is a complex endeavour founded on voluntarily sharing organisational processes and resources—including goal setting, culture, rewards and power (State Government of Victoria, 2005a, p.37). Lewis and colleagues lend support to this position, while also observing that the meaning has taken on new dimensions over the course of history. They make the point that although inter-agency and community collaboration extends back to the charitable societies of the nineteenth century, contemporary collaborations take time and applied effort, and necessarily 'reach for deeper and more fundamental' interactions (Lewis et al., 2012, p.37).

> **Collaboration**
> Cooperatively working together to achieve a mutual goal.

Brody (2005) identifies four types of collaboration:

* Short-term ad hoc collaborations: formed out of the need for organisations to work together in response to a crisis.
* Medium-term coalitions: built around common interests in a campaign or project.
* Federations: involving the establishment of semi-independent, ongoing relationships in which organisations retain autonomy.
* Consortiums: partnerships formed in order to jointly deliver services.

Brody further observes: 'A good collaborative process builds a series of progressively deeper and more comprehensive agreements among the participants' (Brody, 2005, p.397). This process involves:

1 Initial agreement over the common need to be addressed.
2 Decision about how to effectively work together.
3 Information sharing.
4 Formation of a common vision.
5 Development of implementation strategies.

Source: Brody, 2005

Catherine Foster Alter (2009, pp.436–7) discusses inter-organisational collaborations in terms of purpose and identifies four types; these are summarised in Box 10.2.

BOX 10.2

Forms of inter-organisational collaboration

Obligational: Informal, loosely connected collaborations that are essentially formed to share resources. They are based on reciprocity, often arise out of friendship and personal networks, and can be short or long term. A longer-term example is a practitioner network or community of practice that meets regularly to share skills and knowledge.

Promotional: More formal partnerships, or consortiums, often involving pooling of resources, formed to achieve a common end that cannot be accomplished with the resources of the individual organisations. Because they are task- and outcome-focused, a high degree of centralisation and coordination is required. They can be short or long term. A short-term example is organisations coming together for political strength to challenge a policy decision, or lobbying for legislative change.

Systemic: Formal partnerships with integration of resources to jointly provide services. These often involve common plans, parallel management structures and co-location of staff. They are usually long term. An example is a multi-service complex, which might include a police family violence response team, specialist family violence support services, sexual assault counselling and community nursing services.

Consolidated: Highly formalised partnerships that are essentially mergers. These represent the extreme end of the collaboration scale, and technically exceed collaboration, as the organisations have amalgamated.

Foster Alter warns that evidence to date indicates that successful, effective and efficient inter-organisational collaborations are expensive in terms of time, effort and skills, even though they are often formed with the intention of stretching resources.

Collaborating in teams

Team work is endemic to health and human services practice. The majority of workers practice in intra-organisational teams. The first management position of many executive level managers, who began their career as practitioners at the coalface, was as team leader. But even though working in teams may be familiar ground, managers must exercise caution about assuming that teams are necessarily ideal structures to work within, to lead, or for achieving successful client outcomes (Weber & Pockett, 2011). Martin-Rodriguez et al. (2005, p.132) observe that team work is hard work: success requires a range of interpersonal and relational skills, including 'willingness to collaborate, trust in each other, mutual respect and communication', together with supportive organisational conditions through human resource management and leadership, and appropriate systemic support in the organisational environment. These conditions are not always present, and most of us can relate negative experiences in teams (Hughes & Wearing, 2013).

Weber and Pockett (2011, pp.275–6) explain that teams are defined by collaboration. They are formed with the purpose of enhancing performance and success for the team members, the organisations that contextualise them, and ultimately the clients that receive the team's services. Teams are micro-organisations; when they are functioning optimally members share a common goal, form plans together, and value each other's contributions. They operate with their own hierarchy and lines of authority, and they have formal and informal systems of communication and interplays of power. As small and intense work spaces, teams can intensify and exacerbate stressful power relationships. It is necessary to keep this in mind if you are a manager—whether a team leader or at upper levels—who has supervisory responsibility for a number of teams. Preventing power issues before they manifest is preferable, though no matter how well you prepare, management challenges are inevitable in the confined and confining spaces of teams. Effective and open communication, clarity of roles, tasks, lines of accountability, and critical awareness of the use and operation of power will contribute significantly to overcoming these tensions. So too will meaningful engagement with individual team members, in balance with the ultimate purpose and goal for the team's existence—its core work.

Many teams within organisations are focused around a single area of work, professional discipline or program area. But there are other types of teams that are comprised of practitioners from multiple professional areas, organisational contexts and professional skill-bases, who gather to achieve a common outcome (whether this is a client outcome, a multi-agency project or community-driven cause). These teams are frequently categorised as multidisciplinary, interdisciplinary and transdisciplinary (Hughes & Wearing, 2013).

D'Amour and colleagues (2005) explain that a **multidisciplinary team** is structured by various professions working in coordination for a prescribed time period to achieve a defined outcome, yet doing so independently, or alongside one another. Multidisciplinary teams are common in healthcare settings, where a team of medical specialists, nursing staff and social workers work together on a particular case (Hughes & Wearing, 2013): an example might be the services that come together in coordinated case management. A defining feature of multidisciplinary teams is the lack of emphasis on members working together and sharing decision-making; rather the focus is directed at optimising goal achievement. These teams are usually organised hierarchically, with the member holding the highest professional status considered by default to be the main authority and team leader (Finlay, 2000, cited in Weber & Pockett, 2011).

Interdisciplinary teams place more importance on collaboration and cooperation; there is common intention to integrate areas of practice and share ownership and responsibility (D'Amour et al., 2005; Weber & Pockett, 2011). The commitment to working together in a participatory way will often be over a longer duration than for the multidisciplinary team. Dyer (2003, p.186) explains that 'organisational support and infrastructure that promotes work interdependence, increases self-management, and increases responsibility on the part of team members for group performance' is required.

The restructure of the Department of Human Services discussed in the previous chapter is an example of a strategy to enable interdisciplinary team work for providing coordinated and integrated services to clients across a number of service areas, such as housing, youth justice and disability. Interdisciplinary teams require a high degree of trust and mutual respect, and members need to be prepared and willing to take on board the

Multidisciplinary team
Comprised of members with diverse professional qualifications; formed to achieve a defined goal. Collaboration is not emphasised, unless directly relevant to the achievement of the common goal.

Interdisciplinary team
Professionals from different work areas who work together closely in a collaborative and cooperative way, sharing responsibility and decision-making.

principles and practices of other professional areas. This is not always readily achieved, as you may be aware. It can be particularly difficult when teams are comprised of members from a range of organisations that have varying expectations, management structures and funding requirements (Weber & Pockett, 2011).

Transdisciplinary team
Transcends professional or disciplinary boundaries to achieve innovative practice through knowledge and skill exchange, and the formation of new approaches.

Professional jurisdictions are deliberately and purposefully transcended in **transdisciplinary teams**, which seek to push the boundaries of collaboration. In these practice groupings significant emphasis is placed on 'consensus seeking and the opening up of professional territories' (D'Amour et al., 2005, p.120). The transdisciplinary team requires members to let go of professional borders and embrace the wisdom of other disciplines and areas of practice (Dyer, 2003), with the ultimate goal of formulating new and innovative approaches. A transdisciplinary team might include members from child protection, housing, education, business, allied health and local government sectors. The goal of a transdisciplinary team, for example, might be to design and implement an integrated response in a local setting that will holistically address the education, health, welfare and employment needs of young sole parents facing child protection, housing, education and substance abuse issues.

In all of these team formations, communication plays a critical role, whether multi-, inter- or transdisciplinary. The success or otherwise of the team in achieving its intended outcomes rests in significant ways on the skill and capacity for members to communicate with one another. Communication facilitates cooperation and, importantly, needs to be sufficiently functional to allow issues within the team to be expressed and addressed.

The role of leadership and how it is exercised is another crucial factor in team success. While some formations (such as multidisciplinary teams) tend to default to a professional hierarchy to establish the leadership role, others (such as interdisciplinary and transdisciplinary teams) can provide space for a more egalitarian process, with leadership shared between team members at various periods, and according to the task at hand. Weber and Pockett (2011, p.281) highlight the importance of 'listening to the point of view of others, being open to different problem-solving styles and approaches, and being flexible ... by not demonstrating a "my way is the best way" attitude'.

Before proceeding to the next section, where we consider another dimension of communication, you might wish to pause and reflect on some of the questions below.

REFLECTION EXERCISE

1   What would you expect from a collaborator?
2   What do you believe are your responsibilities as a collaborator?
3   Develop a definition of a collaborative partnership.
4   How might you begin a collaborative process?
5   Do you have experience working in either a multi-, inter- or transdisciplinary team, or perhaps a combination of these? If so, did you find the experience collaborative? What were some of the positives and negatives of this way of working?
6   What strategies would you use to lead each of these types of teams?

Communication and context

The practitioner profiles included earlier in this chapter, and throughout the entire text, illustrate how fundamental communication is for successful management and leadership. In our own research, effective communication was identified as a key factor in the resolution of management issues, and poor communication was seen as contributing to the failure to resolve a problem (Berends & Crinall, forthcoming).

Up to this point we have conceptualised communication as a process involving the exchange of information between two or more entities. Jeffrey Ford takes this a step further to argue that organisations are in effect 'networks of conversations' (O'Flynn, 2008, pp.185–7). In Ford's view, all organisational processes (for example, budgeting, inducting, planning, leading, evaluating) are not simply activities that involve exchanges of information—communication—they are accumulations of communications that have taken place over time and in a variety of contexts; and are therefore, in effect, extended, multi-layered, complex conversations. As such, the interactions between past and present meanings and contexts directly and indirectly determines how those employed within the organisation carry out the tasks that are connected with their roles.

In Ford's schema, conversations are carried and directed through formal and informal organisational structures, which are fundamentally information- or communication-handling systems. Think back to Chapter 3, when we talked about the way organisational culture is conveyed through symbols and practices that communicate the values and norms of a workplace. These conversations are enfolded with history and meaning. The authority of a CEO is frequently supported by narratives of their exercise of power, such as the extent of their personal sacrifice to establish, or save, the organisation. Equally, less positive stories may circulate about poor interpersonal behaviours, or failure to deliver on targets or promises. These stories then impact on the way workers build narratives about themselves and their work teams, how they position themselves, who they form alliances with, and the nature of their own exchanges; vertically and horizontally.

Linkage
In Chapter 4 we discussed communication as a core responsibility and function of management and leadership, highlighting its essential role in organisational success.

REFLECTION EXERCISE

Reflect on how power and influence are deployed through functional and multi-directional communication processes. Consider processes that rely on management and leadership, decision-making and planning.

Think about a recent organisational decision that affected your area of work that was somewhat controversial. Who communicated the arguments for and against? How were these arguments conveyed? In which and how many directions did the information flow? Whose voices were heard? How was the final decision made, and by whom? How did you find out about the decision and the consequent impact on your area of work? Was the decision well received? Why, or why not?

If organisations can be understood as networks of communication, or conversations, so too can communities. As described above, communities are defined by the meanings generated in the exchanges between members, as well as how the group or community identity is expressed to those outside the community. Taylor and colleagues describe the idea of heritage narrative structures, which are founded on the community's values, traditions and attitudes. These stories establish coherence, and include dominant, competing and subversive stories.

> Heritage narrative structures are the stories communities tell about themselves; they help define the community for members and distinguish it from other communities … they reflect the patterns of stratification and power structures in the community.
>
> Source: Taylor et al., 2013, p.1105

Engaging and collaborating

Regardless of why a community comes together, whether it's due to place, function or concept, there are essential processes that make it possible for it to form as a collective, with a shared identity. Brown and Isaacs identify six core processes, which in their experience are fundamental to the formation of community: capability, commitment, contribution, continuity, collaboration and conscience. (You can read more about these 'six Cs' of community engagement in the State Government of Victoria report (2005a) that is listed in the readings at the end of this chapter.)

We have translated these processes into 'conditions' and include two additional facets: 'communication' and 'diversity' (although evident in the descriptions by Brown and Isaac of the six core processes, they are not separately addressed). This gives us eight conditions for community engagement, articulated in Table 10.1.

TABLE 10.1 Eight core conditions for community engagement

Capability	Skills, knowledge and personal qualities to enable renewal and reinvention of the future. Capacity for 'great conversations about things that matter'.
Commitment	Fairness, transparency, honesty and equity to enable mutuality and voluntary shared participation 'beyond self-interest'.
Contribution	Opportunity and encouragement for all to share their diverse talents towards achieving a common goal.
Continuity	Practices and processes that allow information and knowledge about the community to be sustained and handed on. One way of achieving this is through sharing and rotating roles.
Collaboration	Building 'reliable interdependence' through a 'web of mutual trust'; free flow of information and strengthening of interpersonal relationships.
Conscience	Shared ownership and agreement on ethical standards by the collective.
Communication	Maintenance and promotion of open, transparent information channels flowing in multiple directions, not simply from one source to another. All possible efforts made to ensure shared understanding of intended meanings.
Diversity	Fostering and inclusion of a multitude and variety of voices and abilities with shared commitment to a common ground.

Source: adapted from Brown & Isaacs 1994; State Government of Victoria, 2005a

REFLECTION EXERCISE

Drawing on the above conditions for engagement, reflect on whether and how each of these are evident in the following places:

1   within your own workplace
2   between your organisation and your community stakeholders
3   in practitioner profiles that you have read so far.

Are there further conditions that you would add to this list?

As the practitioner profiles in this book emphasise, it is important for numerous reasons to ensure your organisation is engaged in productive dialogue with community stakeholders. In previous chapters we have noted that effective service delivery requires knowledge and understanding about the communities in the organisational environment—about their needs, and where these needs are not being met. Engagement with the community facilitates inclusiveness, sensitivity and responsiveness to diversity. When we discussed planning and change management we acknowledged that productive relationships with competitors, and other services in your environment, can enhance service delivery options and mitigate duplication.

A cohesive community network of stakeholders can also be a source of political support in the face of funding cuts or service system reforms that are driven from the top down. That said, Taylor and colleagues deliver a note of caution worth heeding: an organisational leadership position does not necessarily translate to success in a community leadership role. Community leaders tend to be 'active across the community, have external links, and community-wide vision' (Taylor et al., 2013, p.1105), which may mean that workers lower on the organisational hierarchy are better placed than the leader of their organisation to undertake leadership roles in the community. Additionally, it is important to emphasise that community engagement is not simply about an organisation being better informed about which services to deliver, or to gain political support for itself; genuine engagement must be equally directed at strengthening the community and building resilience.

REFLECTION EXERCISE

Spend a few moments brainstorming why community engagement might be important:

1   for your organisation
2   for the communities in your network.

Drawing on her work with the Canadian Council for International Collaboration, Jacquie Dale is optimistic that community engagement through public dialogue has the potential to build wisdom and reshape democratic communities by 'marrying values to information to produce wiser policy that is in the interest of all communities, however large or small that community may be' (Ford, 1999, p.485).

Dale proposes working towards engagement through conversations in which parties think about, reflect on and challenge assumptions together, with the aim of building

Linkage
Simon Ruth's profile in Chapter 2 describes his organisation's community engagement practice, which involves fifteen community advisory groups.

Linkage
In Chapter 9 we discussed the importance of focusing on assets and strengths, as well as understanding the needs of communities when conducting community audits.

Linkage
One of the recommended further readings in this chapter (Taylor et al., 2013) offers further insight into requirements for the development of effective community partnerships to achieve health outcomes.

ideas that are based on mutual understandings. For this to be achieved, she highlights four necessary principles:

- Establish equality among participants and exclude coercive influences.
- Listen with empathy.
- Bring assumptions into the open by taking 'deep dives' into underpinning beliefs.
- Encourage a diversity of perspectives.

Dale, 2011, p.363

Dale also suggests a hierarchy of goals that structure the engagement process, which she refers to as the 'Ladder of engagement' (inspired by Arnstein's concept of the ladder of citizen participation—see Dale, 2011, p.389). Figure 10.1 offers an adapted illustration of this process.

FIGURE 10.1 The sequence of engagement

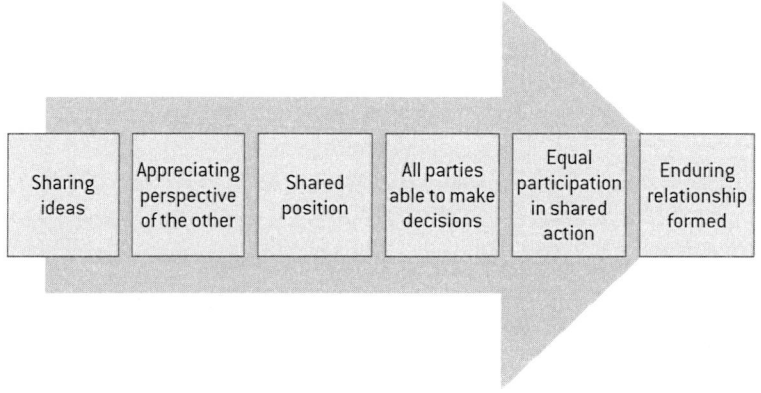

Source: adapted from Dale, 2011, p.369

Our final practitioner profile for this chapter offers insight into the complexity of communication, collaboration and community engagement. What can you take away from Terry Huriwai's practice wisdom about culturally appropriate approaches to communication and engagement?

PRACTITIONER PROFILE 10.4

TERRY HURIWAI

ADVISER, MATUA RAKI, NATIONAL ADDICTION WORKFORCE DEVELOPMENT PROGRAMME, NEW ZEALAND

Position

My role is to facilitate workforce and service development in the addiction sector so that we have effective, welcoming and complexity-capable services. I've worked in various roles in the sector for over twenty years and this experience allows me to utilise relationships and sector knowledge in my work.

The breadth of my current work includes involvement in national and regional policy-making, training (including cultural competence), service development through leading or facilitating discussions with service and organisational leaders, supporting a group of Māori leaders in the sector via information sharing and, at the individual level, mentoring and supporting practice and research.

Because Māori feature in addiction (alcohol and other drug as well as gambling) and mental-health-related problems, Matua Raki has a clear role to support Māori addiction services and practitioners as well as enhancing the capability of non-Māori to make a difference for Māori and their whānau (kin).

A typical day

In my role, no one day is the same. Depending on the project, I may be in any part of the country attending meetings or engaged in training. Even training is not the same as I may be working with a single service, across services within the sector, as well as services from different sectors. Because effective workforce development is carried out in the context of supportive service systems and leadership, the role of Matua Raki requires flexibility to work across different levels of organisational infrastructure nationally, regionally and locally.

One of the things I do daily wherever I am is data management. Scanning my emails to prioritise replies; scanning local and international news, reports and literature relevant to the sector for potential distribution to our Māori leadership group and wider if appropriate; and reading relevant literature or policy to maintain my relevance to the sector I serve. Lately our leadership group has been receiving articles on change management, service modelling and consultation documents from organisations outside of health, as well as best practice guidelines etc.

Growing and sustaining effective Māori services and practitioners (who operate from within a Māori paradigm) and also working to enhance Māori responsiveness by non-Māori sometimes requires different approaches. Recognition of and planning for opportunities to ensure cultural competence is a part of best practice, and ongoing rather than an 'add-on'.

Challenges

Challenges are those one would expect in leadership roles and generally include information management; building motivation in the sector; cultivating leadership in the sector; facilitating communication across the sector; promoting and maintaining best practice and encouraging innovation and action.

In an environment of shrinking resources, workforce development is often relegated to the 'nice to have' rather than the 'must have', so Matua Raki works with organisations and services to ensure best practice is promoted and maintained, and that the right people are part of the sector in spite of these limitations.

Another challenge is working in a system where there appears to be waning support for Māori services or Māori-centric models of working. There is a definite relationship between service development and configuration, models of care and the workforce. It is essential that those of us working in workforce development understand and can influence how services are planned, implemented and evaluated. Working to support a marginalised part of the workforce (Māori) in what many would still consider to be a racist system requires some perseverance.

Matua Raki believes in facilitating more than just training, and promotes the shaping of systems and leadership so any training can be sustained and the return on investment can be evaluated and, if and where necessary, refined to achieve better results. A challenge is finding the balance between working where energy is at the flax roots and working top-down where processes can be cumbersome and addiction is but one of a number of workforce priorities.

(continued)

Lessons learnt

The biggest lesson that I have learnt is that there is always something new to learn.

A close second is that communication is the message received not the message sent. This has taught me to listen and learn and, in that space, understand that one size does not fit all and that it is up to me to ensure I am relevant to the sector and community we serve.

I wish I would have had formal training as a manager, particularly in human resource management, financial control and strategic planning—I, like many, learnt on the job. I think we were leaders who still thought we were working with clients rather than leading colleagues and organisations. Some of us came through that relatively unscathed; others did not do so well. Given the rapidly changing health and social service sectors, this change is a constant that leaders have to cope with. Part of my role is cultivating future and even current leadership so they can navigate these waters. There is an argument that a manager is a manager but in the addiction sector you have to know something of addiction, have a sense of what well-being is for people and, more importantly, have a passion for the people we work with.

Skills and qualities

I am a caretaker—I'm keeping the seat warm till the real person gets here. Obviously as part of workforce development we are often encouraging services and practitioners to succession plan. Below is a list of some of the skills and knowledge needed to do my role.

- Knowledge of the addiction (and increasingly the mental health) sector
- Experience of working in the addiction sector
- Strategic worldview—perseverance and adaptability/flexibility
- Analytical skills
- Advocacy and mediation skills
- Relationship management skills—able to operate across different levels of the system, roles and situations
- Hopeful—a belief that we can make a difference as a sector; our role in the workforce centre is to guide and facilitate services and practitioners to achieve that
- Understand concepts such as Tu rangatira (self-determination, ability to make informed choices) and mana (prestige, influence or status), and operationalise them in our work with Māori and non-Māori (for example, mana enhancing and protecting practice and encouraging self-management)
- To be able to work with Māori services, practitioners and those who influence and shape the delivery of services for Māori
- To be able to work with others and as part of a team
- A sense of humour and able to practice self-care
- Able to manage time and priorities (perhaps an ability to delegate)
- Good communication skills (written and verbal)
- Confidence and commitment to the kaupapa (theme, program) of growing and sustaining robust Māori practice and a flourishing Māori-responsive workforce
- Belief in best practice and that we can make a difference in people's lives
- Intuitive and able to recognise and make the most of opportunities
- Inspirational and motivational—as a servant being supported by those in the sector

Effective communication strategies

- Because we have a couple of us in the Matua Raki team off site we make use of video conference and phone conference facilities for internal meetings, however, from time to time we must have face-to-face meetings to move things along and get a greater sense of buy-in to our work and projects.

- Email of course is an essential communication within our team and the sector.

- Increasing use of blogs and social media to communicate with the sector.

- Face-to-face meetings and training. Because of our lack of capacity much of our training is contracted out. One exception is our cultural competence training, which we take a central role in coordinating and delivering.

- In these days of austerity many are encouraged to conduct business with stakeholders by remote via telephone or video conferencing. Experience shows that you have to do the hard yards at the 'front-end' to build a relationship and trust. This often takes time. For those of us with experience in the sector we can build on existing connections. Sometimes national bodies coming in sound like they are delivering edits from on high and then disappear.

- Matua Raki prides itself on being a part of the sector, because building new relationships is founded on existing relationships. When we are working with those we don't have previous relationships with, people often see that we have sector knowledge, experience and that we are there to help. Once these relationships are established then we can work more remotely. Experience in this takes time.

- Certainly working with Māori requires face-to-face contact to establish and maintain connection, however, increasingly, use of technology allows for greater flexibility and is being grasped.

Terry Huriwai makes the point that effective communication requires real presence in real time, at least initially, to allow relationships to build. We conclude this chapter by looking at factors that contribute to effective and ineffective communication.

Effective and ineffective communication

Attention to and awareness of 'good' and 'poor' communication is applicable at group and individual levels—whether you are a direct service worker or a CEO, communicating face-to-face or virtually, with clients, peers and colleagues, staff under your supervision, communities, or stakeholders. As a manager it is necessary to be aware of any factors that may promote or inhibit respectful and positive communication within the workspace. The checklist in Table 10.2, overleaf, builds on sources of distortion identified by Trevor Tyson, and includes factors associated with the environment within an organisation and those linked to individual personnel. These will, of course, vary according to organisational context.

Effective communication is based on clear, open, respectful and honest exchange. Without these conditions, ineffective or destructive patterns can readily establish themselves in workplaces where high levels of stress and anxiety are associated with everyday work (Tyson, 1998). Unfortunately, communication distortions are common features of the work in many health and human service contexts. Tyson identifies a range of habits that contribute to ineffective communication, as well as skills that promote effective communication. Using these as a basis, we have compiled a list of effective and ineffective communication behaviours in Table 10.3. As the many items listed in the table demonstrate, healthy communication requires awareness and attention to skill development. If you would like to read Tyson's complete chapter on communication, the details are listed in the further readings at the end of this chapter.

TABLE 10.2 Checklist of conditions that shape communication processes within organisations

Physical	Space—appropriate dimensions, not overcrowded or overwhelming	☐
	Furniture—comfortable and conducive to conversation	☐
	Proximity of staff—enabling interaction	☐
	Comfortable noise and temperature levels	☐
	Opportunity for privacy and absence of interruptions	☐
Technological	IT facilities—well maintained and functional	☐
	Audio-visual equipment for video conferencing	☐
	Translation services—access to and use of	☐
	Landline telephone systems—functional	☐
	Assisted communication available where required	☐
	Provision of mobile communication devices for off-site staff	☐
Psychological	Staff morale—engagement levels	☐
	Self-perceptions	☐
	Prejudices and stereotyping	☐
	Concentration and level of interest	☐
	Emotional states	☐
	Power dynamics	☐
Physiological	Health	☐
	Speech and sensory capacity	☐
	Bodily comfort levels	☐
Linguistic	Use of jargon, slang and vernacular	☐
	Accent and brogue	☐
	Ambiguity, mixed messages	☐
	Command of language in use	☐
	Translators—appropriateness and competence with language	☐
	Level of congruence between verbal and non-verbal messages	☐
Cultural diversity	Cultural awareness and competency	☐
	Capacity to find common ground	☐
	Respect for difference	☐
	Inclusiveness and valuing diversity	☐

Interpersonal	Levels of trust between communicators	☐
	Use of body language	☐
	Respect for personal space and boundaries	☐
	Status of relationship between communicators	☐
	Transparent/hidden agendas	☐
	Use of power	☐
Organisational	Staff hierarchy in organisational structure—clear lines of command	☐
	Transparency, accuracy and frequency of communications	☐
	Open and honest communication—encouraged	☐
	Inclusive decision-making	☐
	Meaningful consultation	☐

Source: adapted from Tyson, 1998, pp.82–9

TABLE 10.3 Effective and ineffective communication behaviours

EFFECTIVE COMMUNICATION BEHAVIOUR	INEFFECTIVE COMMUNICATION BEHAVIOUR
Awareness: being alert to conditions that may hinder communication.	Self-absorption: not being aware of context or others; self-focused.
Initiative: acting to mitigate negative and promote positive influences.	Inertia: waiting for others to initiate or take action.
Positivity: promoting positive perspectives; starting exchanges in productive ways—avoiding put-downs, accusations, threats, etc.	Negativity: focusing on the bad, overlooking the good.
Taking responsibility: owning opinions and reactions.	Avoiding responsibility: expecting others to take responsibility for change or action.
Assertiveness: making positive statements about needs, e.g., 'I need' rather than 'I can't'.	Deflecting from self: referring to 'everyone' or others and avoiding ownership when speaking about self, e.g., 'you', 'we'.
Focus: staying on topic, being prepared to deal with the difficult issues.	Deflecting from topic: introducing irrelevant content to divert the discussion and avoid uncomfortable or threatening dialogue.
Active listening: reflecting back to clarify and affirm the message; providing feedback by sharing own opinion.	Analysing: identifying causes and reasons, intellectualising, uninvited problem-solving.
Acceptance: suspending judgment and criticism.	Judging and blaming: making evaluative, rather than descriptive, comments about others. Accusing others, not owning behaviours.
Respect: for sender's viewpoint and values.	Disrespect: put-downs; making patronising and ridiculing statements.
Attentiveness, genuineness and empathy: listening attentively, expressing interest and concern, feeling 'with' rather than 'for'.	Interrupting: cutting the speaker off, imposing own view, failing to listen.

(continued)

TABLE 10.3 Effective and ineffective communication behaviours (*continued*)

EFFECTIVE COMMUNICATION BEHAVIOUR	INEFFECTIVE COMMUNICATION BEHAVIOUR
Objectivity and self-awareness: attention to boundaries, monitoring own language use, non-verbal behaviour and cues from other speaker.	Lack of objectivity and self-awareness: invading personal space, unaware of own body language and non-verbal cues.
Non-competitiveness: fostering a climate of safety, where open exchange can take place.	Competitiveness: seeking to assert dominance, and outdo the other speaker.
Non-aggression: appropriate use of power.	Aggression: inappropriate use of power.
Affirmation: responding warmly and acknowledging others' feelings and beliefs.	'Butting': following a positive statement with a 'but', thereby giving the impression of negating what was said, e.g., 'I agree with you, but …'. 'Shoulding': telling others what they 'should' or 'must' do.
Authenticity: avoiding clichés.	Superficiality: using clichés and dismissive statements that are devaluing, e.g., 'Beggars can't be choosers', 'Takes one to know one'.
Non-defensiveness: allowing others to express negative emotions, including anger. Not taking their expressions personally (this does not mean that assault or violence is condoned).	Defensiveness: reacting to information as if it is an accusation; taking statements personally.
Risk-taking: engaging in authentic, managed self-disclosure.	Denial: suppressing feelings, refusing to share.
Wisdom: maintaining balanced perspective, knowing when to take risks and how to respond and challenge.	Overgeneralising: applying the outcome of a specific event to everything, e.g., 'This always happens'.
Compassionate honesty: being straightforward and upfront without being insensitive or hurtful.	Duplicity: being manipulative, asking questions that mask a hidden agenda or attempt to trap the responder into a particular disclosure.

SUMMARY OF KEY ISSUES

This chapter has emphasised the fundamental role of communication, community engagement and collaboration in organisational management, leadership and practice. All health and human service organisations are required to engage with external stakeholders and communities to varying degrees in order to successfully deliver services. Although this is frequently seen as a way to expand an organisation's resource base, networking and partnership-building are resource intensive in terms of time and skill. Managers and leaders need to be skilled communicators in order to promote a positive workplace culture with an engaged workforce, while at the same time fostering genuine external relationships.

PRACTICE ACTIVITIES

1   Read the list of organisational and personal conditions that shape communication processes in Table 10.2.
    a   Use the check boxes in the right column to mark the conditions that may require attention in your organisation.
    b   What might you add?

2   Reflect on the effective and ineffective communication behaviours in Table 10.3. Identify areas that you might work on personally, and in your organisation.

3   With the practitioner perspectives in mind, and the approaches discussed in this chapter, develop a community engagement strategy for your organisation.

FURTHER READING

Collaboration

Foster Alter, C. (2009). 'Building Community Partnerships and Networks', in Patti, R. J. (ed.), *The Handbook of Human Service Management* (2nd edn), Thousand Oaks: Sage, pp.435–54.

O'Flynn, J. (2008). 'Elusive Appeal or Aspirational Ideal? The Rhetoric and Reality of the "Collaborative Turn" in Public Policy', in O'Flynn, J. & Wanna, J. (eds), *Collaborative Governance. A New Era of Public Policy in Australia?* Canberra, Australia: ANU E Press, pp.181–95.

Community engagement

State Government of Victoria (2005a). *Effective Engagement: Building Relationships with Community and other Stakeholders. Book 1, An Introduction to Engagement*, Melbourne: The Community Engagement Network.

This informative, user-friendly and practical set of materials is available at www.dse.vic.gov.au/effective-engagement.

Communication and collaboration for community engagement

Dale, J. (2011). 'Public Dialogue: Bridging the Gap between Knowledge and Wisdom', in Bird, F. & Westley, F. (eds), *Voices from the Voluntary Sector*, Toronto: University of Toronto Press, pp.361–90.

Taylor, J., Braunack-Mayer, A., Cargo, M., Larkins, S. & Preston, R. (2013). 'A Role for Communities in Primary Prevention of Chronic Illness? Case Studies in Regional Australia', *Qualitative Health Research*, *23*(8), pp.1103–13.

Communication: ineffective and effective communication processes

Tyson, T. (1998). 'Communicating', in *Working with Groups* (2nd edn), South Yarra: MacMillan Education Australia, pp.77–89.

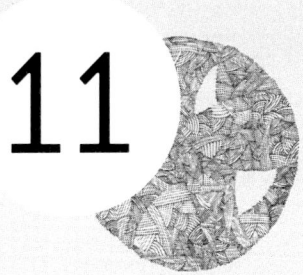

11

Towards Effective Management and Practice in Health and Human Service Organisations

OVERVIEW

This closing chapter encourages the reader to:
- revisit the external context of management in health and human services
- reflect on the emergence and continuing evolution of management challenges in this area
- contemplate a sample of managers' views on 'what matters' in their role
- draw conclusions about keys to successful management and leadership in Australia's health and human service organisations.

This chapter draws together major topics covered in the text. It summarises themes contained in the practitioner profiles on 'what matters' in health and human services management and leadership, and revisits key points addressed throughout the previous chapters.

A context of change

As we have explored, many organisations providing for those experiencing health and social issues were created as a result of community concern and motivation to bring about positive change in the lives of individuals, groups and communities. Over recent decades, the role of government has changed, in terms of funding, service planning and operations, and there has been a decrease in the role of governments as direct service providers. This shift has occurred in association with the introduction of business-oriented strategies to support organisational efficiency and accountability, increased service system regulation through accreditation, and requirements for services to form partnerships and collaborate with government and each other within integrated systems. These reforms present organisations with an array of challenges and threaten the very existence of some services—at least in the forms that have evolved from and with communities. We have focused in this text on a range of organisational types (as outlined in Chapter 2), as many issues facing the NFP sector are relevant to this range of organisations and, therefore, to you, the reader, as a current or future manager and leader in this sector.

The contribution of NFP organisations in Australia

Not-for-profit organisations make a unique and substantial contribution to Australian society, which reflects people's commitment to social well-being and their willingness to work together for the betterment of self and others. As Lyons (2009) noted, NFP contribute to:

- The economy—generating employment and providing services that for-profit firms and governments fail to supply.
- Society—providing expressions of people's capacity to join and work together for themselves (mutuality) and others (altruism); a product of, and also regenerating, social capital.
- The political system—as a vehicle that enables people to participate in the political process by demonstrating what is important; engaging in the most important manifestation of civil society.

With a long history of growth and change, the landscape for organisations continues to evolve, and there are many different structures and systems of governance, which is reflective of a complexity of funding arrangements and associated pressures.

Organisations face increased scrutiny into the effectiveness and quality of the services that they deliver, and more stringent accountability regimes. There are concerns about the capacity of services to deliver, alongside fears that the vibrancy of organisations, their diversity, ethos, capacity for responsiveness to the particular needs of their clients and communities, and their advocacy functions, are being diminished. The complexity of funding and reporting arrangements may lead to unanticipated outcomes, including a change in values, service access and commitment to social well-being.

A National Compact

In 2010, the Australian Government launched a National Compact in recognition of these concerns and of the need for a systematic and transparent process regarding the government's relationship with the NFP sector. The compact is a set of conditions between government and organisations that is based on the belief that having a strong independent sector is essential, and that the country will benefit from clarity regarding the roles of government and organisations (Commonwealth of Australia, 2013). Principles of the code that underpins the National Compact are included in Box 11.1.

Government and the not-for-profit sector

The National Compact was developed following extensive consultation with a broad range of NFP organisations and, together, the sector and Government agreed on the following shared principles:

- We believe a strong independent sector is vital for a fair, inclusive society. The immense contribution the sector and its volunteers make to Australian life should be acknowledged and valued.
- We aspire to a relationship between the Government and the NFP sector based on mutual respect and trust.
- We agree that authentic consultation, constructive advocacy and genuine collaboration between the sector and the Government will lead to better policies, programs and services for our communities.
- We believe the great diversity within Australia's not-for-profit sector is a significant strength, enabling it to understand and respond to the needs and aspirations of the nation's varied communities, in collaboration with those communities.
- We commit to enduring engagement with marginalised and disadvantaged Australians, in particular, Aboriginal and Torres Strait Islander people and their communities.
- We recognise the value of our multicultural society and we will plan, design and deliver culturally responsive services.
- We share a desire to improve life in Australia through cultural, social, humanitarian, environmental and economic activity. To achieve this, we need to plan, learn and improve together, building on existing strengths and making thoughtful decisions using sound evidence.
- We share a drive to respond to the needs and aspirations of communities through effective, pragmatic use of available resources.
- We recognise concerted effort is needed to develop an innovative, appropriately resourced and sustainable sector.
- We acknowledge the need to develop measurable outcomes and invest in accountability mechanisms to demonstrate the effectiveness of our joint endeavours.
- Ultimately, the National Compact and this Code will bring about mutual benefits for the sector and Government through an improved relationship, better designed policies, more effectively implemented service delivery and stronger public communication and community ownership.

Source: extract from the *Code of Best Practice for Engagement with the Not-for-Profit Sector* (Commonwealth of Australia, 2013, p.5). Licensed from the Commonwealth of Australia under a Creative Commons Attribution 3.0 Australia Licence.

This code of engagement reflects an interest in addressing challenging aspects of the relationship between government and NFP that range from understandings about organisations' independence to the usefulness of streamlining reporting requirements. It seeks to develop useful ways of working together while retaining a degree of separation that will maintain the values underpinning community organisations.

As with all 'contracts' of this nature, the National Compact is subject to broader developments, and it was suspended following the change of government in late 2013. In addition, it does not account for State and Territory Government perspectives on their relationship with non-government organisations. The National Compact illustrates one approach to working with organisations, as well as the significant effect external forces have on the context for service provision.

What matters for good management

Within this practice and policy context, the particular challenge for managers and leaders is twofold: to maintain the values, nature, quality and extent of the contribution of health and human service to individual and social well-being; while incorporating a business orientation to organisational practice and responding to an ongoing cycle of policy change. Let us briefly revisit the constellation of knowledge, skills and values important for management in health and human service organisations.

Management in today's health and human services requires:

*   Knowledge, skills and strategies for working with internal and external organisational processes, managing change and engaging with diverse stakeholders (funders, providers, service users, the broader community).
*   Notions of effectiveness and organisational success that are consistent with the values held by stakeholders and with professional ethics.
*   A willingness to support and engage with innovative approaches and a capacity to work productively with uncertainty, within a flexible and functional operational framework.

As we have acknowledged throughout this text, management in health and human service organisations is a broader and more complex endeavour than management in business, as in the latter 'values' tend to be fundamentally defined in terms of volume of work and monetary gain, and position descriptions tend to be more tightly circumscribed. The unique constellation of stakeholder demand and accountability, obligations to professional ethics, and fluid practice environment produces a long list of 'what matters' in managing health and human services; raising ongoing challenges and opportunities. With this understanding, we have explored areas of management practice deemed important *and* challenging by health and human services managers and leaders. Our focus reflects the diverse and inter-related nature of the capacities that are required in today's practice environment. Figure 11.1 is a simple representation of the areas we have explored, which have been informed by research and practice wisdom.

As you will recognise, the areas of expertise are many and diverse. Managers will excel at some and struggle with others, but the important thing is to aspire to better management in an ongoing cycle of action, reflection and change—utilising and benefiting from the contributions of other stakeholders. This includes fellow managers (in practice and policy situations) as well as consumers and members of the broader community.

FIGURE 11.1 What matters for management in health and human service organisations

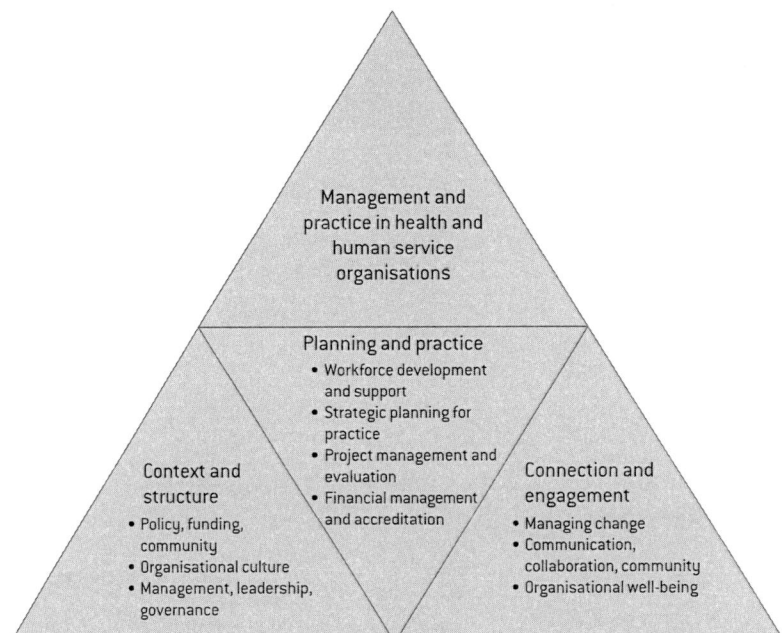

The nature of good management

Organisational culture is the cornerstone of effective and ethical operations. The development and maintenance of shared values and goals are fostered by well-informed strategies for planning, financial management, staff development and communication. For success, these must be complemented by participatory approaches and inclusive practices that ensure power and authority are employed and engaged with productively and not misused. The emphasis on business principles in new public management, which are reflected in funding decisions and understandings of service effectiveness, means conflict is likely within and across organisations, and this can extend into the policy arena. Managers and leaders must anticipate and respond to these challenges in an ongoing climate of change, while remaining true to their understandings of 'what matters' in practical terms. This requires a unique combination of business acumen and professional integrity, combined with clarity of purpose, and ability to communicate with and listen to the many stakeholders in health and human service delivery. The practitioners who have contributed to this text eloquently describe the skills and qualities involved. A sample of their comments is shown in Box 11.2.

A sample of 'what matters' to managers in health and human service organisations

Clear leadership, direction and modelling have been important in providing some stability and confidence within the organisation. *Geoff Soma*

Managers need: advanced knowledge of policy and practice; strong interpersonal and communication skills that build and maintain relationships; finance and business skills; and a passion for promoting community and organisational health and well-being. *Cheryl Sobczyk*

The decision-making process is complex and often the extra time taken to consider the available options, debate a decision with a colleague and potentially identify suitable alternatives, is beneficial for all concerned. *Leanne Coupland*

You have to believe in what you do and work to continually improve at doing it. *Daryl Fitzgibbon*

There is an argument that a manager is a manager, but in the addiction sector you have to know something of addiction, have a sense of what well-being is for people and, more importantly, have a passion for the people you work with. *Terry Huriwai*

A lesson I have learnt over time is to respect, listen, learn and build from the power and potential of local relationships, knowledge and experience. *Sharon Fisher*

It is important to engage constructively with all stakeholders and maintain those relationships through times when differences become difficult. *Jenny Smith*

My approach is consultative, ethical and culturally responsive. *Sue Carswell*

You need to be able to listen. Not only to government, but to staff and consumers. *Simon Ruth*

Management requires a significant amount of people and practical skills. *Geoff Soma*

Keep your staff happy, and trust them. *Vanessa Bleier*

There is sometimes extensive and unsurpassable distance between concrete and conceptual thinking. *Marie Feeley*

The [manager] needs to embrace organisational change, as the health environment is constantly shifting to meet new strategies and priorities. *Melissa Elliott*

Fostering good management

Our research highlights the breadth of demand and complexity of management and leadership in health and human service organisations, which involves many tasks and functions, and requires skills, flexibility and capacity to respond in planned and emergent ways. Managers and leaders face a dual challenge: how to provide and resource services in the present, while at the same time positioning the organisation for survival and growth in the future. Attention and energy must be concentrated on the everyday practical tasks of running an organisation and delivering effective services, while the issues of most concern relate to the 'paucity' of the present and trying to ensure a viable, and possibly better resourced, future (Wagner & Spence, 2003). This requires working paradoxically: maintaining a core vision and delivering effective services according to existing agreements, while adapting and responding to constantly changing circumstances (Corrigan & Garman, 1999; Dixon, 1999).

The resolution of diverse management issues can be significantly facilitated by good communication processes, mutually respectful relationships between management and staff, participatory approaches, and functional teamwork, combined with commitment to thorough planning. Clarity about staff responsibilities and reporting, inclusive approaches and shared leadership roles combine to assist in establishing productive and transparent power relationships that enable an organisation to operate effectively and successfully.

Transformational approaches to leadership are essential (for example, Liebler et al., 2008, in Ray, 2010). Fostering a culture that shares with and supports staff to take risks, and to identify, develop and implement strategies for addressing issues and problems, enhances organisational functionality, health and growth. This necessitates finding a balance between confident leadership, good management and effective communication (Dixon, 1999; Yukl, 1999), in tandem with an inclusive practice approach founded on practising power *with* workers, horizontally and vertically across all levels of the organisation.

A final word

Working with people in challenging and evolving situations requires skills, commitment, knowledge, critical self-awareness and support. In preparing this text, our goal has been to clarify and address 'what matters' for health and human service management from theoretical and practice perspectives. As this arena continues to change, it is essential that managers and leaders are encouraged to take on the required skills, gather the necessary knowledge, and pursue engagement with stakeholders that will enable the provision of services matched to need. We hope our work proves useful in this domain.

Glossary

ACCREDITATION
A process used to assess whether the quality of services provided meets approved standards of care.

ACTION PLAN
Details of the specific tasks required to translate objectives into actions, generated and acted upon by teams and/or individuals at practice level.

ADMINISTRATIVE MANAGEMENT
A theory of management that proposes that efficiency and effectiveness are achieved through the application of particular principles and practices across the whole organisation.

ANTICIPATED CHANGE
Change which is planned for in advance.

BABBAGE PRINCIPLE
A term coined in 1974 by Harry Braverman, based on the ideas of Charles Babbage that assigning and distributing work tasks by matching degree of difficulty with skill level is efficient and productive. In other words, skilled and highly paid workers should only be allocated demanding tasks, while those who are lower paid and less skilled should be given easier tasks

BALANCE SHEET
A summary of the financial balances at a specific time, often the end of the financial year; used to guide decisions about whether activities operating at a loss can be supported by other areas.

BUDGET
A quantified financial plan for a defined period of time; describes the cost implications of activities by clarifying the expenditure required and resources available.

BUREAUCRATIC MANAGEMENT
A theory of management based on the ideas of Max Weber, which proposes that the most effective and efficient way to run an organisation is to have a hierarchical structure, with clear role definitions and rigid lines of accountability.

BUSINESS PLAN
Examines the financial situation of the organisation, anticipating the financial resources required to implement the strategic plan and using this to forecast performance over a defined period.

BUSINESS PROFILE
Develops a picture of the work of the organisation in relation to its environment by looking at clients, services, suppliers, partners and assets.

CHANGE DRIVERS
Internal or external factors that cause an organisation to make changes to services, structure, policy or operations.

CHANGE MANAGEMENT
A systematic and structured process of moving people and organisations from one state to a desired future state.

COLLABORATION
Cooperatively working together to achieve a mutual goal.

COMMUNICATION
An exchange of information between parties using a shared language. Communication may be conveyed in a variety of forms: verbal, sensory, physical, emotional, technological, etc.

COMMUNICATION STRATEGY
A process involving identifying and mapping project stakeholders and mechanisms in order to engage support, thereby enabling project success.

COMMUNITY AUDIT APPROACH
A survey method that seeks information about community perceptions of need, demographic details and other services to assist in determining the most appropriate and beneficial programs and services for the community.

COMMUNITY ENGAGEMENT
Practices undertaken by an organisation with the aim of forming meaningful connections with the communities and stakeholders it interacts with.

COMMUNITY OF INTEREST
A community that forms because of a shared interest, whether in a physical location (for example, a community of students) or not (for example, groups that 'meet' via social media).

COMMUNITY OF PLACE
A form of geographic community that is defined by ongoing interactions of the members due to their proximity.

COMMUNITY OF PRACTICE
A type of community of interest with a specific focus on learning through sharing skills, building knowledge and improving practice in an area of mutual interest.

COMMUNITY SERVICE ORGANISATIONS (CSO)
Umbrella term covering a range of non-profit health and human service organisations that provide services to the community. Includes NGO, NFP, QANGO and GONGO.

COMMUNITY SERVICES WORKFORCE
According to the Australian Institute of Health and Welfare the major services in this workforce involve residential aged care and other residential care, childcare, and other social support and assistance.

CORPORATE CULTURE
The official culture of the organisation that is represented in formal elements that are promoted through documents, websites and displays.

DISCRIMINATION
Disadvantaging a person because of their personal characteristics or situation, which can include race, sex, sexual preference, age, physical or mental disability, family responsibilities or political opinion.

DIVERSITY MANAGEMENT
Actions designed to support an inclusive approach to employment and to foster awareness and acceptance of various backgrounds of staff.

ECOLOGICAL SYSTEMS THEORY
Proposes that understanding human development and behaviour requires looking at the person in the context of the interrelated systems within their environment.

EMERGENT CHANGE
Occurs as a result of external factors, or arises with little warning. There is usually no (or limited) opportunity for influencing the nature of the change, or planning for its implementation.

EMERGENT PLANNING
A 'ground-up' approach to planning that involves embracing opportunities and incorporating them into a planning cycle. The process is responsive, reflective, iterative, evaluative and inclusive.

EMPOWERMENT EVALUATION
A capacity-building approach in which stakeholders are supported to develop skills and resources that enable effective project planning, implementation and review.

EQUITY
An important concept that impacts on the configuration of services according to fundamental views regarding equality, ethics and efficiency in health care.

EVALUATION
A process of systematic enquiry to assess the value and merit of an activity.

EVIDENCE-BASED PRACTICE
The integration of research evidence with practice expertise.

FINANCIAL MANAGEMENT
Processes including the allocation and use of financial and material resources, activities leading to funds acquisition, and accounting for and reporting on resource utilisation.

FORCE FIELD ANALYSIS
A method for identifying and analysing the degree of influence of the forces for and against a proposed change event, with the purpose of reducing resistant forces.

FORECASTING
The use of past experience to estimate the future availability of funds, while accounting for contextual factors.

FORMATIVE EVALUATION
A form of enquiry to determine the extent to which a project has been implemented as planned and provide directions for future development.

GANTT CHART
A horizontal bar chart developed by Henry Gantt in the early 1900s that visually represents the scheduling of a project according to task, time, order of tasks, and key milestones.

GEOGRAPHIC COMMUNITY
A community that comes together because of, or is defined by, physical location.

GOVERNANCE
Governance is not about day-to-day management, but about *overseeing* the management of an organisation; providing guidance to ensure an organisation has good management and leadership and that it honours its values.

GOVERNMENT-OPERATED NON-GOVERNMENT ORGANISATIONS (GONGO)
Organisations that may be established by government but run separately, so the organisation maintains a level of independence and may qualify for government funding.

HAWTHORNE EFFECT
The view that people will adjust their behaviour because they are receiving positive attention from others whom they judge to be superior. In particular, research subjects will alter their behaviour because they are being studied, rather than because of variables in their environment.

HEALTH WORKFORCE
Comprises people employed in health occupations in health service industries. There are many types of occupations; major groups include nurses, medical professionals, allied health workers and social workers.

HORIZONTAL COMMUNICATION
Communication between people who are at the same level, for example, colleagues and peers.

HORIZONTAL EQUITY
The equal provision of services among people with equal levels of need.

HUMAN RELATIONS MANAGEMENT
Human relations management theory asserts that the psychosocial needs of workers must be addressed in order to maximise their performance. It was developed in reaction to the scientific management principles of Taylorism.

HUMAN RESOURCE MANAGEMENT
Involves strategies for managing people to maintain a strong alignment between workforce characteristics and organisational goals. Areas include staff recruitment and development, staff welfare and workforce renewal.

HUMAN SERVICES WORKFORCE
A term used to describe the diverse field of workers employed across community and health services, sometimes referred to as 'the caring professions'.

IMPLEMENTATION PLANNING
A process that addresses contextual factors, gathers resources, and clarifies the time frame for a project to be operational.

INCREMENTAL BUDGET
A budget based on the previous year's budget, with the assumption that income is stable and only a slight adjustment is necessary, to account for inflation.

INDUSTRIAL ORGANISATION
A group of employees and employers, a trade union, or any other group established for people who work in a particular industry, trade or profession.

INTENDED CHANGE
Purposeful change that arises from anticipated events and organisational planning processes.

INTERDISCIPLINARY TEAM
Professionals from different work areas who work together closely in a collaborative and cooperative way, sharing responsibility and decision-making.

LEADERSHIP
Different from management, leadership involves seeing future directions, seeking opportunities and providing a sense of purpose, as well as guiding and motivating people to achieve goals.

LIKERT SCALE
A survey tool that measures opinions about a particular issue. Respondents are provided with a defined range of options, usually five (for example: strongly disagree, disagree, neutral, agree and strongly agree). These are then collated and analysed.

LINE-ITEM BUDGET
Commonly used for projects and programs, this details the staff and material resources (time and money) needed for activities. The four categories are generally staffing, direct costs, program costs and organisational overheads.

LOGIC MODELLING
A diagrammatic representation of the framework for a project, which is developed by those involved in project development and typically includes aims, activities, outputs and impacts/outcomes.

MANAGEMENT

Involves purposeful planning, organising people, systems and resources, supporting and supervising workers, communicating with stakeholders, making decisions, monitoring progress, evaluating results and revising plans to improve future outcomes.

MANAGEMENT FUNCTIONS

The fundamental management processes. These establish the purpose of a management role and circumscribe management tasks, roles and skills.

MANAGEMENT ROLE

A formally or informally defined position that has responsibility for performing a management function.

MANAGEMENT SKILLS

The ability and capacity to carry out tasks and functions pertaining to a management role.

MANAGEMENT TASKS

Specific activities relating to management in an organisational setting. Although often seen as the work of managers, all workers are required to perform management tasks to some degree.

MANAGERIAL ETHICS

Obligations and duties regarding internal and external stakeholders, board members, clients and the broader community.

MARKET RESEARCH APPROACH

Gathering and analysing organisational data to determine whether client needs are being effectively met.

MASLOW'S HIERARCHY OF NEEDS

A theory of human development coined by Abraham Maslow, which proposes that human beings must satisfy a series of needs in order to progress across their life course. There are five stages of need, which must be achieved in ascending order, beginning with physiological needs (food, warmth and shelter). The final stage, which fewer people attain, is self-actualisation.

McDONALDIZATION

A concept that identifies four dominant mechanisms current in organisational management, based on fast-food industry principles: efficiency, calculability, predictability and control.

MECHANISTIC ORGANISATIONS

Organisations, often large, with a hierarchical structure, rigid rules, procedures and lines of accountability, and centralised decision-making.

MULTIDISCIPLINARY TEAM

Comprised of members with diverse professional qualifications; formed to achieve a defined goal. Collaboration is not emphasised, unless directly relevant to the achievement of the common goal.

NEED

A subjective assessment of a problem that is influenced by community standards.

NEW PUBLIC MANAGEMENT (NPM)

Major reform of the public sector toward a market-oriented model, whereby services need to be more responsive to citizens and politicians, and to demonstrate the delivery of desired outcomes within an efficient organisational framework.

NOT-FOR-PROFIT (NFP) AND NON-GOVERNMENT ORGANISATIONS (NGO)

Organisations that do not have shareholders; all income is expended in the provision of services or used to improve the organisation.

OPERATIONAL PLAN

A sub-set of the strategic plan that is focused at the individual program or project level.

OPERATIVE CULTURE

The actual culture of the organisation that is evident in staff behaviour and physical aspects of the work environment.

ORGANIC ORGANISATIONS

In many ways the antithesis of the mechanistic organisation, these are often small and flat structured, with open communication, and flexible decision-making processes to support emergent developments.

ORGANISATIONAL CLIMATE

Shared perceptions among staff about the psychological impact the workplace has on their well-being, as determined by views about how the organisation deals with areas that are personally important to staff.

ORGANISATIONAL CULTURE

A system of shared meaning that distinguishes the organisation from other workplaces. This culture is evident in the policies, practices, attitudes and rituals of the organisation.

ORGANISATIONAL ETHICS

Principles and rules of behaviour established to uphold the values of an organisation.

ORGANISATIONAL POLICIES

General statements intended to communicate expectations and guide staff behaviour.

OUTCOME EVALUATION

The review of short- and longer-term impacts and outcomes of a project to measure the extent to which intended results have been attained.

OUTPUT EVALUATION

An assessment of whether intended project activities have been delivered.

PANOPTICON
An architectural structure designed by Jeremy Bentham in the 18th century that enabled a single unseen observer to oversee the activities of many. Most significantly, the Panopticon created the psychological effect of being under constant surveillance, while never being able to see the observer or to know when they are watching.

PARTICIPATORY MANAGEMENT
A management approach that encourages consultation and genuine participation in organisational decision-making across all levels.

PARTICIPATORY PLANNING
A process that involves various stakeholders in decision-making and the design and implementation of a plan.

PEOPLE SKILLS
Capacity to be self-aware, empathic, inclusive and to effectively communicate with a wide range of people.

PERFORMANCE APPRAISAL
Formal, systematic review of staff performance by employee and their manager; has bearings on decisions about staff development and career direction.

PLANNED CHANGE
Change that is implemented through a managed planning process.

POLICY STASIS
The continued application of an existing policy, which may persist despite external factors indicating that the policy needs amendment.

POWER
Ability to exercise will and influence actions. The force that drives and emerges in the exchange from one state to another.

PRE-CLASSICAL PERIOD
Time before management was formalised as a separate domain of work.

PROFESSIONAL CODE OF ETHICAL CONDUCT
An official guide to the values and standards of a professional group.

PROFIT AND LOSS STATEMENT
A summary of income and expenses for a period (usually monthly, quarterly or annually) to monitor how a project, program or organisation is tracking against the budget plan.

PROGRAM
A complex, integrated system with discrete goals and its own budget.

PROGRAM PLAN

A sequence of strategies, tasks and resources organised into a coherent framework designed to attain a shared goal; the key elements in this process are 'planning' and 'action'.

PROJECT

A unique, one-off effort, with a defined budget, time frame and set of requirements.

PROJECT PLAN

Similar to a program plan, except it's for a specific project. The plan provides a detailed account of the project's aims, objectives, background, activities, stakeholders, resource implications and timeline.

PROJECT TIMELINE

A diagram that maps project activities by time.

PROPOSAL WRITING

The steps involved in preparing a submission for an external funding round to match the requirements and expectations of funding guidelines and priorities.

QUASI-AUTONOMOUS NON-GOVERNMENT ORGANISATIONS (QANGO)

Organisations that are semi-independent from government. They may have an independent board that includes government representatives.

SCIENTIFIC MANAGEMENT

A management approach that is based on the belief that scientific research can aid organisational efficiency and productivity.

SERVICE PROVISION

The practices, methods and modes by which an organisation offers services to clients.

SITUATIONAL LEADERSHIP

Situational leadership argues that to be effective, managers must select a style or strategy according to the presenting situation.

STAFF CONDITIONS

Normally founded on basic conditions set by government, and augmented with conditions put forward by professional associations. Conditions are set through negotiations between employers and staff representatives.

STAKEHOLDER ANALYSIS

A process that identifies who, out of significant individuals and groups affected by a proposed change, is likely to support the change and who might resist.

STANDARD

An explicit statement of the level of care consumers should be able to expect from services.

STRATEGIC PLAN
An organisation's blueprint for future operations over a defined period of time.

SUMMATIVE EVALUATION
An assessment of the extent to which desired outcomes have been achieved.

SUPERVISION
A process involving manager and employee, where the manager allocates and monitors work activities, provides support for work-related challenges, and fosters employee development through mentoring, advice and opportunities for skill development.

SYNERGY
The interaction of two or more entities that results in a greater outcome than is achievable by the individual components.

TAYLORISM
The principles of scientific management developed by Frederick Taylor, based on the idea that work processes can be completed more efficiently if they are broken into small, specialised tasks. Taylorism resulted in the development of the factory production line.

THEORY X AND THEORY Y MANAGEMENT TYPES
Theory X managers assume workers are fundamentally lazy, only motivated by financial reward, and in need of constant supervision. Theory Y managers believe workers are self-motivated, can be left unsupervised and ultimately strive for self-actualisation in work.

TOTAL QUALITY MANAGEMENT
A process of improvement that stems from the premise that service quality should be defined by the needs and wishes of clients. Initiated by leaders in the organisation and involves all members, including clients.

TRANSDISCIPLINARY TEAM
Transcends professional or disciplinary boundaries to achieve innovative practice through knowledge and skill exchange, and the formation of new approaches.

UNIONS
Organisations that represent their worker-members, and aim to preserve or improve workplace conditions. Union staff play an intermediary role during workplace negotiations and provide general advice and support for their members.

UNPLANNED CHANGE
Change that results from unanticipated events, and for which no planning process is implemented.

UTILITARIANISM
The belief that the most ethical stance is to achieve the greatest good for the greatest number of people.

VALUES
Beliefs and behaviours that are held in high regard by an organisation.

VERTICAL COMMUNICATION
Communication between people who are in a hierarchical relationship, for example, supervisor and supervisee, CEO and program manager, team leader and service delivery workers.

VERTICAL EQUITY
The unequal provision of services among people according to their unequal levels of need.

WELFARISM
Attitudes and policies supporting the establishment of a welfare state.

ZERO-BASED BUDGET
A budget that is determined prior to each fiscal year; expenditure must be justified regardless of current or past financial conditions. Planned expenditure generally needs to be completed within the funding period.

252

Bibliography

Aldgate, J., Healy, L., Malcolm, B., Pine, B., Rose, W. & Seden, J. (2007). *Enhancing Social Work Management. Theory and Best Practice from the UK and USA*, London and Philadelphia: Jessica Kingsley Publishers.

Allison, M. & Kaye, J. (2005). *Strategic Planning for Nonprofit Organizations: A Practical Guide and Workbook* (2nd edn), New Jersey: John Wiley & Sons.

Anheier, H. (2005). *Nonprofit Organizations. Theory, Management, Policy*, United Kingdom: Routledge.

Antonakis, J., Avolio, B. J. & Sivasubramaniam, N. (2003). 'Context and Leadership. An Examination of the Nine-Factor Full-Range Leadership Theory Using the Multifactor Leadership Questionnaire', *The Leadership Quarterly, 14*, pp.261–95.

Armstrong, B. K., Gillespie, J. A., Leeder, S. R., Rubin, G. L. & Russell, L. M. (2007). 'Challenges in Health and Health Care for Australia', *Medical Journal of Australia, 187*, pp.485–9.

Armstrong, M. (2011). *How to Be an Even Better Manager* (8th edn), United Kingdom: KoganPage.

Arnstein, S. R. (1969). 'A Ladder of Citizen Participation', *Journal of the American Planning Association, 35*(4), pp.216–24.

Aronson, J. & Smith, K. (2011). 'Identity Work and Critical Social Service Management: Balancing on a Tightrope?' *British Journal of Social Work, 41*, pp.432–48.

Aryee, S., Chen, Z. X. & Budhwar, P. S. (2004). 'Exchange Fairness and Employee Performance: An Examination of the Relationship between Organizational Politics and Procedural Justice', *Organizational Behavior and Human Decision Making Processes, 94*, pp.1–14.

Austin, D. M. (2002). *Human Services Management. Organizational Leadership in Social Work Practice*, New York: Columbia University Press.

Austin, M. J. & Solomon, J. R. (2009). 'Managing the Planning Process', in Patti, R. J. (ed.), *The Handbook of Human Services Management* (2nd edn), Thousand Oaks, California: Sage, pp.321–37.

Austin, M. J., Regan, K., Sample, M. W., Schwartz, S. L. & Carnochan, S. (2011). 'Building Managerial and Organizational Capacity in Nonprofit Human Service Organizations through a Leadership Development Program', *Administration in Social Work, 35*(3), pp.258–81.

Australian Association of Social Workers (2010). *Code of Ethics*, retrieved from www.aasw.asn.au/document/item/740

Australian Bureau of Statistics (2006). *A Picture of the Nation. 2070.0*, retrieved from www.ausstats.abs.gov.au/ausstats/subscriber.nsf

Australian Bureau of Statistics (2009). 'Not-for-Profit Organisations, Australia, 2006–07' (re-issue), Catalogue no. 8106.0.

Australian Bureau of Statistics (2012). '4125.0—Gender Indicators, Australia', Jan. 2012, retrieved from www.abs.gov.au/ausstats/abs@.nsf/Lookup/by+Subject/4125.0~Jan+2012~Main+Features~Labour+force~1110

Australian Community Workers Association (2012). *Code of Ethics*, retrieved 10 Sep. 2012, from www.acwa.org.au/resources/code-of-ethics

Australian Government (2012). 'Health Workforce Australia', retrieved Mar. 2013, from www.hwa.gov.au

Australian Government Fair Work Ombudsman (2013). *Discrimination*, retrieved Jun. 2013, from www.fairwork.gov.au/employment/discrimination/Pages/default.aspx?friendlyURL=1&discrimination

Australian Institute of Health and Welfare (2009). *Health and Community Services Labour Force 2006. National Health Labour Force. Number 42. Cat. no. HWL 43*, Canberra: Australian Government, retrieved from www.aihw.gov.au/WorkArea/DownloadAsset.aspx?id=6442458396

Australian Institute of Health and Welfare (2011). 'Australia's Welfare 2011. Australia's Welfare No. 10. Cat. no. AUS 142', retrieved from www.aihw.gov.au/WorkArea/DownloadAsset.aspx?id=10737420628

Australian Institute of Health and Welfare (2012a). 'Australia's Health 2012. Australia's Health no. 13. Cat. no. AUS 156', Canberra: AIHW.

Australian Institute of Health and Welfare (2012b). *Health Workforce*, Canberra: Australian Government, retrieved from www.aihw.gov.au/health-workforce

Australian Productivity Commission (2006). 'Australia's Health Workforce, Research Report', Canberra.

Australian Productivity Commission (2010). 'Contribution of the Not-for-Profit Sector. Research Report', Canberra: Australian Government.

Baeza, J. I. & Lewis, J. M. (2010). 'Indigenous Health Organizations in Australia: Connections and Capacity', *International Journal of Health Services, 40*, pp.719–42.

Barraket, J. (2008). *Strategic Issues for the Not-for-Profit Sector*, Australia: UNSW Press.

Bartol, K. (2008). *Management Foundations: A Pacific Rim Focus* (2nd edn), Australia: McGraw-Hill.

Bartol, K., Tein, M., Matthews, G., Sharma, B. & Scott-Ladd, B. (2011). *Management. A Pacific Rim Focus*, Australia: McGraw-Hill.

Bennet, S., Agyepong, I. A., Sheikh, K., Hanson, K., Ssengooba, F. & Gilson, L. (2011). 'Building the Field of Health Policy and Systems Research: An Agenda for Action', *Public Library of Medicine, 8*(8), e1001081.

Berends, L. & Crinall, K. (forthcoming). 'Managers' Perspectives on What Matters in Health and Human Services Management'.

Berends, L. & Roberts, B. (2012). 'Implementation Effectiveness of an Alcohol Screening Intervention Project at Two Hospitals in Regional Victoria, Australia', *Contemporary Drug Problems, 39*, pp.289–309.

Berglund, C. (2012). *Ethics for Health Care* (4th edn), Australia: Oxford University Press.

Bess, G. (2009). 'Practitioners' Views on the Future of Human Services Management', in Patti, R. J. (ed.), *The Handbook of Human Services Management* (2nd edn), Thousand Oaks, USA: Sage, pp.473–81.

Bird, F. & Westley, F. (eds) (2011). *Voices from the Voluntary Sector. Perspectives on Leadership Challenges*, Toronto: University of Toronto Press.

Bishop, S. W. (2007). 'Linking Nonprofit Capacity to Effectiveness in the New Public Management Era: The Case of Community Action Agencies', *State and Local Government Review, 39*(3), pp.144–52.

Black, N. & Gruen, R. (2005). *Understanding Health Services*, Glasgow: Open University Press.

Blanchard, K. & Johnson, S. (1993). *The One-Minute Manager*, London: Harper Collins.

Blanchard, K., Zigarmi, P. & Zigarmi, D. (1986). *Leadership and the One Minute Manager*, London: Harper Collins.

Bowen, S. & Zwi, A. B. (2005). 'Pathways to "Evidence-Informed" Policy and Practice: A Framework for Action', *PLoS Medicine, 2*(e166).

Brody, R. (2005). *Effectively Managing Human Service Organizations* (3rd edn), Thousand Oaks, California: Sage.

Brown, J. & Isaacs, D. (1994). 'Merging the Best of Two Worlds. The Core Processes of Organizations as Communities', in Senge, P., Kleiner, M. A., Roberts, C.,

Ross, R. B. & Smith, B. J. (eds), *The Fifth Discipline Fieldbook*, London: Nicholas Brealey Publishing, pp.509–17.

Bryson, J. M. (2004). *Strategic Planning for Public and Nonprofit Organizations* (3rd edn), San Francisco: John Wiley & Sons.

Burns, T. & Stalker, G. (1961). *The Management of Innovation*, London: Tavistock.

Butcher, J. R. (2011). 'An Australian Compact with the Third Sector: Challenges and Prospects', *Third Sector Review, 17*(1), pp.35–58.

Buykx, P., Humphreys, J. S., Tham, R., Kinsman, L., Wakerman, J., Asaid, A. & Tuohey, K. (2012). 'How do Small Rural Primary Health Care Services Sustain Themselves in a Constantly Changing Health System Environment?' *BMC Health Services Research, 12*(81), retrieved from www.biomedcentral.com/1472-6963/12/81

Cameron, E. & Green, M. (2012). *Making Sense of Change Management. A Complete Guide to the Models, Tools and Techniques of Organizational Change* (3rd edn), United Kingdom & USA: Kogan Page.

Carlopio, J., Andrewartha, G. & Armstrong, H. (2001). *Developing Management Skills: A Comprehensive Guide for Leaders* (2nd edn), Frenchs Forest NSW: Pearson Education Australia.

Carson, E., Chung, D. & Day, A. (2009). 'Evaluating Contracted Domestic Violence Programs', *Standardisation and Organisational Culture. Evaluation Journal of Australasia, 9*, pp.10–19.

Carson, E. & Kerr, L. (2012). *Marketisation of Human Service Delivery: Implications for the Future of the Third Sector in Australia*, Paper presented at the ISTR Conference, Siena, Italy. http://c.ymcdn.com/sites/ www.istr.org/resource/resmgr/wp2012/ marketisation_implications_f.pdf

Chernew, M. (2009). 'Research and Reform: Toward a High-Value Health System', *Health Services Research, 44*(5 pt 1), pp.1445–8.

Clegg, S., Kornberger, M. & Pitsis, T. (2011). *Managing and Organizations. An Introduction to Theory and Practice* (3rd edn), London: Sage.

Commonwealth of Australia (2001). 'Report of the Inquiry into the Definition of Charities and Related Organisations', retrieved from www.cdi.gov.au/html/ report.htm

Commonwealth of Australia (2010). *CHC08 Community Services Training Package Qualifications Framework*, Canberra, Australia: Commonwealth of Australia.

Commonwealth of Australia (2013). *Code of Best Practice for Engagement with the Not-for-Profit Sector. Engaging Today for a Better Tomorrow. National Compact. Working Together*, Canberra, retrieved from Office for the Not-for-Profit Sector website at www.notforprofit.gov.au

Community Services and Health Industry Skills Council (2012). *CHC80108 Vocational Graduate Diploma of Community Sector Management*, Canberra, Australia: Commonwealth of Australia.

Connell, R., Fawcett, B. & Meagher, G. (2009). 'Neoliberalism, New Public Management and the Human Service Professions: Introduction to the Special Issue', *Journal of Sociology, 45*(4), pp.331–8.

Corrigan, P. W. & Garman, A. N. (1999). 'Transformational and Transactional Leadership Skills for Mental Health Teams', *Community Mental Health Journal, 35*(4), pp.301–12.

Coulshed, V., Mullender, A., Jones, D. N. & Thompson, N. (2006). *Management in Social Work* (3rd edn), New York: Palgrave Macmillan.

Cree, V. (2010). *Sociology for Social Workers and Probation Officers* (2nd edn), Hoboken: Routledge.

Creed, A. (2011). *Organisational Behaviour*, Australia: Oxford University Press.

Crinall, K. & Laming, C. (2012). 'Walking Together for Safer Communities with Local Action Supported by Family Violence Policy Reforms', in Gunstone, A. (ed.), *Reconciliation in Regional Australia: Case Studies from Gippsland*, Melbourne: Australian Scholarly Publishing, pp.89–107.

Crinall, K., Manning, D., Feeley, M. & Glavas, A. (2010). '"The Power of Pyjamas": Everything Effects Everything Else: Power, Perception and Hidden Forms of Restrictive Practice in Shared Supported Accommodation', paper presented at the From Theory to Practice; Context in Praxis, 8th Action Learning, Action Research and 12th Participatory Action Research World Congress, Melbourne.

Cummins, T. G. & Worley, C. G. (1997). *Organization Development and Change* (6th edn), Ohio, USA: South-Western College Publishing.

Daft, R. L. & Lengel, R. H. (1998). *Fusion Leadership. Unlocking the Subtle Forces that Change People and Organizations*, San Francisco: Berrett-Koehler.

Dale, J. (2011). 'Public Dialogue: Bridging the Gap between Knowledge and Wisdom', in Bird, F. & Westley, F. (eds), *Voices from the Voluntary Sector*, Toronto: University of Toronto Press, pp.361–90.

D'Amour, D., Ferrada-Videla, M., Martin-Rodriguez, L. & Beaulieu, M. (2005). 'The Conceptual Basis for Interprofessional Collaboration: Core Concepts and Theoretical Frameworks', *Journal of Interprofessional Care, 19*(s1), pp.116–31.

Department of Health (2012). *Psychiatric Disability Rehabilitation and Support Services Reform Framework*, Melbourne: Victorian Government.

Department of Planning and Community Development (2011). *Community Sector Workforce Capability Framework—Tool Kit*, Melbourne, Australia: Victorian Government, Department of Planning and Community Development.

Diversity Council of Australia (2012). 'Why Diversity', retrieved Sep. 2012, from www.dca.org.au/why-diversity.html

Dixon, D. L. (1999). 'Achieving Results through Transformational Leadership', *Journal of Nursing Administration, 29*(12), pp.17–21.

Donovan, F. & Jackson, A. (1991). *Managing Human Service Organisations*, Australia: Prentice Hall.

Drucker, P. (1990). *Managing the Nonprofit Organization. Principles and Practices*, New York: Harper Collins.

D'Urbano, T. (2004). *Survey of Organisations in the Human Services Field for a Proposal to Develop a Masters in Human Services Management*, Gippsland Research and Information Service. Monash University. Churchill.

Dwyer, J., Stanton, P. & Thiessen, V. (2004). *Project Management in Health and Community Services. Getting Good Ideas to Work*, Melbourne: Allen & Unwin.

Dyer, J. A. (2003). 'Multidisciplinary, Interdisciplinary, and Transdisciplinary Educational Models and Nursing Education', *Nursing Education Perspectives, 24*(4), pp.186–8.

Eadie, D. C. (2006). 'Planning and Managing Strategically', in Edwards, R. L. & Yankey, Y. A. (eds), *Effectively Managing Nonprofit Organizations*, Washington DC: NASW Press pp.375–88.

Edwards, M., Howard, C. & Miller, R. (2001). *Social Policy, Public Policy. From Problem to Practice*, NSW: Allen & Unwin.

Egan, R. & Hoatson, L. (1999). 'Desperate to Survive: Contracting Women's Services in Melbourne', *Australian Feminist Studies, 14*(30), pp.405–14.

Ermha (2010). *Ermha Annual Report 2010*, Victoria, Australia: Eastern Region Mental Health Association.

Ethics Resource Center (May 2009). 'Definitions of Values', retrieved

5 Sep. 2012, from www.ethics.org/resource/definitions-values

Fawcett, B. & Hanlon, M. (2009). 'The "Return to Community": Challenges to Human Service Professionals', *Journal of Sociology, 45*(4), pp.433–44.

Field, R. (2010). 'Planning and Budgeting', in Gray, I., Field, R. & Brown, K. (eds), *Effective Leadership, Management and Supervision in Health and Social Care*, Exeter, UK: Learning Matters Ltd, pp.120–41.

Finkelman, A. W. (2006). *Leadership and Management in Nursing*, New Jersey Pearson Prentice Hall.

Fisher, E. A. (2009). *Motivation and Leadership in Social Work Management: A Review of Theories and Related Studies, 33*(4), pp.347–67.

Fisher, W. F. (1997). 'DOING GOOD? The Politics and Antipolitics of NGO Practices', *Annual Review of Anthropology, 26*, pp.439–64.

Fleming, J. (2008). 'Health Care Workforce', in Taylor, S., Foster, M. & Fleming, J. (eds), *Health Care Practice in Australia. Policy, Context and Innovations*, Melbourne: Oxford University Press, pp.103–30.

Follett, M. P. (1951). *Creative Experience*, New York: Peter Smith.

Ford, J. (1999). 'Organizational Change as Shifting Conversations', *Journal of Organizational Change Management, 12*(6), pp.480–500.

Foster Alter, C. (2009). 'Building Community Partnerships and Networks', in Patti, R. J. (ed.), *The Handbook of Human Service Management* (2nd edn), Thousand Oaks: Sage, pp.435–54.

Foucault, M. (1979). *Discipline and Punish: The Birth of the Prison*, England: Peregrine Books.

Foucault, M. (1983). 'On the Genealogy of Ethics', in Dreyfus, H. L. & Rabinow, P. (eds), *Michel Foucault. Beyond Structuralism and Hermeneutics* (2nd edn), Chicago: The University of Chicago Press, pp.229–52.

Foucault, M. (1991). 'What is Enlightenment?' in Rabinow, P. (ed.), *The Foucault Reader*, London: Penguin Books, pp.32–50.

Foucault, M. (1992). 'The Subject and Power', in Dreyfus, H. L. & Rabinow, P. (eds), *Michel Foucault, Beyond Structuralism and Hermeneutics*, Chicago: University of Chicago Press, pp.208–28.

Fox, E. M. & Urwick, L.F. (eds) (1973). *Dynamic Administration: The Collected Papers of Mary Parker Follett*, London: Pitman.

Gardner, F. (2006). *Working with Human Service Organisations. Creating Connections for Practice*, Australia: Oxford University Press.

Gilson, L., Hanson, K., Sheikh, K., Agyepong, I. A., Ssengooba, F. & Bennet, S. (2011). 'Building the Field of Health Policy and Systems Research: Social Science Matters', *Public Library of Medicine, 8*(8), e10001079.

Ginsberg, L. H. (ed.) (2008). *Management and Leadership in Social Work Practice and Education*, USA: Council on Social Work Education.

Ginsberg, L. H. & Keys, P. R. (1995). *New Management in Human Services* (2nd edn), USA: NASW Press.

Gippsland Research and Information Service (2004). 'Survey of Organisations in the Human Services Field for a Proposal to Develop a Masters in Human Services Management', Churchill, Victoria, Australia: Monash University.

Government of Western Australia Department of Communities (2010). *Parenting WA Strategic Framework*, Perth: Western Australian Government vol. 2013, retrieved from www.communities.wa.gov.au/Documents/Parents%20Families%20Education%20Care/PWA-strategic-framework.pdf

Gray, I., Field, R. & Brown, K. (2010). *Effective Leadership, Management and Supervision in Health and Social Care*, Exeter: Learning Matters.

Hafford-Letchfield, T. (2006). *Management and Organisations in Social Work*, Exeter: Learning Matters.

Hafford-Letchfield, T., Leonard, K., Begum, N. & Chick, N. F. (2008). *Leadership and Management in Social Care*, London: Sage.

Hansard (2013). 'Debates of the Legislative Assembly for the Australian Capital Territory', Daily Hansard, edited proof transcript, 22 Aug. 2012, accessed 5 Sep. 2013 from www.regnet.anu.edu.au/sites/default/files/Debates%20Educ%20right.pdf

Harris, J. (2007). 'Looking Backward, Looking Forward: Current Trends in Human Services Management', in Aldgate, J., Healy, L., Malcolm, B., Pine, B., Rose, W. & Seden, J. (eds), *Enhancing Social Work Management: Theory and Best Practice from the UK and USA*, London: Jessica Kingsley Publishers, pp.17–34.

Harris, M. F., Harris, E., Roland, M. (2004). 'Access to Primary Health Care: Three Challenges to Equity', *Australian Journal of Primary Health, 10*, pp.21–9.

Hasenfeld, Y. (ed.) (2010). *Human Services As Complex Organizations* (2nd edn), USA: Sage.

Hassan, A. & Wimpfheimer, S. (2012). 'Human Services Management Competencies. A Guide for Public Managers', USA: The National Network for Social Work Management.

Healy, K. (2009). 'A Case of Mistaken Identity: The Social Welfare Professions and New Public Management', *Journal of Sociology, 45*(4), pp.401–18.

Healy, K. & Lonne, B. (2010). *The Social Work and Human Services Workforce: Report from a National Study of Education, Training and Workforce Needs*, Strawberry Hills, NSW: Australian Learning and Teaching Council.

Heath, C. & Heath, D. (2011). *Switch. How to Change when Things Are Hard*, London: Random House.

Heller, R. (1998). *Managing Change*, London: Dorling Kindersley.

Hemmelgarn, A. L., Glisson, C. & James, L. R. (2010). 'Organizational Culture and Climate. Implications for Services and Interventions Research', in Hasenfeld, Y. (ed.), *Human Services As Complex Organizations* (2nd edn), USA: Sage, pp.229–50.

Herman, R. D. & Heimovics, R. D. (1989). 'Critical Events in the Management of Nonprofit Organizations: Initial Evidence', *Nonprofit and Voluntary Sector Quarterly, 18*(2), pp.119–32.

Hinchcliff, R., Greenfield, D., Moldovan, M., Westbrook, J. I., Pawsey, M., Mumford, V. & Braithwaite, J. (2012). 'Narrative Synthesis of Health Service Accreditation Literature', *British Medical Journal Quality and Safety, Online* (Oct. 2012).

Hoefer, R. (2009). 'Preparing Managers for the Human Services', in Patti, R. J. (ed.), *The Handbook of Human Services Management* (2nd edn), Thousand Oaks, USA: Sage, pp.483–501.

Holosko, M. J. (2009). 'Social Work Leadership: Identifying Core Attributes', *Journal of Human Behavior in the Social Environment, 19*(4), pp.448–59.

Houlbrook, M. (2011). 'Critical Perspectives on Results-Based Accountability: Practice Tensions in Small Community-Based Organisations', *Third Sector Review, 17*, pp.45–68.

Hudson, M. (2009). *Managing without Profit* (3rd edn), Sydney, Australia: UNSW Press.

Hughes, C. M., Lapane, K., Watson, M. C. & Davies, H. T. O. (2007). 'Does Organisational Culture Influence Prescribing in Care Homes for Older People? A New Direction for Research', *Drugs and Aging, 24*, pp.81–93.

Hughes, D. (2009). *Liquid Leadership*, West Sussex, UK: Capstone.

Hughes, M. & Wearing, M. (2013). *Organisations and Management in Social Work* (2nd edn), London: Sage.

Jackson, A. & Donovan, F. (1999). *Managing to Survive. Managerial Practice in Not-for-Profit Organisations*, St Leonards, Australia: Allen & Unwin.

Johnson-Abdelmalik, J. (2011). 'The Legitimacy of Ideas: Institutional Foundations of the Non-Profit Community Welfare Sector', *Third Sector Review, 17*, pp.5–27.

Jones, A. & May, J. (1992). *Working in Human Service Organisations: A Critical Introduction*, Melbourne: Longman Cheshire.

Kemmis, S. and McTaggart, R. (1988). *The Action Research Planner*, 3rd edn, Geelong, Victoria: Deakin University Press, p.11.

Kettner, P. M., Moroney, R. M. & Martin, L. L. (2013). *Designing Effectiveness-Based Programs. An Effectiveness-Based Approach.* (4th edn), Thousand Oaks, California: Sage.

Kotter, J. P. (2011a). 'Leading Change: Why Transformation Efforts Fail', in Harvard Business School (ed.), *HBR's 10 Must Reads on Change Management*, Massachusetts, USA: Harvard Business School, pp.1–16.

Kotter, J. P. (2011b, originally published 1990). 'What Leaders Really Do', in Harvard Business Review (ed.), *On Leadership*, Boston, Massachussetts: Harvard Business Review Press, pp.37–56.

KPMG (2007). *Survey of the Community-Managed Housing and Support Workforce Final Report*, Melbourne: KPMG.

Laming, C., Crinall, K., Hurley, J., Patten, S., Goodall, D., Yarram, D., McDonald, P. (2011). *The Gippsland CommUNITY Walk against Family Violence: Evaluation Report*, Churchill, Australia: Monash University.

Larkin, H. (2012). 'Smart Money Management', *Trustee: The Journal for Hospital Governing Boards, 65*, 13–14, pp.19–20.

Lauffer, A. (2011). *Understanding Your Social Agency* (3rd edn), Thousand Oaks, California: Sage.

Lawler, J. (2007). 'Leadership in Social Work: A Case of Caveat Emptor?' *British Journal of Social Work, 37*(1), pp.123–41.

Lawler, J. & Bilson, A. (2010). *Social Work Management and Leadership. Managing Complexity with Creativity*, London and New York: Routledge.

Leggat, S., Bartram, T. & Stanton, P. (2006). 'People Management in Victorian Community Health Services: An Exploratory Study', *Australian Journal of Primary Health, 12*(3), pp.59–65.

Lehmann, J. (2005). 'Human Services Management in Rural Contexts', *British Journal of Social Work, 35*, pp.355–71.

Lewis, J. A., Packard, T. R. & Lewis, M. D. (2012). *Management of Human Service Programs* (5th edn), USA: Brooks/Cole Cengage Learning.

Liang, Z., Howard, P. F., Koh, L. C. & Leggat, S. (2012). 'Competency Requirements for Middle and Senior Managers in Community Health Services', *Australian Journal of Primary Health* (PY12041).

Lukes, S. (2005). *Power. A Radical View* (2nd edn), Hampshire: Palgrave Macmillan.

Lyons, M. (2001). *Third Sector. The Contribution of Nonprofit and Cooperative Enterprises in Australia*, NSW: Allen & Unwin.

Lyons, M. (2009). 'The Nonprofit Sector in Australia: A Fact Sheet', *National Roundtable of Nonprofit Organisations*, retrieved from www.philanthropy.org.au/pdfs/papersreports/NonprofitFactsheet094ed.pdf

Mackay, K. (1991). *Community Management*, Melbourne, Australia: Victorian Council of Social Services & Victoria Law Foundation.

MacLean, S., Berends, L., Hunter, B., Roberts, B. & Mugavin, J. (2012). 'Factors that Enable and Hinder Implementation of Projects in the Alcohol and Other Drug Field', *Australian and New Zealand Journal of Public Health, 36*(1), pp.61–8.

Maddison, S. & Edgar, G. (2008). 'Into the Lion's Den: Challenges for Not-for-Profits in Their Relationship with Government', in Barraket, J. (ed.), *Strategic Issues for the Not-for-Profit Sector*, Sydney, Australia: UNSW Press, pp.188–211.

Magnabosco, J. L. (2006). 'Innovations in Mental Health Services Implementation: A Report on State-Level Data from the U.S. Evidence-Based Practices Project', *Implementation Science*, 1, retrieved from www.implementationscience.com/content/1/1/13

Manning, S. S. (2003). *Ethical Leadership in Human Services. A Multi-Dimensional Approach*, USA: Pearson Education.

Martin-Rodriguez, L., Beaulieu, M., D'Amour, D. & Ferrada-Videla, M. (2005). 'The Determinants of Successful Collaboration: A Review of Theoretical and Empirical Studies', *Journal of Interprofessional Care, 19*(s1), pp.132–47.

Mason, R. (2008). 'DO EVERYTHING, BE EVERYWHERE', *Australian Feminist Studies, 23*(58), pp.485–99.

Mayers, R. S. (2004). *Financial Management for Non-Profit Human Service Organizations* (2nd edn), Springfield, Illinois: Charles C. Thomas.

McDonald, C. (1999a). 'Internal Control and Accountability in Non-Profit Human Service Organisations', *Australian Journal of Public Administration, 58*(1), pp.11–22.

McDonald, C. (1999b). 'Human Service Professionals in the Community Services Industry', *Australian Social Work, 52*(1), pp.17–25.

McDonald, C., Craik, C., Hawkins, L. & Williams, J. (2011). *Professional Practice in Human Service Organisations*, Australia: Allen & Unwin.

McGhee, P. & McAliney, P. (2007). *Painless Project Management*, New Jersey: John Wiley & Sons.

McGuire, M. (2006). 'Collaborative Public Management: Assessing What We Know and How We Know It', *Public Administration Review, 66* (Special Issue, Dec. 2006), pp.33–43.

McIntosh, P. (2010). *Action Research and Reflective Practice*, London and New York: Routledge.

Menefee, D. (2009). 'What Human Services Managers Do and Why They Do It', in Patti, R. J. (ed.), *The Handbook of Human Services Management* (2nd edn), California, USA: Sage, pp.101–16.

Mickan, S. & Rodger, S. (2000). 'Characteristics of Effective Teams. A Literature Review', *Australian Health Review, 23*, pp.201–8.

Miner, J. T., Miner, L. E. & Griffith, J. (2011). *Collaborative Grantseeking. A Guide to Designing Projects, Leading Partners, and Persuading Sponsors*, USA: Greenwood.

Mooney, G. (2003). *Economics, Medicine and Health Care* (3rd edn), England: Pearson Education Limited.

Mor Barak, M. E. & Travis, D. J. (2010). 'Diversity and Organizational Performance', in Hasenfeld, Y. (ed.), *Human Services As Complex Organizations* (2nd edn), USA: Sage, pp.341–78.

Morgan, G. (2006). *Images of Organization* (updated edn), Thousand Oaks, California: Sage.

Mosley, J. E, Maronick, M. P. & Katz, H. (Spring 2012). 'How Organizational Characteristics Affect the Adaptive Tactics Used by Human Service Nonprofit Managers Confronting Financial Uncertainty', *Nonprofit Management & Leadership, 22*(3), pp.281–303.

Moynihan, D. P. & Pandey, S. K. (2005). 'Testing How Management Matters in an Era of Government by Performance Management', *Journal of Public Administration Research and Theory, 15*(3), pp.421–39.

Mugavin, J. & Berends, L. (Jan. 2013). 'Older Wiser Lifestyles (OWL) Program Evaluation. Final Report', Fitzroy, Victoria: Turning Point Alcohol & Drug Centre.

Munn, P. (2003). 'Factors Influencing Service Coordination in Rural South Australia', *Australian Social Work, 56*(4), pp.305–17.

Office of the Anti-Discrimination Commissioner Tasmania (undated). 'Industrial Activity', retrieved from www.antidiscrimination.tas.gov.au/__data/assets/pdf_file/0007/95353/adc_industrialactivity.pdf

O'Flynn, J. (2008). 'Elusive Appeal or Aspirational Ideal? The Rhetoric and Reality of the "Collaborative Turn" in Public Policy', in O'Flynn, J. & Wanna, J. (eds), *Collaborative Governance. A New Era of Public Policy in Australia?* Canberra, Australia: ANU E Press, pp.181–95.

O'Flynn, J. & Wanna, J. (eds) (2008). *Collaborative Governance. A New Era of Public Policy in Australia?* Canberra, Australia: ANU E Press.

O'Leary, R. & Vij, N. (2012). 'Collaborative Public Management: Where Have We Been and Where Are We Going?' *The American Review of Public Administration, 42*(5), pp.507–22.

Osborne, D. & Gaebler, T. (1992). *Reinventing Government: How the Entrepreneurial Spirit is Transforming the Public Sector*, New York: Penguin.

Osborne, S. P. & Brown, K. (2005). *Managing Change and Innovation in Public Service Organizations*, London and New York: Routledge.

Owen, J. (2006). *Program Evaluation: Forms and Approaches* (3rd edn), Crows Nest, NSW: Allen & Unwin.

Owen, J. (2011). *How to Lead* (3rd edn), Harlow, UK: Pearson. Prentice Hall.

Ozanne, E. & Rose, D. (2013). *The Organisational Context of Human Service Practice*, Australia: Palgrave Macmillan.

Packard, T. (2010). 'Staff Perceptions of Variables Affecting Performance in Human Service Organizations', *Non-Profit and Voluntary Sector Quarterly, 39*(6), pp.971–90.

Page, E. S. (2011). *Diversity and Complexity*, Oxfordshire & New Jersey: Princeton University Press.

Parish, S. L., Ellison, J. & Parish, J. K. (2006). 'Managing Diversity', in Edwards, R. L. & Yankey, J. A. (eds), *Effectively Managing Nonprofit Organizations*, Washington: NASW Press, pp.179–94.

Patti, R. (2003). 'Reflections on the State of Management in Social Work', *Administration in Social Work, 27*, pp.1–11.

Patti, R. J. (ed.) (2009). *The Handbook of Human Services Management* (2nd edn), Thousand Oaks, California: Sage.

Pawson, R., Greenhalgh, T., Harvey, G. & Walshe, K. (2005). 'Realist Review: A New Method of Systematic Review Designed for Complex Policy Interventions', *Journal of Health Services Research and Policy, 10* (Supplement 1), pp.21–34.

Pettinger, R. (2004). *Contemporary Strategic Management*, USA: Palgrave Macmillan.

Pine, B. A. & Healy, L. (2007). 'New Leadership for the Human Services: Improving and Empowering Staff through Participatory Processes', in Aldgate, J., Healy, L., Malcolm, B., Pine, B., Rose, W. & Seden, J. (eds), *Enhancing Social Work Management. Theory and Best Practice from the UK and USA*, London: Jessica Kingsley, pp.35–55.

Poindexter, C. C. (2007). 'Management Successes and Struggles for AIDS Service Organizations', *Administration in Social Work, 31*(3), pp.5–28.

Putnis, P. & Petelin, R. (1999). *Professional Communication. Principles and Applications* (2nd edn), Australia: Pearson Education.

Quality Improvement Council (2013). 'Continuous Quality Improvement and Accreditation in Health and Community Services', from www.qic.org.au

Rafferty, A. E., Jimmieson, N. L. & Armenakis, A. A. (2013). 'Change Readiness: A Multilevel Review', *Journal of Management, 38*(1), pp.110–35.

Rainnie, A., Fitzgerald, S., Gilchrist, D. & Morrie, L. (2012). 'Putting the Public First? Restructuring the West Australian Human Services Sector', *International Journal of Employment Studies, 20*(1), pp.104–26.

Randhwa, G. (2007). *Human Resource Management*, India: Atlantic Publishers and Distributors.

Rath, T. (2007). *Strengths Finder 2.0*, New York: Gallup Press.

Ray, N. M. (2010). 'Editorial: Leading and Managing for Improved Health', *Journal of Public Health Management and Practice, 16*(2), pp.91–2.

Reeve, G. (2005). 'Human Services Administration: Managing the Real Complexity', *Public Administration Today, 4*, Jul./Sep.

Robbins, S. P., Bergman, R., Stagg, I. & Coulter, M. (2000). *Management* (2nd edn), Frenchs Forest, NSW: Pearson Education.

Robbins, S. P., Millett, B., Waters-Marsh, T. (2004). *Organisational Behaviour* (4th edn), NSW: Pearson Education Australia.

Sackett, D. L. (1996). 'Evidence Based Medicine: What It Is and What It Isn't', *British Medical Journal, 312*, pp.71–2.

Saldana, J. (2009). *The Coding Manual for Qualitative Researchers*, USA: Sage.

Schein, E. H. (1990). 'Organizational Culture', *American Psychologist, 45*(2), pp.109–19.

Senge, P. M. (1992). *The Fifth Discipline. The Art and Practice of the Learning Organization*, Milson's Point, Sydney: Random House.

Senge, P. M., Roberts, C., Ross, R. B., Smith, B. J. & Kleiner, A. (eds) (1994). *The Fifth Discipline Fieldbook: Strategies and Tools for Building a Learning Organization*, London: Nicholas Brealey Publishing.

Sheikh, K., Gilson, L., Agyepong, I. A., Hanson, K., Ssengooba, F. & Bennet, S. (2011). 'Building the Field of Health Policy and Systems Research: Framing the Questions', *Public Library of Medicine* (8), e1001073.

Smircich, L. (1983). 'Concepts of Culture and Organisational Analysis', *Administrative Science Quarterly, 28*, pp.339–58.

Smith, B. (1992). *Management Development in Australia*, Australia: Harcourt Brace Jovanovich.

Smith, B. (1994). 'Organizations As Communities', in Senge, P. M. (ed.), *The Fifth Discipline Fieldbook*, London: Nicholas Brealey Publishing, pp.507–8.

Smith, S. R. (2010). 'The Political Economy of Contracting and Competition', in Hasenfeld, Y. (ed.), *Human Services As Complex Organizations* (2nd edn), USA: Sage, pp.139–60.

Spooner, C. & Dadich, A. (2008). *Non-Government Organizations in the Alcohol and Other Drugs Sector. Issues and Options for Sustainability*, Australian National Council on Drugs Research Paper No.17, Canberra: Australian National Council on Drugs.

State Government of Victoria (2005a). *Effective Engagement: Building Relationships with Community and other Stakeholders. Book 1, An Introduction to Engagement*, Melbourne: The Community Engagement Network.

State Government of Victoria (2005b). *Effective Engagement: Building Relationships with Community and other Stakeholders. Book 2, The Engagement Planning Workbook*, Melbourne: State Government of Victoria.

State Government of Victoria (2005c). *Effective Engagement: Building Relationships with Community and other Stakeholders. Book 3, The Engagement Tool Kit.* Melbourne: State Government of Victoria.

State Government of Victoria (2011). Department of Human Services.

Human Services: The Case for Change, Melbourne, Victoria: Victorian Government Department of Human Services.

State Government of Victoria (2012). *Psychiatric Disability Rehabilitation and Support Services Reform Framework*, Consultation Paper.

State Government of Victoria (2013a). *What is Community Engagement?* retrieved 7 Jul. 2013, from www.dse.vic.gov.au/effective-engagement/introduction-to-engagement/what-is-community-engagement

State Government of Victoria (2013b). Department of Human Services. 'Organisational Structure', retrieved 11 May 2013, from www.dhs.vic.gov.au/about-the-department/our-organisation/organisational-structure

Stefl, M. E. (2008). 'Common Competencies for all Healthcare Managers: The Healthcare Leadership Alliance Model', *Journal of Healthcare Management, 53*(6), pp.360–73.

Sugarman, B. (1989). 'The Well-Managed Human Service Organization: Criteria for a Management Audit', *Administration in Social Work, 12*(4), pp.17–27.

Summers, N. (2010). *Managing Social Service Staff for Excellence. Five Keys to Exceptional Supervision*, New Jersey & Canada: John Wiley & Sons Inc.

Sun Tzu (1991). *The Art of War* (T. Cleary, trans.), Boston Shambahala Publications.

Taylor, J., Braunack-Mayer, A., Cargo, M., Larkins, S. & Preston, R. (2013). 'A Role for Communities in Primary Prevention of Chronic Illness? Case Studies in Regional Australia', *Qualitative Health Research, 23*(8), pp.1103–13.

Taylor, S., Foster, M. & Fleming, J. (eds) (2008). *Health Care Practice in Australia: Policy, Context and Innovations*, Melbourne: Oxford University Press.

Thomas, N. (2004). *The Concise Adair on Creativity and Innovation*, London: Thorogood Publishing Ltd.

Tolbert, P. S. & Hall, R. H. (2009). *Organizations. Structures, Processes and Outcomes* (10th edn), New Jersey: Pearson Education.

Tremain, S. (ed.), (2005). *Foucault and the Government of Disability*, USA: The University of Michigan Press.

Tyson, T. (1998). *Working in Groups* (2nd edn), South Yarra: Macmillan Education Australia.

Victorian Council of Social Services (2007). *Policies and Procedures: A Guide for Community Management Groups*, Melbourne: Victoria Law Foundation & Victorian Council of Social Services.

Victorian Department of Human Services (2011). 'Our Values', retrieved 5 Sep. 2012, from www.dhs.vic.gov.au/about-the-department/our-organisation/our-values

Victorian Equal Opportunity and Human Rights Commission (2011a). *An Effective Complaint Procedure Checklist*, retrieved from www.victorianhumanrightscommission.com/www/policy-development/complaint-procedure-checklist

Victorian Equal Opportunity and Human Rights Commission (2011b). *Equal Opportunity in Practice. Policy Template: Workplace Equal Opportunity*, retrieved from www.victorianhumanrightscommission.com/www/index.php?option=com_k2&view=item&layout=item&id=1432&Itemid=854

W. K. Kellogg Foundation (1997). *W.K. Kellogg Evaluation Handbook*, retrieved from www.wkkf.org

W. K. Kellogg Foundation (updated Jan. 2004). *Logic Model Development Guide*, Michigan, USA: Kellogg Foundation.

Wagner, K. (2012). '5 Ways to Teach Physicians about Financial Management', *Healthcare Financial Management, 66*, 42.

Wagner, R. (2005). 'Partnerships and Collaboration as Paucity Management Practices in Rural and Regional Community-Based Human Service

Organisations', *Third Sector Review, 11*(1), pp.85–101.

Wagner, R. & Spence, N. (2003). 'Paucity Management Practices in Australian Nonprofit Human Service Organisations', *Third Sector Review, 9*(1), pp.119–35.

Wagner, R., Spence, N. & van Reyk, P. (2000). *Management and Leadership Responsibilities in Community Organisations: A Report on a Study Conducted by the Association of Children's Welfare Agencies and the Workbased Learning Unit at University of Western Sydney.*

Wandersman, A., Snell-Johns, J., Lentz, B. E., Fetterman, D. M., Keener, D. C., Livet, M., Imm, P. S. & Flaspohler, P. (2005). 'The Principles of Empowerment Evaluation', in Fetterman, D. M. & Wandersman, A. (eds), *Empowerment Evaluation. Principles in Practice*, New York: The Guilford Press, pp.27–41.

Wanna, J. (2008). 'Collaborative Government: Meanings, Drivers and Outcomes', in O'Flynn, J. & Wanna, J. (eds), *Collaborative Governance. A New Era of Public Policy in Australia*, Canberra, Australia: ANU E Press, pp.3–12.

Weber, Z. & Pockett, R. (2011). 'Working Effectively in Teams', in O'Hara, A. & Pockett, R. (eds), *Skills for Human Service Practice* (2nd edn), South Melbourne, Australia: Oxford University Press, pp.274–93.

Weeks, W. (1994). *Women Working Together. Lessons from Feminist Women's Services*, Melbourne, Australia: Longman Cheshire Pty Ltd.

Weinbach, R. W. (2007). *The Social Worker As Manager. A Practical Guide to Success* (5th edn), USA: Pearson Education Inc.

Weinbach, R. W. & Taylor, L. M. (2011). *The Social Worker As Manager: A Practical Guide to Success* (6th edn), Boston, MA: Allyn & Bacon.

Wilcoxson, L. & Millett, B. (2000). 'The Management of Organisational Culture', *Australian Journal of Management & Organisational Behaviour, 3*(2), pp.91–9.

Willis, E., Young, S. & Stanton, P. (2005). 'Health Sector and Industrial Reform in Australia', in Stanton, P., Willis, E. & Young, S. (eds), *Workplace Reform in the Healthcare Industry. The Australian Experience*, New York: Palgrave Macmillan, pp.13–29.

Wimpfheimer, S. (2004). 'Leadership and Management Competencies Defined by Practicing Social Work Managers', *Administration in Social Work, 28*(1), pp.45–56.

Yoowinna Wurnalung Healing Service Strategic Business Plan, 2009–2011 (not published).

Yukl, G. (1999). 'An Evaluation of Conceptual Weaknesses in Transformational and Charismatic Leadership Theories', *Leadership Quarterly, 10*, pp.285–305.

Zavattaro, S. M. (2012). 'Management Movements and Phases of the Image: Potential for Closing the Loop', *Administration & Society, 45*(1), pp.97–118.

Index